Clinical Aspects of Helicobacter Pylori Infection

Clinical Aspects of Helicobacter Pylori Infection

Editor: Jordan Phillips

AMERICAN
MEDICAL PUBLISHERS
www.americanmedicalpublishers.com

AMERICAN
MEDICAL PUBLISHERS
www.americanmedicalpublishers.com

Cataloging-in-publication Data

Clinical aspects of helicobacter pylori infection / edited by Jordan Phillips.
p. cm.
Includes bibliographical references and index.
ISBN 978-1-63927-985-2
1. Helicobacter pylori infections. 2. Helicobacter pylori infections--Treatment.
3. Helicobacter pylori infections--Diagnosis. 4. Helicobacter pylori. I. Phillips, Jordan.
RC840.H38 C55 2023
616.330 14--dc23

American Medical Publishers,
41 Flatbush Avenue,
1st Floor, New York,
NY 11217, USA

ISBN 978-1-63927-985-2 (Hardback)

Contents

Preface

The purpose of the book is to provide a glimpse into the dynamics and to present opinions and studies of some of the scientists engaged in the development of new ideas in the field from very different standpoints. This book will prove useful to students and researchers owing to its high content quality.

Helicobacter pylori (H. pylori) refers to a type of bacteria that causes stomach infection. It is the leading cause of peptic ulcers, as well as gastritis and stomach cancer. This infection is common in children and its signs and symptoms are nausea, weight loss, loss of appetite, bloating, etc. The risk factors of H. pylori infection are associated with living situations and environment, including not having access to a consistent source of clean water and living with someone who has an H. pylori infection. Upper endoscopy, breath test and stool test are used to diagnose this infection. There are certain antibiotics that are utilized for treating H. pylori infection, including metronidazole, clarithromycin and amoxicillin. This book elucidates the concepts and innovative management strategies with respect to Helicobacter pylori infection. It will prove to be immensely beneficial to students and researchers in this field. Most of the topics introduced in this book cover clinical aspects of Helicobacter pylori infection.

At the end, I would like to appreciate all the efforts made by the authors in completing their chapters professionally. I express my deepest gratitude to all of them for contributing to this book by sharing their valuable works. A special thanks to my family and friends for their constant support in this journey.

Editor

1

Particulars of the *Helicobacter pylori* Infection in Children

Florica Nicolescu

1. Introduction

Helicobacter pylori (*H. pylori*) is an important pathogen in human gastroenterology. *H. pylori* is commonly acquired during early childhood and it is more common among people in developing countries. Globally, over 50% of the population is infected with this bacteria, being practically evenly distributed between the two genders, in spite of a few studies showing a slight predisposition in males.

The clinical consequences of *H. pylori* infection in children are yet to be fully understood. *H. pylori* infection in children differs from the same infection in adults, both in terms of the percentage of infected individuals, symptoms, degree of complication towards peptic ulcer disease or malignancy, the gastric areas affected, the degree of compliance to therapeutic management or bacterial resistance to treatment.

2. Context

Helicobacter pylori (H. pylori) is a Gram - negative bacillus responsible for one of the most commonly diagnosed infections, namely gastritis, in humans worldwide. [1]

In 1983 Robin Warren, an Australian pathologist, described an S-shaped bacteria for the first time, that was found in the gastric mucosa. Together with Barry Marshall, they managed to isolate thid micro-organism from biopsy samples taken during endoscopy, and called it *Campylobacter pyloridis*, to be called *H. pylori* later on. [2]

Although the presence of bacteria in the stomach had been known as early as the 19th century, these microbes were considered simply a consequence of gastric mucosa contamination from food intake and not colonizing species in the true sense of the word. The current in thinking had been so controversial from the very beginning, that, about 30 years later, when *H. pylori* was discovered and proposed as the causative agent for gastritis and peptic ulcer disease, the scientific community rejected and even ridiculed the new theory. Survival of microbes in the acidic pH conditions of the stomach was considered impossible.

In one of the boldest scientific approaches of the last century, Barry Marshall self-administered an *H. pylori* dose in 1984. Although the researcher physician expected to develop peptic ulcer disease in the coming months, the symptoms emerged much sooner: only 3 days later, Marshall displayed dizziness, halitosis and vomiting, and in another 8 days, pangastritis was diagnosed endoscopically, meaning inflammation of a large areas of the stomach.

Shortly after the publication of results in Warren and Marshall's research, *H. pylori* was also detected in biopsy specimens taken during digestive endoscopy performed in children with chronic gastritis and / or duodenal ulcers; at the same time, resolution of gastric pathology in children was also demonstrated with bacterial eradication. [3] Overall, these discoveries have demonstrated the important role of *H. pylori* in gastric pathology both in adults and children.

The discovery of *H. pylori*, the demonstration of causality between the infection and gastric pathology and improvement of the bacteria eradication methodology increased the living quality for a large number of patients. If, in the past, peptic ulcer disease surgery used to be one of the most common forms of surgery performed, management of ulcers by eradication of *H. pylori* is so effective nowadays that very few patients require surgery. The merit of Warren and Marshall's pioneering research was awarded the Nobel Prize for medicine in 2005.

Goals of current and future research of *H. pylori* equally require better understanding of immune-pathogenics of gastric disease associated with *H. pylori* infection, clarification of modes of transmission, as well as improving the safety and effectiveness of vaccines for prevention of *H. pylori* infection.

Children are different from adults regarding *H. pylori* infection, in terms of the prevalence of the infection, the complication rate, the almost complete absence of gastric malignancy, age-specific issues, with diagnostic tests and medication as well as a higher rate of resistance to antibiotics. The former and other differences as well can explain why some of the recommendations for adults cannot be applied to children. [4]

3. Description of *H. pylori*

Phylogenetic classification of *H. pylori* is: *Helicobacter* genus, *Helicobacteraceae* family, *Campylobacterales* order, *Proteobacteria* subdivision.

H. pylori is a Gram - negative type bacterium, able to colonize the gastric mucosa in the majority of the population in the context of very low pH and low partial pressure of oxygen (pO_2). *H. pylori* has a curved shape and is 2-4 microns long and 1 micron wide. It displays 2-6 flagella of about 3 microns in length, ensuring it high mobility. [5] Optimal development of this organism requires reduced O_2 pressure, high humidity, 37° C temperature and neutral pH. The metabolism of the microbe can process glucose but not any other sugars.

The bacterium displays a range of extraordinary adaptations needed for survival in the extreme conditions of the gastric environment. *H. pylori* is one of the most efficient animal species, capable of degrading urea. The abundance of the *urease* enzyme allows rapid urea hydrolysis in the gastric environment, with release of bicarbonate and ammonia, which neutralize the gastric pH and provide for the optimum conditions for bacterial life. At the same time, the ammonia generated is used in the metabolism of the bacterium for the synthesis of amino acids. [6] Initially, the *urease* enzyme is solely localized in the cytoplasm, however, in the case of exposure to acid *in vivo*, autolysis of the cell wall takes place and release of the enzyme, which is subsequently fixed on the *H. pylori* surface. At the same time, increased motility allows the bacterium to penetrate and become fixed in the layers of the gastric mucosa. [7]

Outside the host organism, however, *H. pylori* is fragile and unable to survive when stored at low and ultra-low temperatures as compared with other intestinal bacteria. Although healthy individuals' manner of infection of is not yet fully understood, it is assumed that transmission is largely by direct contact of individuals and less by contaminated objects.

4. The rate of *H. pylori* infection

H. pylori infection global rate differs by region, ethnicity, age, and socio-economic level of the population. The percentage of infected individuals is higher in disadvantaged socio-economic categories and increases with age. Large infection percentages (about 80%) may be found in Asian countries, in Eastern and South-Eastern Europe, in Latin America, whereas much smaller percentages (about 40%) are characteristic to Western countries. [8-10]

Regardless of the geographic area analysed, one finds that *H. pylori* infection is usually acquired in early childhood both in developed and developing countries.

5. Prevalence

Overall, about one third of the population is infected with *H. pylori*, and the frequency increases with age.

In general, the prevalence is higher in developing countries, and the infection is contacted at an early age. The incidence is 3-10% of the population every year in developing countries, as compared to 0.5% in developed countries. [11]

The prevalence of *H. pylori* infection is not only lower in industrialized countries than in developing countries, but the incidence of *H. pylori* infection, gastric cancer, peptic ulcer disease and related diseases are also declining. Worldwide, more than 1 billion people are estimated to be infected with *H. pylori*. [4]

6. Possibility of transmission

H. pylori does not tolerate increased O_2 partial pressure, high temperatures or nutrients poor environments outside the host organism. In other words, *H. pylori* is excellently adapted to gastric existing parameters, but it is a fragile organism, non-viable outside the host. One study highlights the possibility for *Helicobacter pylori* infection from a water supply. For these reasons, although the exact *H. pylori* mode of transmission is not completely understood, the type of transmission is accepted by primarily direct contact of healthy individuals with an infected person. Transmission of infection may also be the result of transport vectors.

H. pylori isolated strains are found more often in staff performing endoscopies than the general population.

H. pylori has been isolated and cultivated from faeces, indicating the possibility of faecal-oral transmission. Also, *H. pylori* was found in the oral cavity in both saliva and the plaque, suggesting oral-oral transmission variant. Therefore, transmission of *H. pylori* can occur by oral-oral, faecal-oral transmission or a combination thereof. [12]

Horizontal transmission is favoured by overcrowding found in densely populated human communities. This version is the most likely in the case of infection transmission among family members. Thus, children of *H. pylori* infected mothers run an 8 times higher risk of acquiring the bacterium. [13]

7. Diagnosis of *H. pylori*

Correct diagnosis of *H. pylori* is possible through a wide range of working methods. However, the opportunity to diagnose *H. pylori* and the working method chosen should be evaluated according to the specificity of each case.

H. pylori infection generated symptoms is nonspecific, including abdominal pain, gastro-oesophageal reflux with or without heartburn, halitosis, vomiting or hematemesis.

Because symptoms caused by *H. pylori* are general (nonspecific), the *H. pylori* infection may overlap with another digestive or abdominally located disorder. Therefore, the primary purpose of investigating gastrointestinal symptoms should be elucidating their real ethyology and not just determining the presence of *H. pylori* infection. This consideration is especially important in the case of *H. pylori* infection in children under the age of 12, because the latter are unable to accurately describe the location, nature or intensity of their discomfort. [14]

Assessment of patients infected with *H. pylori* should pay particular attention to anorexia and weight loss, pallor or laboratory tests to identify anaemia, vomiting, abdominal pain or pain associated with meals and night-time, as well as to any descriptions of gastrointestinal haemorrhage.

In children suspected of *H. pylori* infection, history should include the following:

- Abominable pain nature, location, frequency, duration, severity, exacerbation and alleviating factors;
- The intestinal transit and description of the stool;
- Appetite, diet, changes in weight;
- Halitosis, vomiting and description of the gastric material;
- Ulcer disease or gastrointestinal disorders (e.g. Crohn's disease) running in the family;
- Medications (on-prescription and OTC);
- Previous diagnostic tests and gastrointestinal tract specific therapy.

Physical examination of an asymptomatic *H. pylori* infected child usually ends in confusing results. In children with chronic gastritis, duodenal and peptic ulcer, important findings include epigastric tenderness or gastrointestinal bleeding (e.g., positive guaiac stools, tachycardia, pallor).

Children with peptic ulcer can develop complications (e.g., severe blood loss in the gastrointestinal tract, perforation, obstruction) and may show signs of hemodynamic instability or signs of acute abdomen. Children with long-term peptic ulcer caused by *H. pylori* may become anaemic from undetected and asymptomatic chronic bleeding. In such children, the following should be considered:

- The child's overall appearance;
- Assessment of perfusion, paying special attention to the child's mental status, heart rate, pulse as well as *refill of capillaries*.
- Evaluation of *the child's skin as well as* conjunctivae in order to check pallor.
- Careful cardiac and pulmonary scrutiny.
- Abdomen inspection, auscultation and palpating.
- Making a rectal exam and the guaiac test of the stool. [4]

For accurate diagnosis of *H. pylori* infection, several methods are available with varying degrees of accuracy:

7.1. Histopathological methods

Isolation and cultivation of *H. pylori* in biopsy specimens taken during endoscopy is the golden standard in diagnosing the infection. In addition, this method also has the advantage of providing information about tissue pathology as caused by *H. pylori* infection. Since distribution of *H. pylori* concentration on the gastric mucosa is not uniform but has rather the appearance of distinct lower or higher concentration islands, taking at least 2 biopsies is recommended, one of the gastric body and the other from the antrum. [15]

7.2. Breath analysis

Diagnosis of *H. pylori* infection may also be performed by breath analysis after oral administration of a urea solution. If the urea used is provided with a ^{13}C- labelled carbon atom, this isotope dosage can be performed, but the method is both very precise and demanding in terms of the equipment involved. Alternatively, unmarked urea can be administered to qualitatively detect the presence of *H. pylori* by identification of NH_3 (ammonia) in the air expired. [4]

7.3. Immunological methods

H. pylori infection causes emergence of specific antibodies: anti - *H. pylori* antibodies (IgA and IgG) in serum, blood, urine and / or saliva. Although cheap and fast, detection of these antibodies is not relevant to assess the current status of infection or success of the eradication therapy. Because of immunological memory, antibodies may persist for months and years even in the host organism after eradication of the infection. [16-18]

7.4. Detection of antigens

Identification of *H. pylori* antigen in faeces is an accurate way of establishing the diagnosis, as a non-invasive method and easier to apply in children than administration of urea solution or endoscopy.

In addition, the method has the advantage that even after the passage of five days from sample harvest, diagnosing *H. pylori* is as accurate. Thus, sampling of biological material can be performed without the active participation of children and their visit to the medical centre, as the sample may be dispatched by courier. [4]

Colonization of gastric mucosa by *H. pylori* does not automatically mean onset of the disease, but the infection correlates with increased risk of infection during the onset of peptic ulcers and gastric cancer. The materialization of this risk depends on a summation of factors related to the genome of the bacterium, the host and environmental factors.[19]

A wide range of extra-gastrointestinal disorders are thought to be associated with *H. pylori* infection, e.g. otitis media, upper respiratory tract infections, periodontitis, food allergies, Sudden Infant Death Syndrome (SIDS). However, there is currently no convincing scientific evidence regarding the causal relationship between *H. pylori* infection and such disorders.

Symptoms associated with *H. pylori* infection may be absent even in some cases where the presence of *H. pylori* was proved by histological analysis. In other cases however, infection is followed by the occurrence of peptic ulcer and its complications. The general pathology of *H. pylori* includes phenomena such as dyspepsia and refractory anaemia. [15]

8. Incriminatory factors

To determine their causal relationship with *H. pylori* infection, epidemiological studies have addressed various factors such as a bacterial cause, the host, genetic and environmental factors. Data are related to the spread of infection from person to person (e. g. dental plaque), but the origin and the mode of transmission is incomplete known. [4]

H. pylori infection causes include the following:

- We can observe that the transmission of *H. pylori* is possible person to person.

Groups of infection are under observation, particularly within families of infected children. Possible routes are faecal-oral, oral-oral and gastro-oral. Mother to child transmission has been suggested in a study analysing DNA of *H. pylori* strains. [20] Studies have shown identical *H. pylori* strains in mothers and their younger children. Maternal symptoms of nausea and vomiting and pacifier use were associated with the risk of *H. pylori* infection in children.

Cervantes et al. participated a study performed at the US-Mexico border and they have shown that a younger brother is 4 times more prone to *H. pylori* infection if the mother was *H. pylori* infected, compared to an uninfected mother. Younger brothers are 8 times more likely to acquire the infection if an older brother had persistent *H. pylori* infection. [13]

Absence or poor personal hygiene may also play a role. Increase in *H. pylori* infection may be observed in developing countries, which may reflect the combined effects of poor living conditions, poor hygiene and overcrowded cities.

The status of *H. pylori* infection in the United States, a comparatively higher socio-economic setting, shows that the higher the social and economic level, the lower the incidence of *H. pylori* infection, a finding that may reflect also the same factors as those mentioned in the case of developing countries.

- In the clinical manifestations of *H. pylori* infection the bacterial factors may play an important role. Patients infected with *H. pylori* may have two basic phenotypes reported the presence or absence of cytotoxin vacuole.

Inflammation is more pronounced in people with cytotoxin - positive infection, confirmed at endoscopy, than in those infected with *H. pylori* cytotoxin - negative.

As far as bacterial factors are involved, presence of two fundamental phenotypes has been shown in *H. pylori* infected patients, i.e. vacuolating cytotoxin positive and negative, respectively. Endoscopy performed on cytotoxin-positive infected patients has proved inflammation more marked than in patients where the cytotoxin was absent.[13]

The significance of host dependent factors has been demonstrated by such observations as the fact that adults are less capable of solving acute infections than children.

A different such factor may be the presence of hypochlorhydria in the host, which allows specific *H. pylori* colonization of the stomach.

In addition, *H. pylori may only persist if the* metaplastic epithelium of the stomach is atrophied.[4]

- One study highlights the possibility for *H. pylori* infection from a water supply. [21]
- Transmission of infection may also be the result of transport vectors. [22]
- *H. pylori* isolated strains are found more often in staff performing endoscopies than the general population.

9. Pathophysiology

H. pylori organisms are spiral Gram - negative bacteria, highly mobile due to their multiple unipolar flagella. They are microaerophilic powerful urease producers. These organisms inhabit the mucus adjacent to the gastric mucosa.

Important adaptive features improve survival of the organism in an acidic environment include its shape and motility, its low oxygen needs, its adhesion molecules serving a feeding role in certain gastric cells and *urease* production. Bacterial *urease* converts urea to ammonia and bicarbonate, therefore neutralizing gastric acid and providing protection from a hostile environment. Some of the lipopolysaccharides of the organism mimic the Lewis blood group antigens structure. This molecular mimicry also helps the survival of *H. pylori* in the unfavourable gastric environment. [23]

H. pylori generates disease triggers, including *urease*, vacuolating cytotoxin, catalase and lipopolysaccharide (LPS). *Urease* is a potent antigen inducing increased production of immunoglobulin G and immunoglobulin A. Expression of vacuolating cytotoxin generating inflammatory cytokines may be associated with more pronounced inflammation and marked tendency of disease triggering.

The most important virulence factor in *H. pylori* infection is cytotoxin - associated antigen (CagA). A person infected with CagA -negative strains is likely to develop chronic gastritis and have little chance to develop peptic ulcer disease or gastric cancer.

On the other hand, infection with CagA -positive strains greatly increases the risk of peptic ulcer and gastric cancer. Movement of CagA protein into gastric epithelial cells leads to rearrangement of the host cytoskeleton, alters signalling cell and disturbs the cell cycle control. [24]

In children with *H. pylori* infection, who have peptic ulcer disease, *in situ* expression of CagA is increased and may play an important role in the pathogenesis of peptic ulcer disease. [25]

The bacteria *H. pylori* localises in the stomach, induces inflammatory cytokines formation and causes gastric inflammation. People with *H. pylori* gastritis associated with increased gastric acid gastritis are prone to peptic ulcer disease. [26] In contrast, people infected with *H. pylori* associated with corpus gastritis, with decreased gastric acid production are more prone to developing gastric atrophy (intestinal metaplasia and gastric adenocarcinoma).

The infection with *H. pylori* has been associated with iron deficiency anaemia. The two main assumptions underlying this theory are iron sequestration because of antral *H. pylori* infection and decrease of non- hemin iron absorption caused by hypochlorhydria.

H. pylori infection and its association with gastric malignancies have been well described in several epidemiological studies. [27] However, the evolution from inflammation to cancer remains unclear.

There exists a model describing the progressive evolution of *H. pylori* infection to hypochlorhydria, chronic gastritis, atrophic gastritis, dysplasia, intestinal metaplasia and gastric cancer. [28, 29, 30, 31]

A newer hypothesis suggests that *H. pylori* infection may protect against self - inflammatory diseases such as asthma or inflammatory bowel disease. For instance, epidemiological data suggest that infection with *Helicobacter pylori* is less common in patients with inflammatory bowel disease, which leads to research for defining potential mechanisms underlying these clinical findings. [27]

10. Morbidity

Most *H. pylori* infected children are asymptomatic. Antral gastritis is the most common manifestation in children. Duodenal and gastric ulcers may be associated with *H. pylori* gastritis in adults, but is less common in children. The risk of gastric cancer, including non - Hodgkin lymphoma (i.e. associated to the lymphoid tissue mucosa MALT]) and adenocarcinoma is increased in adults.[4]

The relationship between *H. pylori* gastritis and recurrent abdominal pain (RAP) is controversial. The incidence of *H. pylori* gastritis in patients with RAP is not significantly higher than the incidence of *H. pylori* infection in the general population. Although certain studies have shown an improvement in symptoms in children with RAP and *Helicobacter pylori* gastritis after eradication therapy for *H. pylori*, data from a recent double-blind controlled trial have not confirmed this finding. [32]

According to the North American Society for Paediatric Gastroenterology, Hepatology and Nutrition no results were sufficiently reliable to support routine testing for *H. pylori in* children with RAP. [33]

Data published so far highlight an association between *H. pylori* infection and gastrointestinal symptoms in children, but no association has been found between RAP and *H. pylori* infection. Conflicting evidence has been found however concerning the association of *H. pylori* infection with epigastric pain. [34]

There are studies suggesting that *H. pylori* protects the human body from developing gastroesophageal reflux disease, while others affirm a causal association between them. Analysis of studies in conducted in adults has found no association between *H. pylori* eradication and development of new cases of gastroesophageal reflux disease in dyspeptic patients. [35]

According to a pediatric retrospective study, there was a significantly higher prevalence of reflux esophagitis in *H. pylori* infected children. [36]

H. pylori infection was also associated with extraintestinal manifestations such as short stature, immune thrombocytopenic purpura and migraine, with different levels of causation. [37, 38]. This infection is also associated with coronary diseases, iron-deficiency anemia and hepatobiliary diseases among others. [39, 40, 41, 42, 43, 44]

11. Dissemination (population category)

The predominance *H. pylori* infection is increased in black, Hispanic, Asian, and Native American populations.

The infection with *H. pylori* affect more than a half of the world's population, which is acquired almost always within the first 5 years of life [45]. In the developed world, the prevalence rates vary from 1.2% to 12.2% [46-49]. In developing countries, the prevalence rates are much higher. The serological prevalence rates of *H. pylori* were 45% among Indian children [40,51]. In Bolivia and Alaska, at the age of 9 years, the seroprevalence was 70% and 69%, respectively [52]. The seroprevalence in preschoolers in Brazil was found to be 69.7% [53]. An age-related increase of the prevalence of *H. pylori*, irrespective of the economic state of the country, was observed by several independent studies across the world [47-51, 54, 55].

In a study of Prof Dr Sibille Koletzko et al [15] was presented that during the first years of life in both developing and industrialized countries the *H. pylori* infection is usually acquired.The epidemiology of *H. pylori* infection in children, in Europe and North America has changed in recent decades. In the northern and western European countries are founding low incidence rates, resulting in prevalence far below 10% in children and adolescents. In contrast, the infection is still common in certain geographic areas such as southern or eastern Europe, Mexico, and certain immigrant populations from South America, Africa, and most Asian countries, and aboriginal people in North America. The different prevalence of infection and the corresponding effect on health care resources in industrialized compared with developing countries require different recommendations with respect to testing and treating children. These guidelines apply only to children living in Europe and North America, but not to those living in other continents, particularly in developing countries with a high *H. pylori* infection rate in children and adolescents and with limited resources for health care [15].

Infection rates are similar in men and women alike.

Many study present that less than 10% of children under 12 years of age are infected in developed countries, but seropositivity increases with age, to a rate of 0.3-1% per year. Seropositivity studies in developed countries in adults showed a prevalence of 30-50%.

In the US, estimated prevalence is 20% for people under 30 and 50% for persons over 60. In developing countries, prevalence rates are much higher. *H. pylori* serological prevalence rates have been 15% and 46% for Gambian children under 20 months and 40-60 months, respectively. [56]

12. Laboratory methodology

An important study of Prof Dr Sibille Koletzko et al was presented by using the testing guidelines recently provided by the European Society for Paediatric Gastroenterology Hepatology and Nutrition (ESPGHAN) and the North American Society for Paediatric Gastroenterology, Hepatology and Nutrition (NASPGHAN) for *H. pylori* infection in children [15]. These recommendations are:

- The primary purpose of clinical investigation of gastrointestinal symptoms is to determine the primary cause of the symptoms, and not the presence of *H. pylori* infection only.
- Diagnostic tests for *H. pylori* infection are not recommended in children with functional abdominal pain. Currently, in the absence of ulcer disease, there is insufficient evidence to justify a causal relationship between *H. pylori* gastritis and abdominal symptoms. Therefore, cases of abdominal pain consistent with diagnostic criteria for functional pain should not be investigated for *H. pylori,* unless upper endoscopy is conducted during diagnostic, in search of some organic disease.
- In children with first-degree relatives with gastric cancer, *H. pylori* testing may be considered.
- In children with refractory iron deficiency anaemia in whom other causes have been excluded, *H. pylori* testing can be considered.
- There is insufficient evidence that *H. pylori* infection is causally linked with otitis media, respiratory tract infections, periodontal diseases, food allergies, sudden infant death syndrome, idiopathic thrombocytopenic purpura and short stature.
- To confirm eradication in children selected with disease complicated by peptic ulcer or lymphoma and in children who remain symptomatic.

For diagnostic tests to be applied, the recommendations are as follows:

- For the diagnosis of *H. pylori* infection during esophagogastroduodenoscopy (EGD), it is recommended to obtain gastric biopsy samples (antrum and corpus gastritis).
- It is recommended that the initial diagnosis of *H. pylori* infection rely on positive histopathology examination and a rapid *urease* positive test or a positive culture.
- The ^{13}C - urea breath test (UBT) is a non-invasive test to determine successful eradication of *H. pylori.*
- A positive enzyme immunoassay (ELISA) for the detection of *H. pylori* antigen in the stool is a noninvasive test to determine whether *H.pylori* has been eradicated. Several methods are available for detection of the *H. pylori* antigen in stool, such as the enzyme immunoassay test (EIA) based on polyclonal or monoclonal antibodies and immunochromatographic tests (the so-called rapid tests).

Stool tests are generally much more convenient in children than UBT. Neither storage of evidence at room temperature for up to 5 days nor freezing them for months or even years appears to influence the accuracy of the stool tests. So far, only EIA based on monoclonal antibodies has equalled UBT accuracy.

- Tests relying on antibody detection (IgG, IgA) against *H. pylori* in the blood serum, urine and saliva are not viable for use in the clinic setting.
- Physicians are recommended to wait for at least 2 weeks after end of the proton pump inhibitors (IPP) therapy and for 4 weeks after end of antibiotics before conducting biopsy and non-invasive tests (UBT, stool test) for *H. pylori.*

It should be noted that these guidelines only apply to children in Europe and North America, not in other continents, particularly developing countries, with a high rate of paediatric *H. pylori* infection and limited health resources.

Another studies / tests

- Imaging studies are not useful in the diagnosis of *H. pylori* infection. They can be useful in patients with complicated diseases (e.g., ulcer, gastric cancer, MALToma).
- Urea breath test: The patient ingests a test meal containing carbon-13 (^{13}C) labelled urea, which is a nonradioactive isotope. *H. pylori urease* activity produces ^{13}C-labelled carbon dioxide, detectable in the breath. A positive result confirms *urease* activity and *H. pylori* infection. This is a highly specific test, sensitive in patients over 6 years of age. It is useful to check eradication of *H. pylori* after treatment. Experience in children 5 years or younger, in infants particularly, is relatively limited and needs further validation.

Detection of *Helicobacter pylori*

The procedure of choice for detecting gastritis, duodenitis and PUD in the paediatric population is upper endoscopy (EGD)

- EGD allows direct visualization of the mucosa, for locating the source of bleeding, to detect *H. pylori* by biopsy, culture and cytology analysis and DNA testing using PCR.
- In addition, a rapid test based on detection of *urease* activity (a *H. pylori* highly specific marker) may be performed. The test, called the *Campylobacter test* (CLO) allows diagnosis of *H. pylori* infection within 24 hours.
- Two modified urea rapid test kits are currently available on the market and reported as more accurate, with shorter reaction time and of better value for money than the CLO test.
- Endoscopy in children may reveal a nodular appearance in the gastric antrum resulting from lymphoid hyperplasia [34]. Approximately 50% of affected children have displayed endoscopic evidence of changes of *H. pylori* gastritis.

The appearance of an active ulcer is round or oval lesion in shape, the perforated base being smooth and white, with a red and oedematous surrounding mucosa. In *H. pylori* infection, the most common site for ulcer is the duodenal bulb.

Biopsy obtained from the prepiloric antrum has the highest yield in *H. pylori* infection. Often, tissue samples are also obtained from the body and the transition areas of the stomach, especially when the patient has recently taken acid suppressing medications.

- Endoscopic biopsy is indicated for the following reasons:
- Histological examination of gastric tissue;
- Rapid *urease* test (e.g. CLO test)
- Culture of organisms;
- PCR test for identification of *H. pylori* DNA
- Histological findings include infiltration of a substantial number of plasma cells and lymphocytes into the gastric mucosa and Giemsa, Diff-Quick visible bodies or haematoxylin and eosin. Sensitive colouring of a small number of bacteria is possible with a silver staining method such as Genta or Warthin-Starry.

Stages

- Multiple stages in the progression of the disease are well described in the literature, although no stages system for *H. pylori* infection has been established.
- The first step is chronic gastritis, followed by a second step, atrophic gastritis. The third step is intestinal metaplasia, which can evolve to dysplasia. The last step in this process is gastric adenocarcinoma.
- This is a very slow process (which may take decades, for example), and can stop at any step because gastric cancer probably requires several other factors to grow, not just *H. pylori* infection.

Treatment measures of *Helicobacter pylori* infection

Let us mention the new treatment rules recommended for the following patient groups [15]:

- In the presence of *H. pylori*-positive PUD, eradication of the microorganism is recommended.
- On detection of *H. pylori* infection by biopsy based methods in the absence of PUD, *H. pylori* treatment may be considered. The decision to treat *H. pylori* associated gastritis without duodenal or gastric ulcer is subject to the clinician's judgment and deliberation is undertaken with the patient and family, taking into account potential risks and benefits of treatment for the patient.
- In *H. pylori* infected children, whose next of kin suffer from gastric cancer, treatment can be offered.
- The "test - and-treat" strategy is not recommended for children. The main purpose of the tests is to diagnose the cause of the clinical symptoms.

Currently practiced therapeutic approach takes the following into account:

- *H. pylori* acquired resistance to antibiotics, which requires bacterial strain susceptibility testing to a certain class of antibiotics in geographic areas where resistance is seen in encountered in a percentage of patients;
- Success rate in eradication of infection is directly dependent on the dose and duration of medication administered. In practice however, this is less apparent because of lower compliance in long cures and because of adverse effects (vomiting, nausea, malaise) in high doses;
- Bismuth (Bi^{3+}) salts preparations are effective but difficult to accept by children because of their bad taste;
- Therapeutic management aims not at eradication of *H. pylori* infection only but also at resolution of the pathology is determines (gastritis, reflux, dyspepsia etc.) and therefore triple therapy may be associated with prokinetics and hygienic-dietary regime to spare digestion;
- Unwanted side effects of the antibiotics cure can be reduced by administration of probiotic preparations that restore normal intestinal flora.

The following treatments should be implemented [15]:

- First line eradication regimens are: triple therapy with a PPI + amoxicillin + imidazole, or PPI + amoxicillin + clarithromycin + amoxicillin or bismuth salts + imidazole or sequential therapy. Sequential therapy involves dual therapy with a PPI and amoxicillin for 5 days, successively followed by five days of triple therapy (a PPI with clarithromycin and metronidazole / tinidazole). In fact, this scheme may be considered as quadruple therapy provided in a sequential manner. It is speculated that the initial use of amoxicillin reduces bacterial load and provides protection against resistance to clarithromycin.
- Clarithromycin antibiotic susceptibility testing is recommended prior to clarithromycin triple therapy in areas / populations definable as clarithromycin highly resistant (> 20%) to *H. pylori.*
- The recommended period for triple therapy is 7-14 days. Costs, compliance and adverse effects should be taken into account.
- A reliable non-invasive test for eradication is recommended at least 4-8 weeks after treatment.

In cases of treatment failure, the following 3 options are recommended:

- EGD with culture and sensitivity tests, including alternative antibiotics if not performed prior to standard treatment.
- *Insitu* fluorescence hybridization (FISH) on paraffin-embedded biopsies, if clarithromycin susceptibility testing was not performed before standard therapy.
- Therapy changing by addition of an antibiotic, using various antibiotics, as well as addition of bismuth, and / or increase of the dose and / or treatment duration.

If not possible to perform a primary culture, the following regimens are suggested as second-line or rescue therapy [15]:

- Quadruple therapy consists of metronidazole + amoxicillin + PPI + bismuth. In most guidelines, quadruple therapy is the recommended second-line therapy, but this is a complicated regimen to administer. In addition, bismuth salts are not universally available.
- Triple therapy consists of PPI + levofloxacin (moxifloxacin) + amoxicillin. Regimen evaluation using fluoroquinolones, including levofloxacin, as second-line therapy in children is limited. In studies in adults, the treatment seems to be effective.

Although studies during ideal therapy duration for second-line treatment are not conclusive, a longer treatment duration is recommended, up to 14 days.

Other procedures

- Surgical procedures are rarely needed in treatment of patients with *H. pylori* infection. However, the ulcer, surgery may be required for certain complications unresponsive to medical treatment, including difficult to treat abdominal pain, gastric outlet obstruction, perforation and severe bleeding.
- Consultations pediatric gastroenterologists: For evaluation, endoscopy and biopsy to confirm *Helicobacter pylori* infection and rule out other causes for abdominal pain or bleeding;
- Surgeon - For intervention in patients with severe or intractable pain or bleeding or patients with intestinal perforation or obstruction of the gastro-intestinal tract;
- Radiologist - For patients requiring upper gastrointestinal imaging with contrast-enhanced studies.

Hygienic-dietary regime

A sparing digestive hygienic-dietary regime is recommended, including meals and snacks every 3-4 hours with correct chewing and avoidance of food aggressors. Foods such as fruit juices and certain dairy products may have a modest bacteriostatic effect on *H. pylori*. Active principles (sulforaphane and indole-3-carbinol) of the Brassicaceae family are also included here.

- Two randomized, placebo-controlled studies have evaluated the effect of probiotic food as an adjunct to standard triple therapy for eradication of *H. pylori* infection in children and have had conflicting results [58, 59].
- In a recent prospective study in adults, it was suggested that the addition of vitamin C to a regimen of *H. pylori* with amoxicillin, metronidazole, and bismuth can significantly increase the *H. pylori* eradication rate [60].

13. Medicines used in *H. pylori* eradication therapy [61-73]

Antibiotics, beta-lactamases

Beta-lactamases used to treat *H. pylori* infected patients are stable in an acidic environment, binding to proteins in bacterial cell walls, inducing direct lysis in the wall, and inhibiting cell wall synthesis.

Amoxicillin (Amoxil®, Polymox®, Trimox®, Wymox®)

Bacterially active against *Helicobacter pylori*. Available as GTT 50mg/ml; susp.125, 200, 250, or 400mg/5ml; caps 250 and 500 mg chewable tablets and 125, 200, 250, or 400mg.

Antibiotics, macrolides

Macrolides used to treat *H. pylori* infection are stable in the stomach, entering the bacterial cell, binding to receptors on the ribosomal subunits and inhibiting bacterial protein synthesis.

Clarithromycin (Biaxin®, Fromilid®)

This displays bactericidal activity against *H. pylori* antimicrobial spectrum similar to that of erythromycin but stable in acid and with fewer adverse gastrointestinal effects. Available as 125 or 250mg/5ml granules for suspension and 250 or 500 mg film-coated tablets.

Antibiotics, antiprotozoans

Used in the treatment of *H. pylori* infected patients, this antibiotic generates intracellular products affecting bacterial DNA.

Metronidazole (Flagyl®, Protostat®)

Metronidazole diffuses well into all tissues, is stable in an acidic environment, and provides bactericidal activity against *H. pylori*. Available as ex tempore 50 sau100mg/5ml suspension, 250 or 500mg tablets and 375 mg capsules.

Antibiotics, tetracyclines

Tetracyclines bind to ribosomal subunits and inhibit protein synthesis of susceptible bacteria. Use in paediatric patients should be limited in cases where other antibiotic regimens fail.

Tetracycline hydrochloridum (Achromycin®, Sumycin®, Terramycin®)

Bacteriostatic but may be bactericidal in high concentrations. Also available as 250 or 500mg tablets, 100, 250, or 500 mg capsules, and 125mg/5ml suspension.

H^2 receptor antagonists

H_2 receptors are located on acid-producing parietal cells. Blocking the action of the histamine suppresses gastric acid secretion.

Ranitidine (ranitidinum) or Famotidine (famotidinum)

H_2 antagonists prescribed for 8 weeks, when most *H. pylori* associated ulcers are cured. H_2 blockers have no antibacterial effect, therefore antibiotics should be used to eradicate *H.*

pylori. Available as 15mg/ml syrup, 75, 150, or 300 mg tablets, as well as effervescent tablets 150mg.

Proton Pump Inhibitors

This class of medicinal products includes acid inhibitors more potent than H_2 receptor antagonists; they block the secretion of gastric acid proton pump (Na + / H +-ATP-ase), the final common path of the secretion. This class is recommended as part of a regimen of medications in symptomatic patients with *H. pylori* infection. Similar to H_2-receptor blocking treatment, proton pump inhibitor (PPI) treatment only does not eliminate the *H. pylori* infection, but increases the bacteriostatic activity against *H. pylori*.

Examples of trade names depending on the active substance:

- Omeprazole: Omeprazole®, Prilosec®, Omez®, Omeran®, Ulto® (available within 10, 20 or 40 mg per tablet)
- Esomeprazole: Nexium®, Emanera®, Helide®, Esomeprazole Sandoz® (20 or 40 mg)
- Pantoprazole: Controlo®, Nolpaza® (20 or 40 mg per tablet)
- Lansoprazol: Prevacid®, Lanzul® 30mg

Proton Pump Inhibitors are potent gastric acid blockers. For best effectiveness, to be administered before the first meal of the day. Enteric film-coated granules in capsules, they ensure adequate bioavailability. For children unable to swallow whole capsules, the grains are opened and put in acid substances (e.g. apple juice), which is preferable to administer to the lower bioavailability suspension. Available as 10 or 20 mg SR capsules and granules for suspension *per os* 20 or 40 mg/package.

Lansoprazole (Prevacid®)

Potent gastric acid blocker. Best administered just before the first meal of the day. Enteric film-coated granules in capsules, ensuring adequate bioavailability. For children unable to swallow the intact capsules, granules are placed in acid substances (e.g., applesauce or apple juice), preferable to the administration of lower bioavailable suspension. Available as capsules with 15 or 30 mg retard release and 15 mg or 30mg/package granules for suspension *per os*.[75-85]

Bismuth

Bismuth subsalicylate and bismuth subcitrate have complementary effects with most antimicrobials. Bismuth disrupts enzymatic activity in bacterial cell walls. Bismuth is particularly effective in the lysis of the cell wall of the microorganism when close to the gastric epithelium and relatively inaccessible to most antimicrobial agents.

Bismuth subsalicylate (Pepto-Bismol®)

These lyse bacterial cell walls, prevent microorganism adhesion to epithelium and inhibit *urease*.

Available as 262 mg chewable tablets (bismuth subsalicylate) and 262mg or 525mg/15ml solution.

Bismuth subcitrate (De - Nol®) acts similarly. The patient should be warned against normal black stools during the treatment administration.

Patient care

In children with *H. pylori* and complications of the peptic ulcer disease (PUD), including bleeding, severe pain, perforation, or obstruction, care must include the following [86-106]:

- Attention to the airway, breathing and circulatory status
- Monitoring of fluid resuscitation, with consideration for transfusion
- Careful nasogastric lavage in stabilization of upper gastro-intestinal bleeding
- Antacid therapy with proton pump inhibitors (PPIs), maximum dosage
- Appropriate consultation with specialists in endoscopy or other procedures
- In children with stress-induced PUD, the treatment of the severe disease or traumatic injury
- additional outpatient care includes monitoring the patient's symptoms, assessment of patient tolerance to treatment regimen, and follow-up tests to confirm the effectiveness of the treatment. The tests should be conducted at least 6 weeks and preferably 3 months after treatment.

Outpatient treatment of patients

- Patients should avoid all irritating drugs, including anti-inflammatory drugs (NSAIDs), aspirin, and preparations with corticosteroid
- It is necessary for the treatment of iron deficiency anaemia.

Prophylactic measures

- The transmission mode of *H. pylori* infection is not fully understood.
- Data from epidemiological studies suggest that the following measures may be helpful to reduce transmission:
- Policies supporting improvement of living conditions, particularly in developing countries;
- For all patients with chronic symptoms of the gastro-intestinal tract, appropriate reference for definitive diagnosis and treatment, which may also help to prevent exposure of family members and close contacts.[103-111]
- *H. pylori* infection vaccines: several studies performed with *urease* -based vaccines have shown limited efficacy in humans. Vaccines based on recombinant CagA-VacA-0AP proteins display good immunogenicity of CagA - based cow - 0AP good immunogenicity and safety profile in phase I, but no subsequent efficacy studies have been reported. No further results from clinical trials on *H. pylori* vaccines have been reported in recent years. Currently, there is no authorised anti - *H. pylori* vaccine [74].

***H. pylori* Complications**

- PUD - perforation, gastrointestinal bleeding

- Iron deficiency anaemia
- Malignancies of:- The gastric mucosa associated to lymphoid tissue (MALT) - Adenocarcinoma of the gastric corpus, and the antrum
- Gastric outlet obstruction
- Increased sensitivity to enteric infections such as salmonella and giardiasis because of *H. pylori*-induced hypochlorhydria [92, 96]

14. Prospects study

1. Prospects for the eradication of *H. pylori* infection with multidrug therapy are good, with up to 95% reported efficacy rates.
2. Treatment is often unsuccessful because of lack of patient compliance and antibiotic resistance.
3. When cleaning is completed, long-term reinfection rates are low. Among children living in developing countries or among families with infected members, reinfection rates may be increased.
4. In this moment, the nature of *H. pylori* infection transmission is not fully understood. Therefore, the ability to implement appropriate preventive measures to control the infection is limited.
5. The theory concerning *H. pylori* person-to-person transmission, supported by data from epidemiological studies, may prove useful in promoting policies to improve the living and hygiene conditions and reduce crowdedness.
6. The true effect of educational authorities to reduce transmission of *H. pylori* in the patient's family (e.g., teaching children about proper hygiene and toilet practices) is unknown. However, such efforts may be part of a sensible approach to reducing the transmission of all infection pathogens in the infection of the gastrointestinal tract [109-111].

15. Conclusions

The infection with *H. pylori* is a common problem in pediatric practice and its origin is related with poor socio-econo-mic conditions. Only a small number of children with well-defined clinical syndromes are benefited at present from testing and treatment.

The first line eradication regimens are triple therapy with a PPI, amoxicillin and imidazole, or PPI, amoxicillin, clarithromycin and amoxicillin or bismuth salts and imidazole or sequential therapy.

Each country may need to be adapted the recommendations guidelines to national health care systems, because certain tests or treatment regimens may not be available and /or reimbursed by health insurance programs.

Author details

Florica Nicolescu*

Address all correspondence to: florica.nicolescu@gmail.com

Toxicology Department, "Carol Davila" University of Medicine and Pharmacy, Bucharest, Romania

References

[1] Blecker U. *Helicobacter pylori*-associated gastroduodenal disease in childhood. *South Med J*. Jun 1997;90(6):570-6; quiz 577.

[2] Warren JR, Marshall BJ. Unidentified curved bacilli on gastric epithelium in active chronic gastritis. *Lancet*. 1983;1:1273–5.

[3] Hill R, Pearman J, Worthy P, Caruso V, Goodwin S, Blincow E. *Campylobacter pyloridis* and gastritis in children. *Lancet*. 1986;1:387.

[4] Mutaz I Sultan, Carmen Cuffari, Pediatric *Helicobacter pylori* Infection, *emedicine.medscape.com/article/929452.*

[5] Goodwin CS, McCulloch RK, Armstrong JA, Wee SH. Unusual cellular fatty acid and distinctive ultrastructure in a new spiral bacterium (*Campylobacter pyloridis*) from the human gastric mucosa. *J Med Microbiol*. 1987;19:257–67.

[6] Peterson WL, Graham DY. *Helicobacter pylori*. In: Feldman M, Friedman, Sleisenger MH, Scharschmidt BF, editors. *Sleisenger and Fordtran's gastrointestinal and liver disease pathophysiology diagnosis management*. Philadelphia: WB Saunders Company; 2002. pp. 732–46.

[7] Phadnis SH, Paelow MH, Levy M, Ilver D, Caulkins CM, Conners JB, et al. Surface localization of *Helicobacter pylori* urease and heat shock protein homolog requires bacterial autolysis. *Infec Immun*. 1996;64:905–12.

[8] Opekun AR, Gilger MA, Denyes SM, Nirken MH, Philip SP, Osato MS, et al. *Helicobacter pylori* infection in children of Texas. *J Pediatr Gastroenterol Nutr*. 2000;31:405–10.

[9] Kate V, Ananthakrishanan N, Ratnakar C, Badrinath S. Anti-*H.pylori* IgG seroprevalence rates in asymptomatic children and adults form south India. *Indian J Med Microbiol.* 2001;19:20–5.

[10] Malaty HM, Haveman T, Graham DY, Fraley K. *Helicobacter pylori* infection in asymptomatic children: Impact of epidemiological factors on accuracy of diagnostic tests. *J Ped Gastroenterol Nutr.* 2002;35:59–63.

[11] Rosenberg JJ. *Helicobacter pylori. Pediatr Rev.* Feb 2010;31(2):85-6; discussion 86.

[12] Gold BJ. New approach to *Helicobacter pylori* infection in children. *Curr Gastroenterol Rep.* 2001;3:235–47.

[13] Cervantes DT, Fischbach LA, Goodman KJ, Phillips CV, Chen S, Broussard CS. Exposure to *Helicobacter pylori*-positive siblings and persistence of *Helicobacter pylori* infection in early childhood. *J Pediatr Gastroenterol Nutr.* May 2010;50(5):481-5.

[14] M Rowland, C Imrie, B Bourke, B Drumm, How should *Helicobacter pylori* infected children be managed?, Gut BMJ,1999;45:I36-I39 doi:10.1136/gut.45.2008.i36

[15] Koletzko S, Jones NL, Goodman KJ, et al. Evidence-based guidelines from ESPGHAN and NASPGHAN for *Helicobacter pylori* infection in children. *J Pediatr Gastroenterol Nutr.* Aug 2011;53(2):230-43

[16] Gold BD, Colletti RB, Abbott M, Czinn S, Elitsur Y, Hassall E, et al. *Helicobacter pylori* infection in children: Recommendation for diagnosis and treatment. *J Pediatr Gastroenterol Nutr.* 2000;31:490–7.

[17] Day AS, Sherman PM. Accuracy of office-based immunoassay for the diagnosis of *Helicobacter pylori* infection in children. *Helicobacter.* 2002;7:205–9.

[18] 54. Makristathis A, Hirschl AM, Lehours P, Megraud F. Diagnosis of *Helicobacter pylori* infection. Helicobacter. 2002;9:7–14.

[19] Bahu MG, da Silvaria TR, Maguilnick I, Ulbrich-Kulczynski J. Endoscopic nodular gastritis: An endoscopic indicator of high-grade bacterial colonization and severe gastritis in children with *Helicobacter pylori. J Pediatr Gastroenterol Nutr.* 2003;36:217–22.

[20] Konno M, Fujii N, Yokota S, et al. Five-year follow-up study of mother-to-child transmission of *Helicobacter pylori* infection detected by a random amplified polymorphic DNA fingerprinting method. *J Clin Microbiol.* 43(5):2246-50.

[21] Ahmed KS, Khan AA, Ahmed I, et al. Impact of household hygiene and water source on the prevalence and transmission of *Helicobacter pylori*: a South Indian perspective. *Singapore Med J.* Jun 2007;48(6):543-9.

[22] Grubel P, Huang L, Masubuchi N, Stutzenberger FJ, Cave DR. Detection of *Helicobacter pylori* DNA in houseflies (*Musca domestica*) on three continents. *Lancet.* Sep 5 1998;352(9130):788-9.

[23] Appelmelk BJ, Simoons-Smit I, Negrini R, et al. Potential role of molecular mimicry between *Helicobacter pylori* lipopolysaccharide and host Lewis blood group antigens in autoimmunity. *Infect Immun*. Jun 1996;64(6):2031-40.

[24] Figueiredo C, Machado JC, Yamaoka Y. Pathogenesis of *Helicobacter pylori* Infection. *Helicobacter*. 2005;10 Suppl 1:14-20.

[25] Rick JR, Goldman M, Semino-Mora C, et al. *In situ* expression of cagA and risk of gastroduodenal disease in *Helicobacter pylori*-infected children. *J Pediatr Gastroenterol Nutr*. Feb 2010;50(2):167-72.

[26] Baysoy G, Ertem D, Ademoglu E, et al. Gastric histopathology, iron status and iron deficiency anemia in children with *Helicobacter pylori* infection. *J Pediatr Gastroenterol Nutr*. Feb 2004;38(2):146-51.

[27] Williams MP, Pounder RE. *Helicobacter pylori*: from the benign to the malignant. *Am J Gastroenterol*. Nov 1999;94(11 Suppl):S11-6.

[28] Correa P, Haenszel W, Cuello C, Tannenbaum S, Archer M. A model for gastric cancer epidemiology. Lancet 1975; 2: 58-60.

[29] Correa P. A human model of gastric carcinogenesis. Cancer Research 1988; 48: 3554-3560.

[30] Correa P. Human gastric carcinogenesis: a multistep and multifactorial process. First American Cancer Society Award lecture on cancer epidemiology and prevention. Cancer Research 1992; 52: 6735-6740.

[31] Correa P, Piazuelo MB. The gastric precancerous cascade. Journal of Digestive Diseases 2012; 13(1): 2-9.

[32] Ashorn M, Rago T, Kokkonen J, et al. Symptomatic response to *Helicobacter pylori* eradication in children with recurrent abdominal pain: double blind randomized placebo-controlled trial. *J Clin Gastroenterol*. Sep 2004;38(8):646-50.

[33] Gold BD, Colletti RB, Abbott M, et al. *Helicobacter pylori* infection in children: recommendations for diagnosis and treatment. *J Pediatr Gastroenterol Nutr*. Nov 2000;31(5): 490-7.

[34] Spee LA, Madderom MB, Pijpers M, van Leeuwen Y, Berger MY. Association between *Helicobacter pylori* and gastrointestinal symptoms in children. *Pediatrics*. Mar 2010;125(3):e651-69.

[35] Yaghoobi M, Farrokhyar F, Yuan Y, Hunt RH. Is There an Increased Risk of GERD After *Helicobacter pylori* Eradication?: A Meta-Analysis. *Am J Gastroenterol*. Jan 19 2010.

[36] Moon A, Solomon A, Beneck D, Cunningham-Rundles S. Positive association between *Helicobacter pylori* and gastroesophageal reflux disease in children. *J Pediatr Gastroenterol Nutr*. Sep 2009;49(3):283-8.

[37] Franchini M, Veneri D. Helicobacter pylori-associated immune trombocitopenia, Platelets, 2006;17(2);71-7

[38] Takahashi M, Kimura H, Watanabe K Helicobacter pylori infection in patients with idiopathic short starure. Pediatrics International, 2002;44(3):277-80

[39] Capurso G, Lahner E, Marcheggiano A, Caruana P, Carnuccio A, Bordi C, Delle Fave G, Annibale B. Involvement of the corporal mucosa and related changes in gastric acid secretion characterize patients with iron deficiency anemy associated with Helicobacter pylori infection. Aliment Pharmacol Ther 2001; 15(11): 1753-1761.

[40] Pelicano R, Franceschi F, Saracco G, Fagoonee S, Roccarina D, Gasbarrini A. Helicobacters and extragastric diseases. Helicobacter 2009; 14(Suppl 1): 58-68.

[41] Arnold DM, Bernotas A, Nazi I, Stasi R, Kuwana M, Liu Y, Kelton JG, Crowther MA. Platelet count response to *H. pylori* treatment in patients with immune thrombocytopenic purpura with and without *H. pylori* infection: a systematic review. Haematologica 2009; 94(6): 850-856.

[42] Franceschi F, Navarese EP, Mollo R, Giupponi B, De Marco G, Merra G, Gasbarrini G, Silveri NG. Helicobacter pylori and atherosclerosis. A review of the literature. Recent Progr Med 2009; 100(2): 91-96.

[43] Rogha M, Nikvarz M, Poumoghaddas Z et al. Is Helicobacter pylori infection a risk factor for coronary heart disease? ARYA Atherosclerose 2012; 8(1): 5-8.

[44] Pirouz T, Zounubi L, Keivani H, Rakhshani N, Hormazdi M. Detection of Helicobacter pylori in paraffin-embedded specimens from patients with chronic liver diseases, using the amplification method. Digestive Diseases and Sciences 2009; 54(7): 1456-1459.

[45] Suerbaum S, Michetti P, *Helicobacter pylori* infection. N Engl Med 2002; 347: 1175-86

[46] Rothenbacher D, Bode G, Berg G, Gommel R, Gonser T, Alder G, et al. Prevalence and determinants of *Helicobacter pylori* infection in preschool children: A population based study from Germany. *Int J Epidemiol.* 1998; 27: 135–41.

[47] Opekun AR, Gilger MA, Denyes SM, Nirken MH, Philip SP, Osato MS, et al. *Helicobacter pylori* infection in children of Texas. *J Pediatr Gastroenterol Nutr.* 2000; 31: 405–10

[48] Wizla-Derambure N, Michaud L, Ategbo S, Vincent P, Ganga-Zandzou S, Turck D, et al. Familial and community environmental risk factors for *Helicobacter pylori* infection in children and adolescents. *J Pediatr Gastroenterol Nutr.* 2001; 33: 58–63.

[49] Mourad-Baars PE, Verspaget HW, Mertens BJ, Luisa Merain M. Low prevalence of *Helicobacter pylori* infection in young children in the Netherlands. *Eur J Gastroenterol Hepatol.* 2007; 19: 213–6.

[50] Kate V, Ananthakrishanan N, Ratnakar C, Badrinath S. Anti-*H. pylori* Ig G seroprevalence rates in asymptomatic children and adults form south India. *Indian J Med Microbiol.* 2001; 19: 20–5.

[51] Gold BJ. *Helicobacter pylori* infection in children. *Curr Prob Pediatr.* 2001; 31: 247–66.

[52] Rocha GA, Rocha AM, Silva LD, Samtos A, Bocewicz AC, Queiroz RM, et al. Transmission of *Helicobacter pylori* infection in families of preschool-aged children from Minas Gerais, Brazil. *Trop Med Int Health.* 2003; 8: 987–91.

[53] Malaty HM, Haveman T, Graham DY, Fraley K, *Helicobacter pylori* infection in asymptomatic children: Impact of epidemiological factors on accuracy of diagnostic tests. *J Ped Gastroenterol Nutr.* 2002; 35: 59–63.

[54] Ndip RN, Malange AE, Akoachere JF, MacKay WG, Titanji VP, Weaver LT. *Helicobacter pylori* antigens in faeces of asymptomatic children in the Buea and Limbe health districts of Cameroon: A pilot study. *Trop Med Int Health.* 2004; 9: 1036–40.

[55] Rajindrajith S et al, *Helicobacter pylori* Infection in Children, *Saudi J Gastroenterol*, 2009, 15 (2): 86-94.

[56] Sullivan PB, Thomas JE, Wight DG, et al. *Helicobacter pylori* in Gambian children with chronic diarrhoea and malnutrition. *Arch Dis Child.* Feb 1990;65(2):189-91.

[57] Bujanover Y, Konikoff F, Baratz M. Nodular gastritis and *Helicobacter pylori. J Pediatr Gastroenterol Nutr.* Jul 1990;11(1):41-4.

[58] Lionetti E, Miniello VL, Castellaneta SP, et al. *Lactobacillus reuteri* therapy to reduce side-effects during anti-*Helicobacter pylori* treatment in children: a randomized placebo controlled trial. *Aliment Pharmacol Ther.* Nov 15 2006;24(10):1461-8.

[59] Goldman CG, Barrado DA, Balcarce N, et al. Effect of a probiotic food as an adjuvant to triple therapy for eradication of *Helicobacter pylori* infection in children. *Nutrition.* Oct 2006;22(10):984-8.

[60] Zojaji H, Talaie R, Mirsattari D, et al. The efficacy of *Helicobacter pylori* eradication regimen with and without vitamin C supplementation. *Dig Liver Dis.* Sep 2009;41(9): 644-7.

[61] Ruggiero P. *Helicobacter pylori* infection: what's new. *Curr Opin Infect Dis.* Jun 2012;25(3):337-44.

[62] Bahremand S, Nematollahi LR, Fourutan H, et al. Evaluation of triple and quadruple *Helicobacter pylori* eradication therapies in Iranian children: a randomized clinical trial. *Eur J Gastroenterol Hepatol.* May 2006;18(5):511-4.

[63] Bhasin DK, Sharma BC, Ray P, et al. Comparison of seven and fourteen days of lansoprazole, clarithromycin, andamoxicillin therapy for eradication of *Helicobacter pylori*: a report from India.. *Helicobacter.* Jun 2000;5(2):84-7.

[64] Bonamico M, Strappini PM, Bonci E, et al. Evaluation of stool antigen test, PCR on ORAL samples and serology for the noninvasive detection of *Helicobacter pylori* infection in children. *Helicobacter*. Feb 2004;9(1):69-76.

[65] Booka M, Okuda M, Shin K, et al. Polymerase chain reaction--restriction fragment length polymorphism analysis of clarithromycin-resistant *Helicobacter pylori* infection in children using stool sample. *Helicobacter*. Jun 2005;10(3):205-13.

[66] Bourke B, Ceponis P, Chiba N, et al. Canadian *Helicobacter* Study Group Consensus Conference: Update on the approach to *Helicobacter pylori* infection in children and adolescents - an evidence - based evaluation. *Can J Gastroenterol*. Jul 2005;19(7): 399-408.

[67] Cammarota G, Cianci R, Cannizzaro O, et al. High-dose versus low-dose clarithromycin in 1-week triple therapy, including rabeprazole and levofloxacin, for *Helicobacter pylori* eradication. *J Clin Gastroenterol*. Feb 2004;38(2):110-4.

[68] Chan KL, Zhou H, Ng DK, Tam PK. A prospective study of a one-week nonbismuth quadruple therapy for childhood *Helicobacter pylori* infection. *J Pediatr Surg*. Jul 2001;36(7):1008-11.

[69] Chan KL, Zhou H, Ng DK, Tam PK. A prospective study of a one-week nonbismuth quadruple therapy for childhood *Helicobacter pylori* infection. *J Pediatr Surg*. Jul 2001;36(7):1008-11.

[70] Chong SK, Lou Q, Asnicar MA, et al. *Helicobacter pylori* infection in recurrent abdominal pain in childhood: comparison of diagnostic tests and therapy. *Pediatrics*. Aug 1995;96(2 Pt 1):211-5.

[71] Czinn SJ. *Helicobacter pylori* infection: detection, investigation, and management. *J Pediatr*. Mar 2005;146(3 Suppl):S21-6.

[72] Di Caro S, Franceschi F, Mariani A, et al. Second-line levofloxacin-based triple schemes for *Helicobacter pylori* eradication. *Dig Liver Dis*. Jul 2009;41(7):480-5.

[73] Drumm B. *Helicobacter pylori* in the pediatric patient. *Gastroenterol Clin North Am*. Mar 1993;22(1):169-82.

[74] Graham DY, Rakel RE, Fendrick AM, et al. Practical advice on eradicating *Helicobacter pylori* infection. *Postgrad Med*. Mar 1999;105(3):137-40, 145-8.

[75] El-Omar EM, Oien K, Murray LS, et al. Increased prevalence of precancerous changes in relatives of gastric cancer patients: critical role of *H. pylori*. *Gastroenterology*. Jan 2000;118(1):22-30.

[76] Ernst PB, Gold BD. *Helicobacter pylori* in childhood: new insights into the immunopathogenesis of gastric disease and implications for managing infection in children. *J Pediatr Gastroenterol Nutr*. May 1999;28(5):462-73.

[77] Farrell MK. Dr. Apley meets *Helicobacter pylori*. *J Pediatr Gastroenterol Nutr*. Feb 1993;16(2):118-9.

[78] Feydt-Schmidt A, Kindermann A, Konstantopoulos N, et al. Reinfection rate in children after successful *Helicobacter pylori* eradication. *Eur J Gastroenterol Hepatol*. Oct 2002;14(10):1119-23.

[79] Fiedorek SC, Casteel HB, Pumphrey CL, et al. The role of *Helicobacter pylori* in recurrent, functional abdominal pain in children. *Am J Gastroenterol*. Mar 1992;87(3):347-9.

[80] Francavilla R, Lionetti E, Castellaneta SP, et al. Improved efficacy of 10-Day sequential treatment for Helicobacter *pylori* eradication in children: a randomized trial. *Gastroenterology*. Nov 2005;129(5):1414-9.

[81] Gillen D, el-Omar EM, Wirz AA, et al. The acid response to gastrin distinguishes duodenal ulcer patients from *Helicobacter pylori*-infected healthy subjects. *Gastroenterology*. Jan 1998;114(1):50-7.

[82] Gisbert JP, Luna M, Gomez B, et al. Recurrence of *Helicobacter pylori* infection after several eradication therapies: long-term follow-up of 1000 patients. *Aliment Pharmacol Ther*. Mar 15 2006;23(6):713-9.

[83] Gisbert JP, Perez-Aisa A, Castro-Fernandez M, et al. *Helicobacter pylori* first-line treatment and rescue option containing levofloxacin in patients allergic to penicillin. *Dig Liver Dis*. Apr 2010;42(4):287-90.

[84] Glassman MS. *Helicobacter pylori* infection in children. A clinical overview. *Clin Pediatr (Phila)*. Aug 1992;31(8):481-7.

[85] Gormally S, Drumm B. *Helicobacter pylori* and gastrointestinal symptoms. *Arch Dis Child*. Mar 1994;70(3):165-6.

[86] Graham DY, Shiotani A. The time to eradicate gastric cancer is now. *Gut*. Jun 2005;54(6):735-8.

[87] Guo CY, Wu YB, Liu HL, et al. Clinical evaluation of four one-week triple therapy regimens in eradicating *Helicobacter pylori* infection. *World J Gastroenterol*. Mar 1 2004;10(5):747-9.

[88] Hardikar W, Feekery C, Smith A, et al. *Helicobacter pylori* and recurrent abdominal pain in children. *J Pediatr Gastroenterol Nutr*. Feb 1996;22(2):148-52.

[89] Heldenberg D, Wagner Y, Heldenberg E, et al. The role of *Helicobacter pylori* in children with recurrent abdominal pain. *Am J Gastroenterol*. Jun 1995;90(6):906-9.

[90] Horvitz G, Gold BD. Gastroduodenal diseases of childhood. *Curr Opin Gastroenterol*. Nov 2006;22(6):632-40.

[91] Huang FC, Chang MH, Hsu HY, et al. Long-term follow-up of duodenal ulcer in children before and after eradication of *Helicobacter pylori*. *J Pediatr Gastroenterol Nutr*. Jan 1999;28(1):76-80.

[92] Huebner ES, Surawicz CM. Probiotics in the prevention and treatment of gastrointestinal infections. *Gastroenterol Clin North Am*. June 2006;35:355-65.

[93] Israel DM, Hassall E. Treatment and long-term follow-up of *Helicobacter pylori*-associated duodenal ulcer disease in children. *J Pediatr*. Jul 1993;123(1):53-8..

[94] Judd RH. *Helicobacter pylori*, gastritis, and ulcers in pediatrics. *Adv Pediatr*. 1992;39:283-306.

[95] Khurana R, Fischbach L, Chiba N, et al. Meta-analysis: *Helicobacter pylori* eradication treatment efficacy in children. *Aliment Pharmacol Ther*. Mar 1 2007;25(5):523-36.

[96] Kimia A, Zahavi I, Shapiro R, et al. The role of *Helicobacter pylori* and gastritis in children with recurrent abdominal pain. *Isr Med Assoc J*. Feb 2000;2(2):126-8.

[97] Kiyota K, Habu Y, Sugano Y, et al. Comparison of 1-week and 2-week triple therapy with omeprazole, amoxicillin,and clarithromycin in peptic ulcer patients with *Helicobacter pylori* infection: results of a randomized controlled trial. *J Gastroenterol*. 1999;34 Suppl 11:76-9.

[98] Knippig C, Arand F, Leodolter A, et al. Prevalence of *H. pylori*-infection in family members of *H. pylori* positive and its influence on the reinfection rate after successful eradication therapy: a two-year follow-up. *Z Gastroenterol*. Jun 2002;40(6):383-7.

[99] Koivisto TT, Rautelin HI, Voutilainen ME, et al. First-line eradication therapy for *Helicobacter pylori* in primary health care based on antibiotic resistance: results of three eradication regimens. *Aliment Pharmacol Ther*. Mar 15 2005;21(6):773-82.

[100] Logan RP, Gummett PA, Schaufelberger HD, et al. Eradication of *Helicobacter pylori* with clarithromycin and omeprazole. *Gut*. Mar 1994;35(3):323-6.

[101] Long SS, Pickering LK, Prober CG, eds. *Helicobacter pylori*. In: *Principles and Practice of Pediatric Infectious Diseases*. New York, NY: Churchill Livingstone; 1997:1029-33.

[102] Moshkowitz M, Reif S, Brill S, et al. One-week triple therapy with omeprazole, clarithromycin, and nitroimidazole for *Helicobacter pylori* infection in children and adolescents. *Pediatrics*. Jul 1998;102(1):e14.

[103] Nista EC, Candelli M, Cremonini F, et al. Levofloxacin-based triple therapy vs. quadruple therapy in second-line *Helicobacter pylori* treatment: a randomized trial. *Aliment Pharmacol Ther*. Sep 15 2003;18(6):627-33.

[104] Paoluzi OA, Visconti E, Andrei F, et al. Ten and eight-day sequential therapy in comparison to standard triple therapy for eradicating *Helicobacter pylori* infection: a randomized controlled study on efficacy and tolerability. *J Clin Gastroenterol*. Apr 2010;44(4):261-6.

[105] Parsonnet J. *Helicobacter pylori. Infect Dis Clin North Am.* Mar 1998;12(1):185-97.

[106] Parsonnet J, Hansen S, Rodriguez L, et al. *Helicobacter pylori* infection and gastric lymphoma. *N Engl J Med.* May 5 1994;330(18):1267-71.

[107] Raguza D, Machado RS, Ogata SK, et al. Validation of a monoclonal stool antigen test for diagnosing *Helicobacter pylori* infection in young children. *J Pediatr Gastroenterol Nutr.* Apr 2010;50(4):400-3.

[108] Siberry GK, Iannone R, eds. Formulary: drug doses. In: *The Harriet Lane Handbook.* 15th ed. St Louis, MO: Mosby; 2000:622, 630, 645-6, 674-5, 772-3, 795, 837.

[109] Vinette KM, Gibney KM, Proujansky R, Fawcett PT. Comparison of PCR and clinical laboratory tests for diagnosing *H. pylori* infection in pediatric patients. *BMC Microbiol.* Jan 27 2004;4:5.

[110] Wewer V, Andersen LP, Paerregaard A, et al. Treatment of *Helicobacter pylori* in children with recurrent abdominal pain. *Helicobacter.* Sep 2001;6(3):244-8.

[111] Windle HJ, Kelleher D, Crabtree JE. Childhood *Helicobacter pylori* infection and growth impairment in developing countries: a vicious cycle?. *Pediatrics.* Mar 2007;119(3):e754-9.

2

Helicobacter pylori — Current Therapy and Future Therapeutic Strategies

Rajinikanth Siddalingam and
Kumarappan Chidambaram

1. Introduction

Helicobacter pylori (H pylori) is a spiral-shaped bacterium that is attached to or just above the gastric mucosa. The organism can persist in the stomach indefinitely and may not cause clinical illness for many years after infection [1]. Indeed, a large number of infected patients never develop any symptoms [2, 3]. However, literature has also associated *H pylori* infection with gastritis and gastric malignancies (gastric adenocarcinoma and MALT-lymphoma) [4]. Chronic *H pylori* infection has also been associated with several extra intestinal diseases, such as autoimmune thrombocytopenia, sideropenic anemia and chronic urticaria but the pathogenesis is still not known [5]. *H pylori* gastric infection is one of the most prevalent infectious diseases worldwide with an estimate of 40%-50% of the world population [3]. Remarkable differences are due to geographical, socio-economic and demographic factors [6]. *H pylori* transmission is still not completely understood. In addition, among infected patients, the reasons why only some develop symptoms is still a matter of speculations. Studies suggested that *H.pylori* is also transmitted from domestic animals like cat and sheep, but humans are the primary reservoir of *H pylori* infection [7, 8]. Several tests are available to detect *H pylori* in patients with ulcer or dyspepsia. The more commonly used tests are the evaluation of biopsy specimens during upper gastrointestinal tract (GI)I endoscopy, the detection of serum anti *H pylori* antibodies and breath tests with 13C-labeled urea (9-11) The discovery that most upper gastrointestinal diseases are the consequence of *H pylori* infection that can be treated with antibacterials, is an important medical advance [12]. Although, in the last few decades, *H pylori* eradication has been standardized, occurrence of resistance to therapeutic regimens is a growing problem [3, 14]. The purpose of this paper is to provide an appraisal of the most effective, current treatments available for *H pylori,* and to speculate on the potential for newer approaches in treatment and prophylaxis in future.

2. Epidemiology and prevalence

Humans are the only host for *H.pylori,* which is found in stomach, duodenum, esophagus and rectum on areas of metaplastic gastric epithelium [15]. Other *H.pylori* species have been isolated from the animals [16]. Animal models of *Helicobacter* infection have been developed due to shared characteristics of other *H.pylori* like *H.mustelae* and *H. felis* with *H.pylori. H.pylori* exists the world over and its prevalence in the population increases with age [17, 18] In developed countries, prevalence increases with rate of 1% per year of age, where as it is rare in children, and reaches 70% in the seventh decade [19]. In developing countries, more than 50% children acquire the infection by the age of 10 years, and more than 80% of the population gets infected by the age of 20 years [20-22]. In asymptomatic individuals prevalence of *H.pylori* infection varies from 31%-84% [22]. *H.pylori* infection is chronic and once acquired remains life long, unless eradicated by antibiotics given for some other conditions [22]. Humoral and tissue immune response by the host is usually not sufficient to clear the infection. Though the mode of transmission is not yet well established, most probably it occurs by oral-oral or faeco-oral route and important risk factors are socioeconomic status and age [7, 8]. Overcrowding, poor socio-economic status and poor hygiene are associated with high infection rate. Re-infection rate after eradication is quite high in developing countries due to above mentioned risk factors [23].

Colonization of *H.Pylori* occurs by producing urease and gastric acid inhibitory protein. It can colonize only in gastric type epithelium and cannot stay anywhere else in the GI in the absence of gastric mucosa [24]. Metaplasia, which is present in more than 90% of patients of duodenal ulcer, occurs by replacing the columnar cells, normally covering the duodenal villi, by gastric type epithelium. Adhesion of *H.pylori* to the gastric epithelium occurs by tissue specific proteins. Colonization of the duodenal bulb by *H.pylori* leads to mucosal inflammation which makes it vulnerable to attack by acid or pepsin or bile resulting into ulceration, however, factors leading to gastric metaplasia in the duodenal bulb are not known. Stimulation of the immune system of *H.pylori* contributes to host damage and it evades the immunological clearance [25-2]).

3. Diseases associated with *H.pylori*

H.pylori infection is found to be associated with gastritis, non-ulcer dyspepsia (NUD), duodenal ulcer, gastric ulcer, gastric cancer, gastric lymphoma of mucosa associated lymphoid tissue (MALT) and even coronary heart disease [28, 29]. It has now been well established that *H.pylori* is the cause of almost all duodenal ulcers (DU) and chronic benign gastric ulcers (GU) which are not associated with nonsteroidal anti-inflammatory drugs (NSAID) [30]. More than 95%

of DU and 90% of GU are associated with *H.pylori* infection and there is a dramatic decrease in their relapse rate after the *H.pylori* eradication. Right now there is no convincing evidence that NUD symptoms are due to *H.pylori* infection. Prevalence of *H.pylori* infection is comparable between healthy individuals and patients with the symptoms of NUD. Recurrent abdominal pain in children suggestive of NUD subsides after the eradication of *H.pylori* which indirectly associates *H.pylori* infection with NUD. However, further studies are necessary to eradicate *H.pylori* completely in NUD. [31]

4. Current therapy of *H.pylori* infection

The objective of *H. pylori* treatment is the complete elimination of the organism from the GI of patients and once this has been achieved then the rate of reinfection is low. Development of a successful treatment for *H. pylori* infection has been fraught with difficulty. The survival capabilities of the *H.pylori* organism over a wide pH spectrum within the stomach make the task of eradication difficult [32]. The organism must be eradicated from each of these potential niches and this is a daunting task for any single antibiotic. Initial attempts to cure the infection showed that the presence of antibiotic susceptibility in vitro did not necessarily correlate with successful treatment. It was rapidly recognized that the therapy with a single antibiotic led to a poor cure rate and various antimicrobial mixtures were tried resulting in several effective combinations of antibiotics, bismuth and antisecretory drugs [33, 34].

It is vital that the infection be treated optimally with clinically relevant *H.pylori*– eradication regimens that has an acceptably high eradication rate and without major side effects and with minimal induction of bacterial resistance. The reasonable eradication targets would be ≥90% cure rate on per-protocol analysis, and ≥80% cure rate on intent-to-treat analysis [35]. Such goals have not been achieved with antibiotics alone. Because of luminal acidity influences the effectiveness of some antimicrobial agents that are active against *H. pylori.* In order to achieve the desirable eradication rate, the antibiotics are combined with proton-pump inhibitors or ranitidine bismuth citrate. So-called triple therapies, combinations of one anti secretory agent with two antimicrobial agents for 7 to 14 days, have been extensively evaluated, and several regimens have been approved by the Food and Drug Administration (FDA). Combination drug regimens are essential to maximize the chance of eradicating the infection and to minimize the risk of promoting antimicrobial (to metronidazole and clarithromycin) resistance [35].

The most widely used antimicrobials in these regimens are amoxicillin, clarithromycin, metronidazole, tetracycline, and bismuth. Resistance of *H pylori* to the limited range of antibiotics that have efficacy in its treatment can severely affect attempts to eradicate the bacteria. Resistance to tetracycline or amoxicillin is extremely rare [36, 37]. The issue of resistance primarily concerns the nitroimidazoles (metronidazole or tinidazole) and macrolides (clarithromycin) [38, 39]. Prevalence of *H pylori* resistance to metronidazole is approximately 25% in developing countries, because of the frequent use of nitroimidazoles to treat other diseases% [40, 41]. Increasing the dosage of metronidazole administered (e.g., from 1.0

to 1.5 g/day) generally improves the results of therapy when treating metronidazole-resistant *H.pylori* strains. Resistance to clarithromycin is becoming more prevalent in some European countries, where the prevalence may be as high as 17% [40, 41]. The clinical effect of clarithromycin resistance is essentially complete loss of any clarithromycin anti-*H pylori* effect; outcome of therapy can generally be predicted on the basis of what could be expected if only the other antimicrobials in the regimen are used [39].

4.1. First-line therapy of *H.pylori* infection

First-line *H. pylori* therapy should ideally be short, easy to administer, well tolerated and relatively cheap [42]. However, over and above these considerations, the prime objective of any treatment is to eradicate the infection in the maximum number of patients [43]. Some of the best validated first-line treatments for *H pylori* include amoxicillin or clarithromycin-based triple therapies, which consists of a proton pump inhibitor PPI (standard dose twice daily) combined with clarithromycin (500 mg twice daily) and either amoxicillin (1 g twice daily) or metronidazole (500 mg twice daily) for a minimum of 7 days. Bismuth-based quadruple therapies consisting of a histamine receptor antagonist or PPI combined with bismuth, tetracycline, and metronidazole [42, 43]. Another alternative approach is to include ranitidine bismuth citrate (RBC) in place of a PPI in clarithromycin triple therapy. These regimens have the propensity to eradicate 70 to 85% of the infection. However, the regimen, which employs a PPI with clarithromycin and amoxicillin is the most widely endorsed first-line regimen for *H pylori* [42, 43]. Any of the currently available PPIs may be used with equivalent treatment efficacy [44, 45] with the exception of esomeprazole as it is prescribed once daily because it is imperative that the standard dose of a PPI be prescribed twice daily in order to maximize treatment efficacy [46]. RBC is sometimes used in place of a PPI in countries outside the United States with at least equal and perhaps greater efficacy [47]. Metronidazole can be used as an alternative to amoxicillin, particularly in the setting of penicillin allergy or intolerance [42, 43].

Bismuth-based quadruple therapy is another option in penicillin allergic patients which yields similar eradication rates to clarithromycin triple therapies [48, 49]. A recent meta-analysis including five randomized trials reported intention-to-treat (ITT) and per protocol (PP) eradication rates of 79% and 85% for clarithromycin triple therapy and 80% and 87% for bismuth quadruple therapy, respectively [50]. Recently, simplified twice-daily dosing regimens for bismuth quadruple therapy have been successfully used in clinical trials [51].It is worth noting that the dosing of metronidazole used in the various bismuth quadruple therapies has not been consistent across studies. As higher doses of metronidazole (500 mg) may provide better cure rates than lower doses (250 mg), caution must be exercised when interpreting the data from comparative studies and pooled analyses involving quadruple therapies. Although there is no universal standard, there has been a desire to decrease the duration of therapy, particularly in countries outside the United States where treatment durations of at least 7 days have been recommended [42]. Until very recently, the recommended treatment duration in the United States has been 10–14 days due to lower eradication rates with 7-day regimens [52]. However, a large randomized US trial, rabeprazole-based triple therapy for 7 days was found to be as effective as 10 days of therapy (ITT eradication rates of

77% [71%–83%] vs. 78% [72%–84%], respectively) [53]. Based upon these results, 7-day rabeprazole-based triple therapy has been approved by the Food and Drug Administration for use in the United States. However there is some minor disagreement on the duration of treatment; the US guidelines recommend a 14-day course, whereas in Europe, a 7-day course is considered to be sufficient and Canadian and Asia–Pacific guidelines correspond largely to the Maastricht 2–2000 guidelines [54].

4.2. Second-line therapy of *H.pylori* infection

The choice of second-line treatment depends on which treatment approach was used initially, because retreatment with the same regimen is not recommended. If a clarithromycin-based regimen was used initially, a metronidazole-based regimen should be used as follow-up (in combination with a PPI, tetracycline, and bismuth), and vice versa. Prolonging the treatment period to 14 days is probably necessary. Because bacterial resistance to metronidazole or clarithromycin results primarily from previous treatment failures, first-choice treatment should never combine clarithromycin and metronidazole in the same regimen [55]. Second-line therapy has been extensively reviewed by several authors [55-57]. The assessment of *H pylori* sensitivity to antibiotics may be useful only after failure of the second-line therapy [58]

The most widely recommended second-line treatment for persistent *H pylori* infection is quadruple therapy with a PPI (standard dose twice daily), bismuth salt (subsalicylate or subcitrate 120 mg 4 times daily), metronidazole (500 mg thrice daily) and tetracycline (500 mg 4 times daily) for minimum of 7 days. Further failures should be managed by specialists. The Table 1 summarizes the suggested therapeutic regimens for eradication of *H pylori* infection. No other second-line treatment strategies have been widely endorsed; however, -line therapy should be [59] rifabutin-based triple therapy and furazolidone-based triple therapy [59, 60] have been investigated and suggested as alternatives to bismuth quadruple therapy (Table 1). As second-line therapy, the Maastricht 2-2000 Consensus Report suggests a quadruple therapy based on bismuth (120 mg, q.i.d.), tetracycline (500 mg, q.i.d.), metronidazole (500 mg, t.i.d.) and antisecretive agent (PPI, b.i.d.) for a minimum of 7 days [34]. Further trials have shown that replacing the proton pump inhibitor and the bismuth compound of the quadruple therapy by RBC also achieves good results, with an eradication rate ranging between 57%-95% [61, 62]. The failure of second line quadruple therapy is associated with its discontinuation because of high incidence of side effects (6%-68%) [63]. A triple therapy with the combination of levofloxacin, rabeprazole and tinidazole or amoxicillin has been proposed as an alternative to Maastricht. This protocol shows an eradication rate higher than 90% compared to quadruple therapies given for 7 days (63%) with a lower incidence of side effects [64]. Rifabutin has been shown to have a good eradication rate (87%), if administered at a high dose (300 mg) in combination with amoxicillin and PPI, as compared to quadruple therapy. Wong et al [65] showed that a combination of levofloxacin, rifabutin and rabeprazole has a high efficacy with an eradication rate >90%. Furazolidone is also used to replace metronidazole in quadruple therapy [66]. Different *in vivo* studies have confirmed the efficacy of regimens containing a high-dose furazolidone [200 mg, b.i.d.] as the second-line therapy in patients with metronidazole-resistance [66]. Many other combinations have been used with various rates of success.

Bacterial eradication may fail in up to 40% of cases after the suggested second-line regimens. As a consequence, to treat patients who have already undergone the first- and second-line therapies is a common challenge [67]. A recent rifabutin based triple therapy shown eradication rates of 100 and 87.5 % (Per Protocol and Intention-to-Treat analysis) in primary resistance to clarithromycin and tinidazole and 82.2 and 78.5% in secondary resistance [68].

4.3. Third-line rescue therapy for persistent *H.pylori* infection

Patients who fail both first- and second-line therapy are a clinical challenge. New modified eradication regimes involve the substitution of antibiotics used with other drugs, such as rifabutin, levofloxacin, and furazolidone [58-65] These antibiotics should be considered for third-line treatment. Currently, no widely endorsed treatment regimens are available, for persons with persistent *H.pylori* infection despite two or more previous courses of antibiotics (third-line therapy). A number of third-line regimens such as bismuth quadruple therapy, rifabutin-based triple therapy, levofloxacin-based triple therapy furazolidone-based triple therapy and Doxycycline-based therapy have been investigated and shown in Table 2.

The new fluoroquinolone, levofloxacin, has shown an excellent activity against a variety of Gram-positive and Gram-negative organisms which are resistant to the established agents Matsuzaki et al [69] studied several strains and reported that levofloxacin had an excellent and wide spectrum antibacterial activity compared with other fluoroquinolones and antibiotics tested [69]. A previous study has shown efficacy and safety of levofloxacin based triple therapy in *H.pylori* infection first-line therapy [70]. Recently, Gatta et.al [71] have proposed a third-line treatment after two eradication failed courses without fluoroquinolones, with standard dose of PPIs (b.i.d.), levofloxacin (250 mg, b.i.d.) and amoxicillin (1 g, b.i.d.) for 10 days. The eradications rates of 76.2% and 84.6% according to ITT and PP anlysis, respectively, have been achieved. The levofloxacin-based treatment could eradicate most of the strains (92.3%) which are resistant *in vitro* to both clarithromycin and metronidazole, but susceptible to levofloxacin. Furthermore, this drug combination, successfully employed as rescue therapy, is well tolerated and has no major side-effects [72].

Rifabutin, a spiropiperidyl derivative of rifamycin, has been shown to exhibit high in vitro activity against *H.pylori* [73, 74]. Furthermore, clinical trials have suggested that rifabutin may be a possible candidate for second or third line eradication combination therapy [75]. Furthermore, rifabutin is chemically stable at a wide pH range [74]. Recently, rifabutin-based rescue therapies (twice-daily standard-dose PPI plus amoxicillin 1 g twice daily or levofloxacin 500 mg once daily plus rifabutin 300 mg daily, for 7 days) have been shown to represent an encouraging strategy for eradication failures because they are effective against *H pylori* strains resistant to clarithromycin or metronidazole [75, 76]. However, rifabutin is very costly, and concerns still remain about the widespread use of this drug because of the possibility for accelerating development of drug resistance. Results of a recent study [59] suggest that a 10-day rescue therapy regimen based on the use of rabeprazole (20 mg twice daily) plus amoxicillin (1 g twice daily) plus levofloxacin (500 mg once daily) is more effective than standard quadruple regimen as a second-line option for *H.pylori* eradication. Additionally, a 7-day quadruple-therapy regimen containing amoxicillin and tetracycline has recently been proven more effective than standard quadruple therapy with metronidazole and tetracycline to rescue failed triple therapy, by overcoming the antimicrobial resistance of *H.pylori* [77-81].

Doxycycline is a widely used tetracycline antibiotic for eradicating several infections. With respect to tetracycline, Doxycycline requires the administration of only two tablets per day, leading to a better compliance in patients undergoing eradication therapies. Furthermore, Heep et.al [82] have found no secondary resistance to doxycycline in *H.pylori* patients who failed one or more eradication therapies. Quadruple regimens represent the most widely used rescue therapy. Induction of metronidazole resistance has suggested a new protocol, namely replacing tetracycline with doxycycline (because it requires the administration of only two tablets per day) and metronidazole with amoxicillin (because its resistance is less 1%), one week quadruple therapy with doxycycline (100 mg, b.i.d.), amoxicillin (1 g, b.i.d.), omeprazole (20 mg, b.i.d.) and bismuth salts (120 mg, two tablets b.i.d). This treatment has proved to be a highly effective third-line 'rescue' therapy, achieving 91% eradication rate in patients harbouring metronidazole and clarithromycin resistant H pylori strains (by ITT analysis) [83]. This regimen shows excellent compliance (99%) with mild side-effects.

1.	Bismuth subsalicylate (120 mg q.i.d) + metronidazole (500 mg t.i.d) + tetracycline (.500 mg q.i.d) + proton pump inhibitor (standard dose b.i.d) for a minimum of 7 days
2.	Levofloxacin (250 mg b.i.d) + amoxicillin (1g mg b.i.d) + proton pump inhibitor (standard dose b.i.d) for 10 days

o.d = once daily; b.i.d = twice daily; t.i.d = three times daily; q.i.d = four times daily

Table 1. Second line therapy regimens of *H.pylori* infection.

1	Rifabutin (300 mg o.d) + amoxicillin (1g b.i.d)+ proton pump inhibitor (standard dose b.i.d) for 10 days
2	Furazolidone 200 mg bid + amoxicillin (1g b.i.d) + proton pump inhibitor (standard dose b.i.d) for 14 days
3	Furazolidone 200 mg bid + tetracycline (1g b.i.d) + proton pump inhibitor (standard dose b.i.d)+ bismuth (140 mg b.i.d) for 7 days
4	Doxycycline (100 mg, b.i.d.) + amoxicillin (1g b..id) + omeprazole (20 mg, b.i.d)+ bismuth salts (120 mg, b.i.d) for 7 days.

o.d = once daily; b.i.d = twice daily; t.i.d = three times daily; q.i.d = four times daily

Table 2. Third line rescue therapy regimens of *H.pylori* infection.

4.4. Failure of therapy

The reasons behind failure of these antibacterial treatments are not very clear, but are likely multifactorial [85-87]. Failure of therapy is most frequently associated with drug resistance and non-compliance, due to complexity of rgimens and associated side effects, e.g., nausea, diarrhea, taste disturbances, mucositis, and pseudo membranous colitis. The continuing emergence of resistance to the conventional antibacterials used to treat *H. pylori* infections is of major concern [85]. Resistance to nitroimidazoles (e.g. metronidazole) is extremely high in the developing world and rates of resistance(>50%) have been described in Western countries [39-41]. Strains of *H. pylori* which are resistant to clarithromycin are also now widespread e.g., 10–17% in most part of Europe [39].

5. Future therapeutic strategies

Resistance in *H. pylori* is anticipated to increase because the currently effective drugs are used to treat many other infections where also develops the drug resistance in body. So there is an urgent need for improvement over current regimens due high resistance over no of antibiotics using in current therapy and moreover current triple and quadruple therapies are may not be desirable for widespread eradication of *H. pylori* infection in future. The next generation of *H.pylori* therapeutic regimens should be simpler, novel and specific. There are some novel approaches available to achieve this goal, such as development of therapeutic vaccine, geonome bsed drug discovery, pathogen –host tissue adhesion inhibitor, and novel site specific drug delivery at specific site of *H.pylori* infection.

5.1. Vaccine development

The success of eradication of *H.pylori* by antibiotic therapy is being hampered by the increasing occurrence of antibiotic resistance *H.pylori* strains and patience compliance. Consequently investigative attention has been focused on development of an effective therapeutic vaccine. From mathematical [88] and animal models [89] of *H. pylori* colonization, the host response has been suggested to play an important role in bacterial growth regulation. Immunization against *H. pylori* may thus be considered as a strategy to deviate the immune response programmed by infection, i.e., the re-direction of a host response from natural infection leading to persistence of infection and gastric disease, to another state in the host response capable of attenuating or eliminating *H. pylori* and its associated gastric inflammatory sequelae. Evidence from both animal models and humans implicate *H. pylori* in the activation of B cell and T cell functions leading to heterogeneous systemic and local antibody responses, lymphoid follicle hyperplasia, and significant recruitment of CD4+and CD8+ T cells [90, 91].

Vaccination against H. pylori has been performed in several animal models. Although several studies showed the benefit of prophylactic as well as therapeutic vaccination in animals, bacterial eradication was not observed in humans [92]. Knockout studies in mice revealed that the Th2 response can be absent but immunization is still possible when using urease as an antigen [93, 94].

A number of novel approaches to delivery of *H. pylori* vaccine have been reported recently. Smythies et.al [95] reported on *H.pylori* vaccination based on a modified polio virus vector where the capsid genes are replaced with *H.pylori* urease B. Poliovirus UreB replicons were co-administered with a recombinant vaccinia virus engineered to express polio virus capsid proteins, resulting in a vaccine which can only undergo one round of infection. Mice which are transgenic for the human poliovirus receptor (C57BL/ 6/DAB) are susceptible to infection with poliovirus via the systemic route. Replicon vaccination resulted in clearance of an established *H.pylori* infection in 73% of mice compared to 31% of vector-immunized controls. Furthermore, immunization prevented an infection from becoming established in 80% of immunized mice. Bacterial ghosts (Gram-negative bacterial cell envelopes, devoid of cytoplasmic envelopes) have also been shown to have good adjuvant properties [96]. *H. pylori* ghosts induced protection in a mouse model without the use of an additional adjuvant, although batch-to-batch variations were observed and improvements are therefore required before this approach could have practical applications [97]. Sodium alginate microbeads have also been tested for controlled release of a model *H. pylori* vaccine [98]. Alginate beads are widely used for encapsulation of drugs, and the mild formulation conditions, and their reported muco-adhesive properties should make them ideal carriers for vaccine antigens. Recombinant urease encapsulated in alginate beads was administered to mice via the subcutaneous, nasal and oral routes. Unexpectedly, only subcutaneous delivery induced a significant antibody response and led to reductions in *H. pylori* colonization (as determined by urease test) indicating that this approach also needs further improvement [98].

DNA vaccines are a potentially attractive approach to vaccination, and a genomic library approach has shown encouraging preliminary results in mice [99]. Two recent studies have investigated the adjuvant properties of CpG motifs in the context of DNA immunization. Interestingly, a prototype immunization construct encoding the UreB subunit which included CpG motifs [100] induced significant increases in the expression of IL-10 and beta-defensins in the gastric mucosa. In an approach that aimed to induce and modulate the immune response by triggering a specific Toll-like receptor (TLR), Sommer et.al [101] immunized C57BL/6 mice with *H. pylori* lysate mixed with a synthetic CpG oligonucleotide targeted at TLR-9 (CpG oligonucleotide 1688). Immunization induced a Th1-biased immune response as expected, and immunized mice had 10-fold reduced levels of *H.pylori* in the gastric mucosa after challenge. Synthetic CpGs have recently been approved for human use as a therapy for genital warts [102], and so given the encouraging results from mice, this approach might also be applicable for a human *H.pylori* vaccine. However, DNA vaccination studies in human volunteers have reported only suboptimal immune responses [103] and it appears that the barriers to DNA uptake may be more difficult to overcome in humans [104]. To return to our original question regarding what we have learned from the mouse model, the data from animal models of *H. pylori* infection support the feasibility of both therapeutic and prophylactic vaccination, for neonates and adults. Furthermore, a variety of routes of application and adjuvants are effective. It is, however, clear that only a better understanding of the underlying immune mechanisms will make it possible to improve efficacy and to address the issue of post immunization gastritis.

5.2. Genome-based drug discovery

The recent availability of the genome sequences of two different isolates of *H.pylori* [105, 106] has provided much stimulus to research aimed at discovering and developing novel therapeutics to eradicate *H. pylori*. *H pylori* is a relatively simple organism with a small genome of *circa* 1.7 × 10^6 nucleotides, varying slightly according to the strain of the organism, and encoding around 1600 genes [107]. Of these, depending on the stringency of the comparison, roughly 55% have homologs of putative known identity in other organisms, while another 10% have database homologs of unknown identity. The remaining 35% are unique to *H pylori* at this time. This complement of 1600-1700 gene contain a relatively small number which encode proteins whose functions are essential to the viability of the bacterium. A genome-based strategy facilitates the expeditious advanced selection of novel lethal targets not used by current antimicrobials, thus providing the opportunity to identify novel classes of antibacterials. In the case of vaccine discovery and development, comparison of two genomes has allowed the identification of a "common set" of *H.pylori* genes, among which genes encode antigens [108].

The principle underlying genome based drug development is to identify those essential proteins which are specific to *H.pylori,* and then to isolate, identify and synthesize a small molecule chemical which inhibits the essential activity of such proteins [105]. This approach is designed both to identify a drug that will work as a monotherapy, which would be specific for *H pylori* and would not interfere with other organisms. In case of *H. pylori* drug discovery, the task is to identify those essential proteins which are specific for and conserved in *H. pylori*. Identification of essentiality involves a process whereby attempts are made to mutate a gene performed using an allelic recombination method via homologous recombination and so" knock-out" its function [106]. If a particular mutant can be generated, the disrupted gene does not code for a biological process that is required for viability in vitro. "Knock-out" mutagenesis experiments with selected members of the "common set" of *H. pylori* genes have allowed the identification of targets for drug discovery in a variety of *H. pylori* physiological functions [107, 108]. These targets include proteins involved in cell envelope synthesis/ integrity, cell division, protein synthesis, nucleic acid biosynthesis, gene expression and regulation, cell metabolism and energetics, as well as proteins encoded by *H. pylori* genes of unknown function [109]. Because many essential proteins are enzymes, it is possible to establish in vitro assays to detect the ability of compounds to interfere with their enzymatic activity. The selected essential protein target is overproduced in *E.coli*, purified, and employed to identify inhibitory compounds by High Throughput Screening [110, 111]. This involves the automated micro assay screening of the ability of large numbers of compounds (>200, 000) to inhibit the enzymatic activity of the target protein. Conformed "hits" are then tested for their ability to selectively kill *H.pylori* in vitro, and to eradicate *H.pylori* infection in an animal model. Lead compounds are subjected to chemical structure-activity relationship studies to improve antibacterial potency and selectivity, as well as solubility, oral bioavailability, duration of action and pharmacokinetic properties [101]. Understanding the mechanism of action of a particular target enzyme or molecular modeling based on three-dimensional crystal structure of the protein, with or without bound inhibitor(s), can be used to facilitate medicinal chemistry studies [112, 113]. As lead compounds are identified, the classical medicinal chemistry and combinatorial chemistry approaches are applied to improve the potency and the desired microbiological properties, with the ultimate goal of producing compounds suitable for human trials.

5.3. Novel drug delivery approaches

One of the reasons for incomplete eradication of *H.pylori* is probably due to the short residence time of antimicrobial agents in stomach so that effective antimicrobial concentration cannot be achieved in the gastric mucus layer or epithelial cell surfaces where *H.pylori* resides [114-116]. Conventional tablets and capsules are, in general used for eradication therapy but these do not remain in stomach for prolonged time therefore it is difficult to reach minimum inhibitory concentration in gastric mucus where *H.pylori* colonize. To overcome the problem, a new concept is proposed based on gstroretentive concept (Floating drug delivery systems and Mucoadhesive drug delivery systems) with site specific drug delivery [117]. It is expected that the topical delivery of narrow spectrum antibiotic through floating and bioadhesive drug delivery system may result in complete removal of organism from stomach.

5.4. Floating drug delivery systems (FDDS)

Floating drug delivery systems have a bulk density less than gastric fluids and so remain buoyant in the stomach without affecting the gastric emptying rate for a prolonged period of time. The FDDS can be divided into effervescent and non-effervescent systems. Effervescent floating dosage forms are matrix type systems prepared with the help of swellable polymers such as methylcellulose and chitosan and various effervescent compounds, such as sodium bicarbonate, tartaric acid, and citric acid. They are formulated in such a way that when comes in contact with the acidic gastric contents, CO2 is liberated and gets entrapped in swollen hydrocolloids, which provides buoyancy to the dosage forms. Non-effervescent floating dosage forms use a gel forming or swellable cellulose type of hydrocolloids, polysaccharides, and matrix-forming polymers like polycarbonate, polyacrylate, polymethacrylate, and polystyrene [118]. The formulation method includes a simple approach of thoroughly mixing the drug and the gel-forming hydrocolloid. After oral administration this dosage form swells in contact with gastric fluids and attains a bulk density of < 1. The air entrapped within the swollen matrix imparts buoyancy to the dosage form. The so formed swollen gel-like structure acts as a reservoir and allows sustained release of drug through the gelatinous mass. While the system floats on the gastric contents, the drug is released slowly at the desired rate from the system. After release of drug, the residual system is emptied from the stomach. The FDDS greatly improve the pharmacotherapy of the stomach through local drug release, leading to high drug concentrations at the gastric mucosa for eradicating *H.pylori* from the submucosal tissue of the stomach, making it possible to treat stomach and duodenal ulcers, and gastritis [119-121].

In our previous study [114] we have developed the floating in situ gelling system of amoxicillin and evaluated in vivo efficiency in Mongolian gerbil model, the result indicated that the floating in situ gel has promising potential for eradicating *H.pylori* infection. In this study the gelled solution floated in stomach for >20 h, and *the in vivo H.pylori* clearance efficiency was 10 time more than that of amoxicillin solution in gerbils model.

Yang et al [119] developed a swellable asymmetric triple-layer tablet with floating ability to prolong the gastric residence time of triple drug regimen (tetracycline, metronidazole, and clarithromycin) in *H.pylori*–associated peptic ulcers using hydroxy propyl methyl cellulose

(HPMC) and poly ethylene oxide (PEO) as the rate-controlling polymeric matrix. The design of the delivery system was based on the swellable asymmetric triple-layer tablet approach. Tetracycline and metronidazole were incorporated into the core layer of the triple-layer matrix for controlled delivery, while bismuth salt was included in one of the outer layers for instant release. According to the authors, the aim of such a device was to obtain a simple regimen for a standard triple therapy. Indeed, they obtained *in vitro* a duration of buoyancy and sustained release of metronidazole and tetracycline over prolong time of period. The rapid effect of the device would be due to the rapidly dissolving layer containing the bismuth salt, which disintegrated within 10–15 min in vitro. However, no in vivo data are available concerning the floating characteristics of the drug delivery system or its effect against *H.pylori*.

Umamaheshwari et al (120) developed several drug delivery systems especially designed to improve efficiency against *H.pylori*. In all of them, they used an antiurease drug, acetohydroxamic acid (AHA), as an active agent against the bacterium. *H. pylori* urease hydrolyses urea present in the gastric juice and extracellular fluid to generate ammonia and bicarbonate, which effectively neutralize an acidic pH in its environment [121, 122]. Thus, urease inhibitors hinder the bacterium to protect itself against low pH and avoid thus the problem of treatment of antibiotic-resistant strains [123].

The same authors developed polycarbonate microballoons by an emulsion (o/w) solvent evaporation technique. In vitro (i.e. in simulated gastric fluid) 74% to 85% of microballoons stayed buoyant up to 12 h and exhibited a sustained drug release profile. In vitro and in vivo growth inhibition studies were performed using cultures of *H. pylori* and *H. pylori*-infected Mongolian gerbils, respectively. Microballoons showed 10 times higher anti-*H. pylori* activity compared with AHA solution [124].

Umamaheshwari et al. [125] developed cellulose acetate butyrate coated floating microspheres of cholestyamine for targeting to *H.pylori* infection In vitro (drug release, buoyancy) and in vivo studies (gastric mucoadhesion in the rat stomach) led the authors to conclude that this drug delivery system possessed both floating and bioadhesive properties, and may be successful in the treatment of *H.pylori*. Katayama et al [126] deveolped a susrtained release liquid preparation of ampicillin using sodium alginate for the treatment of *H.pylori* infection. The gastroretentive property of the device was provided by the ability of sodium alginate to form a firm gel when an acid or di-or trivalent metal ions (Ca^{2+}, Ba^{2+}, Sr^{2+}) were added. The authors expected the solution to be able to spread out, adhere to the gastric mucosa, and release the antibiotic continuously (ampicillin). The alginate formulation gelled in stomach and delivered ampicillin locally in stomach and showed significant anti *H.pylori* effect in rat model.

5.5. Mucoadhesive drug delivery systems (MDDS)

Bioadhesive drug delivery systems are used to localize a delivery device within the lumen to enhance the drug absorption in a site-specific manner. Mucoadhesive drug carrier may prolong the residence time of drug in stomach because they adhere to mucus surface, resulting in an effective localizing drug concentration. Mucoadhesion is a very complex process and several theories have been put forward to explain the mechanism, including electrical, adsorption, and wetting and diffusion theories [127]. Because the mucosal surface is negatively charged, a positive charge on polymer might facilitate the mucoadhesion process. Some of the most promising charged excipients used commonly in these systems include polycarbophil, carbopol, lecithins, chitosan, carboxy methyl cellulose and gliadin, etc. Some investigators have tried a synergistic approach between floating and bioadhesion systems [120, 124, 128]. Among the mucoadhesive formulation, mucioadhesive microspheres have gained considerable attention due to their ability to adhere to mucus layer as well as release drugs locally at the infected cell line.

Nagahara et al [128] formulated mucoadhesive microspheres containing amoxicillin. They dispersed the drug and bioadhesive polymers (carboxyvinyl polymer and curdlan [polysaccharide]) in melted hydrogenated castor oil. They compared these microspheres with an amoxicillin suspension in infected Mongolian gerbils under feeding conditions. The microspheres with an amoxicillin dose of 1.0 mg/kg provided the same clearance rate (20%) as the amoxicillin suspension with a dose of 10 mg/kg. This means that the amoxicillin-microspheres provided 10 times greater anti-*H.pylori* activity than the amoxicillin suspension. Moreover, adhesion of microspheres on the stomach wall was observed (°47% and °20% remained in the stomach after 2 and 4 h, respectively). The authors concluded that these mucoadhesive microspheres containing an appropriate antimicrobial agent should be useful for the eradication of *H. pylori*.

Wang et al. [129] studied positively charged gelatin microspheres as gastric mucoadhesive drug delivery system for eradication of *H.pylori*. Umamaheshwari et.al [130] developed nonoparticles bearing amoxicillin using gliadin polymer rand evaluated in-vivo the anti *H.pylori* efficiency of nanoparicles in gerbil model, results were found to be promising molecule to eradicate of *H.pylori* infection. Radiet et.al [131] developed tetracycline-loaded crosslinked chitosan microspheres to increase the local concentration of the antibiotic in the stomach and, thus eradicate *H.pylori* infection. The microspheres were examined for gastric residence time and local tetracycline concentrations in fasted gerbils. The microspheres were found to reside in the stomach even after 10 h of administration.

Recently, Zhepeng et.al [132] also published a study on mucoadhesive microspheres containing amoxicillin by an emulsification/evaporation method, using ethylcellulose as matrix and carbopol 934P as a mucoadhesive polymer. This work showed that free amoxicillin was rapidly degraded in acidic medium; however, amoxicillin entrapped in the microspheres microspheres kept stable. Furthermore, studies on the *in vivo* clearance of *H.pylori* revealed that, in a single-dosage administration, the mucoadhesive microspheres had a better effectiveness than that of amoxicillin powder.Finally this study showed a complete eradication *of H.pylori* with microspheres in five of six rat stomachs, whereas amoxicillin powder showed four times less effectiveness. The authors found a tendency for an effective anti-*H.pylori* activity induced by mucoadhesive microspheres, but concluded that larger groups of animal are required to confirm these results.

Among all the drug delivery approaches (Dosage forms) described herein, some provide interesting solutions, although many of them present drawbacks. In the particular case of *H.pylori* eradication, the ideal dosage form should, to be really effective, not only stay in the stomach, but also target the bacterium. However, knowledge about this pathogen discovered twenty years ago is still poor. More data are necessary, for example, to identify an "ubiquitous" receptor (i.e. for all *H.pylori* strains) at the surface of the bacterium, which could provide a strong interaction with a ligand [133-135]. Thus, the development of an efficient gastroretentive dosage form against *H. pylori* is closely linked to a better understanding of its pathogenicity mechanisms.

6. Conclusion

Considerable advances have been made in understanding the evolution of the organism and pathogenesis of disease. Although combination therapies have high rates of eradication, the preferred therapy would be one which use a low dose of a single drug with a short duration treatment and without any adverse effect. The sequencing of two strains of *H.pylori* has provided a wealth of data that will be useful in understanding the pathogenesis of disease, microbial evolution and highlight potential therapeutic targets and potential vaccine candidates. In future, it is likely to advance understanding of disease progression and aid in the development of novel therapies. First aspect of research is that genomic studies are arousing considerable interest, and will certainly be followed up in future research for development of new therapies. A second area of research that is becoming increasingly important is the development of novel targeted drug delivery systems for *H.pylori* infection. The floating and mucoadhesive formulation of antibacterial drugs have shown good *H. pylori* clarence effect in both *in-vitro* and in-vivo animal model studies. However, extensive clinical studies are required in human to establish a correlation.

Author details

Rajinikanth Siddalingam and Kumarappan Chidambaram

Department of Pharmaceutical Technology, School of Pharmacy, Taylor's University, Subang Jaya, Kuala Lumpur, Malaysia

References

[1] Warren JR, Marshall B. Unidentified curved bacilli on gastric epithelium in active chronic gastritis. Lancet 1983; 11273-1275.

[2] McColl KEL, Murray L, El-Omar E, Dickson A, El-Nujumi A, Wirz A, Kelman A, Penny C, Knill-Jones R, Hilditch T. Symptomatic benefit from eradicating Helicobacter pylori infection in nonulcer dyspepsia. N Engl J Med 1998; 339 1869-1874.

[3] McNamara D, Buckley M, Gilvarry J, O'Morain C. Does Helicobacter pylori eradication affect symptoms in nonulcer dyspepsia: a five-year follow-up study. Helicobacter 2002 ;7, 317-321.

[4] Suerbaum S, Michetti P. *Helicobacter pylori* infections, New Engl J Med 347: 1175–1186, 2002.

[5] Gasbarrini A, Franceschi F, Armuzzi A, Ojetti V, Candelli M, Torre ES, De Lorenzo A, Anti M, Pretolani S, Gasbarrini G. Extradigestive manifestations of *Helicobacter pylori* gastric infection. Gut 1999; 45, 109-I12.

[6] Malaty HM, Graham DY. Importance of childhood socioeconomic status on the current prevalence of *Helicobacter pylori* infection. Gut, 35:742-745, 1994.

[7] Mitchell H, Megraud F, Epidemiology and diagnosis of *Helicobacter pylori* infection, Helicobacter 2002;7, 1-8–16..

[8] Brown, LM, Thomas, TL, Chang, YS.You, WC, Liu, WD,. Zhang, L, Pee, D, Gail, MH. *Helicobacter pylori* infection in rural China: demographic, lifestyle and environmental factors, Int. J. Epidemiol 2002, 31: 638–645.

[9] Howden CW, Hunt RH. Guidelines for the management of *Helicobacter pylori* infection, Am J Gastroenterol 1998;93:2330-2338.

[10] Drumm B, Koletzko S, Oderda G. *Helicobacter pylori* infection in children: a consensus statement. J Pediatr Gastroenterol Nutr 2000; 30, 207-213.

[11] Graham DY, Qureshi WA. Markers of infection. In: Mobley HLT, Mendz GL, Hazell SL, eds, *Helicobacter pylori:* physiology and genetics. Washington, D.C.: ASM Press, 2001 :499-510.

[12] Schmitz A, Josenhans C, Suerbaum S. Cloning and characterisation of the *Helicobacter pylori* flbA gene which codes for a membrane protein involved in coordinated expression of flagellar genes. J Bacteriol 1997; 179, 987-997.

[13] Nilius M, Malfertheiner P. *Helicobacter pylori* enzymes. Aliment Pharmacol Ther 1996; 10(Suppl 1):65-71.

[14] Graham DY, Klein PD, What you should know about the methods, problems, in terpretations and uses of urea breath tests. Am J Gastroenterol 1991; 86, 1118-1122.

[15] Megraud F. Epidemiology of *Helicobacter pylori* infection: where are we in 1995? Eur J Gastroenterol Hepatol 1995 ; 7, 292-295.

[16] Mendal MA, Goggin PM, Molineaus N, Childhood living conditions and *Helicobacter pylori* seropositivity in adult life. Lancet, 1995 ;332: 896-897.

[17] Noach LA, Rolf TM, Bosma NB. Gastric metaplasia and *Helicobacter pylori* infection. Gut 1993; 34, 1510-1514.

[18] Rahman MM, Mahalanabis D, Sarker SA, Bardhan PK, Alvarez JO, Hildebrand P, Beglinger C, Gyr K. *Helicobacter pylori* colonization in infants and young children is not necessarily associated with diarrhea. J Trop. Pediatr 1998; 44, 283–287.

[19] Robert WF, John C, Helicobacter in the developing world. Microbes and Infection 2003; 5, 705–713.

[20] Dunn BE, Cohen H, Blaser MJ. *Helicobacter pylori*, Clin. Microbiol. Rev, 1997; 10, 720–741.

[21] Go MF. Review article: natural history and epidemiology of *Helicobacter pylori* infection. Aliment Pharmacol. Therapeutics, 2002; 16 (1) 3–15.

[22] Bardhan PK. Epidemiological features of *Helicobacter pylori* infection in developing countries. Clin. Infect. Dis 1997; 25, 973–978.

[23] Lindkvist P, Enquselassie F, Asrat D, Muhe L, Nilsson I, Giesecke J. Risk factors for infection with *Helicobacter pylori*—a study of children in rural Ethiopia. Scand J Infect Dis 1998;30, 371–376.

[24] Mobley HLT. *Helicobacter pylori* urease. In: Achtman M, Suerbaum S, eds, *Helicobacter pylori:* molecular and cellular biology. Wymondham, United Kingdom: Horizon Scientific Press 2001; 155-1570.

[25] Weeks DL, Eskandari S, Scott DR, Sachs G. A H+-gated urea channel: the link between *Helicobacter pylori* urease and gastric colonization. Science 2000;28, 482-485.

[26] Josenhans C, Suerbaum S, *Helicobacter* motility and chemotaxis. In: Achtman M, Suerbaum S, eds. *Helicobacter pylori:* molecular and cellular biology. Wymondham, United Kingdom: Horizon Scientific Press, 2001; 171-184.

[27] Ilver D, Arnqvist A, Ogren J. *Helicobacter pylori* adhesin binding fucosylated histo-blood group antigens revealed by retagging. Science 1998; 279, 373-377.

[28] Rogha M, Nikvarz M, Poumoghaddas Z, Shirneshan K, Dadkhah D, Pourmoghaddas M. Is helicobacter pylori infection a risk factor for coronary heart disease?. ARYA Atheroscler 2012; 8(1): 5-8.

[29] Rogha M, Dadkhah D, Poumoghaddas Z, Shirneshan K, Poumoghaddas M. Association of Helicobacter pylori infection with severity of coronary heart disease et al. ARYA Atheroscler 2012; 7(4): 138-41.

[30] Saad R, Chey WD. A clinician's guide to managing Helicobacter pylori infection. Cleve Clin J Med 2005;72(1) 109-118.

[31] McCarthy C, Patchett S, Collins RM. Long-term prospective study of *Helicobacter pylori* in non-ulcer dyspepsia. Dig Dis Sci 1995', 40, 114-119.

[32] Miehlke S, Bayerdorffer E, Graham DY. Treatment of *Helicobacter pylori* infection. Semin Gastrointest Dis 2001; (1), 167–179.

[33] Ricci V, Zarrilli R, Romano M. Voyage of *Helicobacter pylori* in human stomach: odyssey of a bacterium. Dig Liver Dis 2002; 34 (1)2–8.

[34] Graham DY. Therapy of *Helicobacter pylori*: current status and issues. Gastroenterology 2000; 118, S2–8.

[35] Mégraud F, O'Morain C, Malfertheiner P. on behalf of the Working Party of the European *Helicobacter pylori* Study Group. Guidelines for clinical trials in *Helicobacter*

pylori infection. Statistical annex: statistical aspects of clinical trials in *Helicobacter pylori* infection. Gut 1997; 41, S19–23.

[36] Gerrits MM, Schuijffel D, van Zwet AA, Kuipers EJ, Vandenbroucke-Grauls CM, Kusters JG. Alterations in penicillin-binding protein 1A confer resistance to beta-lactam antibiotics in Helicobacter pylori. *Antimicrob Agents Chemother2002;* 46, 2229–2233.

[37] Kwon DH, Kim JJ, Lee M, et al. Isolation and characterization of tetracycline-resistant clinical isolates of Helicobacter pylori. *Antimicrob Agents Chemother 2000;* 44, 203–3205.

[38] Megraud F. Epidemiology and mechanism of antibiotic resistance in Helicobacter pylori. *Gastroenterology 1998;* 115:1272–1278.

[39] Huang J, Hunt RH. The importance of clarithromycin dose in the management of Helicobacter pylori infection: a meta-analysis of triple therapies with a proton pump inhibitor, clarithromycicn and amoxicillin or metronidazole. *Aliment Pharmacol Ther 1999;* 13:719–729.

[40] Iovene MR, Romano M, Pilloni AO, et al. Prevalence of antimicrobial resistance in eighty clinical isolates of Helicobacter pylori. *Chemotherapy 1999;* 45, 8–14.

[41] Debets-Ossenkopp YJ, Herscheid AJ, Pot RG, Kuipers EJ, Kusters JG, Vanderbroucke-Grauls CM. Prevalence of Helicobacter pylori resistance to metronidazole, clarithromycin, amoxicillin, tetracycline and trovafloxacin in The Netherlands. *J Antimicrob Chemother 1999;* 43:415–511.

[42] Malfertheiner P, Megraud F, O'Morain C, Hungin AP, Jones R, Axon A, Graham DY, Tytgat G. Current concepts in the management of Helicobacter pylori infection, the Maastricht 2-2000 Consensus Report. Aliment Pharmacol Ther 2002;, 16:167-180.

[43] Coelho LG, Leon-Barua R, Quigley EM. Latin-American Consensus Conference on Helicobacter pylori infection. Latin-American National Gastroenterological Societies affiliated with the Inter-American Association of Gastroenterology (AIGE). Am J Gastroenterol 2000; 95, 2688-2691, 2000.

[44] Ulmer HJ, Beckerling A, Gatz G. Recent use of proton pump inhibitor-based triple therapies for the eradication of H pylori: a broad data review. Helicobacter 2003; 8, 95-104.

[45] Vergara M, Vallve M, Gisbert JP, Calvet X. Meta-analysis: comparative efficacy of different proton-pump inhibitors in triple therapy for Helicobacter pylori eradication.Aliment Pharmacol Ther 2003;18:647-654.

[46] Vallve M, Vergara M, Gisbert JP, Calvet X. Single vs. double dose of a proton pump inhibitor in triple therapy for Helicobacter pylori eradication: a meta-analysis. Aliment Pharmacol Ther 2002; 16:1149-1156.

[47] Buzas GM, Jozan J. Eradication of Helicobacter pylori infection in Europe: a meta-analysis based on congress abstracts, 1997-2002. Orv Hetil 2002; 145:2035-2041.

[48] Fischbach LA, van Zanten S, Dickason J. Meta-analysis: the efficacy, adverse events, and adherence related to first-line anti-Helicobacter pylori quadruple therapies. Aliment Pharmacol Ther 2004 ; 20, 1071-1082.

[49] Gene E, Calvet X, Azagra R, Gisbert JP. Triple vs. quadruple therapy for treating Helicobacter pylori infection: a meta-analysis. Aliment.Pharmacol.Ther 2003; 17:1137-1143.

[50] Gene E, Calvet X, Azagra R, Gisbert JP. Triple vs quadruple therapy for treating Helicobacter pylori infection: an updated meta-analysis. Aliment. Pharmacol.Ther 2003;18, 543-544.

[51] Graham DY, Belson G, Abudayyeh S, Osato MS, Dore MP, El-Zimaity HM. Twice daily (mid-day and evening) quadruple therapy for *H. pylori* infection in the United States. Dig Liver Dis 2004 ;36:384-387.

[52] Howden CW, Hunt RH. Guidelines for the management of Helicobacter pylori infection. Ad Hoc Committee on Practice Parameters of the American College of Gastroenterology. Am J Gastroenterol 1998;93:2330-2338.

[53] Vakil N, Lanza F, Schwartz H, Barth J. Seven-day therapy for Helicobacter pylori in the United States. Aliment Pharmacol Ther, 2004;20, 99-107.

[54] Suerbaum S, Michetti P. *Helicobacter pylori* infection. N Engl J Med 2002; 347(15) 1175-1186.

[55] Peitz U, Sulliga M, Wolle K, et al. High rate of post-therapeutic resistance after failure of macrolide-nitroimidazole triple therapy to cure Helicobacter pylori infection: impact of two second-line therapies in a randomised study. *Aliment Pharmacol Ther 2002;*16:315–324.

[56] McLoughlin RM, O'Morain CA, O'Connor HJ. Eradication of *Helicobacter pylori*: recent advances in treatment. Fundam Clin Pharmacol 2005; 19: 421-427.

[57] Gisbert JP, Pajares JM. Review article: *Helicobacter pylori* 'rescue' regimen when proton pump inhibitor-based triple therapies fail. Aliment Pharmacol Ther 2003;16:1047-1057.

[58] Bilardi C, Dulbecco P, Zentilin P, Reglioni S, Iiritano E, Parodi A, Accornero L, Savarino E, Mansi C, Mamone M, Vigneri S, Savarino V. A 10-day levofloxacinbased therapy in patients with resistant Helicobacter pylori infection: a controlled trial. Clin Gastroenterol Hepatol 2004;2:997-1002.

[59] Nista EC, Candelli M, Cremonini F, Cazzato IA, Di Caro S, Gabrielli M, Santarelli L, Zocco MA, Ojetti V, Carloni E, Cammarota G, Gasbarrini G, Gasbarrini A. Levofloxacin-based triple therapy vs. quadruple therapy in second-line Helicobacter pylori treatment: a randomized trial. Aliment Pharmacol Ther2003;, 18:627-633.

[60] Perri F, Festa V, Clemente R, Villani MR, Quitadamo M, Caruso N, Bergoli ML, Andriulli A. Randomized study of two "rescue" therapies for Helicobacter

pyloriinfected patients after failure of standard triple therapies. Am J Gastroenterol 2001; 96:58-62.

[61] Zullo A, Hassan C, Campo SM, Lorenzetti R, Febbraro I, De Matthaeis M, Porto D, Morini S. A triple therapy regimen after failed *Helicobacter pylori* treatments. Aliment Pharmacol Ther 2001; 15: 1193-1197.

[62] Michopoulos S, Tsibouris P, Bouzakis H, Balta A, Vougadiotis J, Broutet N, Kralios N. Randomized study comparing omeprazole with ranitidine as anti-secretory agents combined in quadruple second-line *Helicobacter pylori* eradication regimens. Aliment Pharmacol Ther 2000; 14: 737-744.

[63] Gomollon F, Ducons JA, Ferrero M, Garcia Cabezudo J, Guirao R, Simon MA, Montoro M. Quadruple therapy is effective for eradicating *Helicobacter pylori* after failure of triple proton-pump inhibitor-based therapy: a detailed, prospective analysis of 21 consecutive cases. *Helicobacter* 1999; 4: 222-225.

[64] Watanabe Y, Aoyama N, Shirasaka D, Maekawa S, Kuroda K, Miki I, Kachi M, Fukuda M, Wambura C, Tamura T, Kasuga M.Levofl oxacin based triple therapy as a second-line treatment after failure of *helicobacter pylori* eradication with standard triple therapy. Dig Liver Dis 2003; 35: 711-715.

[65] Wong WM, Gu Q, Lam SK, Fung FM, Lai KC, Hu WH, Yee YK, Chan CK, Xia HH, Yuen MF, Wong BC. Randomized controlled study of rabeprazole, levofl oxacin and rifabutin triple therapy vs. quadruple therapy as second-line treatment for *Helicobacter pylori* infection. Aliment Pharmacol Ther 2003; 17:553-560.

[66] Ebrahimi-Dariani N, Mirmomen S, Mansour-Ghanaei F, Noormohammadpoor P, Sotodehmanesh R, Haghpanah B, Bahrami H. The efficacy of furazolidone-based quadruple therapy for eradication of *Helicobacter pylori* infection in Iranian patients resistant to metronidazole-based quadruple therapy. Med Sci Monit 2003: 9: PI105-PI108.

[67] Isakov V, Domareva I, Koudryavtseva L, Maev I, Ganskaya Z. Furazolidone-based *pylori* resistant to metronidazole. Aliment Pharmacol Ther 2002; 16:1277-1282.

[68] Toracchioa S, Capodicasab S, Sorajac DB, Cellinic L, Marziob L. Rifabutin based triple therapy for eradication of *H. pylori* primary and secondary resistant to tinidazole and clarithromycin. Digestive Liver Disease 2005;37: 33–38.

[69] Matsuzaki K, Koyama H, Chiba A, Omika K, Harada S, Sato Y, et.al. In vitro activities of levofloxacin and other antibiotics against fresh clinical isolates. Jpn J Antibiot 1999;52:571–84.

[70] Cammarota G, Cianci R, Cannizzaro O, Cuoco L, Pirozzi Gasbarrini A, et al. Efficacy of two one-week rabeprazole /levofloxacin-based triple therapies for *Helicobacter pylori* infection. Aliment Pharmacol Ther 2000; 14:1339–43.

[71] Gatta L, Zullo A, Perna F, Ricci C, De Francesco V, Tampieri A, Bernabucci V, Cavina M, Hassan C, Ierardi E, Morini S, Vaira D. A 10-day levofl oxacin-based triple therapy

in patients who have failed two eradication courses. Aliment Pharmacol Ther 2005; 22: 45-49.

[72] Zullo A, Hassan C, De Francesco V, Lorenzetti R, Marignani M, Angeletti S, Ierardi E, Morini S. A third-line levofloxacinbased rescue therapy for *Helicobacter pylori* eradication. Dig Liver Dis 2003; 35: 232-236.

[73] Kunin CM. Antimicrobial activity of rifabutin. Clin Infect Dis 1996;22 :1:S3–13.

[74] Heep M, Beck D, Bayerdorffer E, Lehn N. Rifampin and rifabutin resistance mechanism in *Helicobacter pylori*. Antimicrob Agents Chemother 1999;43:1497–1499.

[75] Perri F, Festa R, Clemente R, Quitadamo M, Andriulli A. Rifabutin-based "rescue therapy" for *Helicobacter pylori* infected patients after failure of standard regimens. Aliment Pharmacol Ther 2000;14:311–316.

[76] Wong WM, Gu Q, Lam SK, et al. Randomized controlled study of rabeprazole, levofloxacin and rifabutin triple therapy vs quadruple therapy as second-line treatment for Helicobacter pylori infection. *Aliment Pharmacol Ther 2003;*17:553–560.

[77] Chi CH, Lin C-Y, Sheu B-S, Yang H-B, Huang A-H, Wu J-J. Quadruple therapy containing amoxicillin and tetracycline is an effective regimen to rescue failed triple therapy by overcoming the antimicrobial resistance of Helicobacter pylori. *Aliment Pharmacol Ther 2003;* 18:347–353.

[78] Gisbert JP, Calvet X, Bujanda L, Marcos S, Gisbert JL, Pajares JM. "Rescue" therapy with rifabutin after multiple *Helicobacter pylori* treatment failures. *Helicobacter,* 2003;8: 90-94.

[79] Canducci F, Ojetti V, Pola P, Gasbarrini G, Gasbarrini A. Rifabutin-based *Helicobacter pylori* eradication 'rescue therapy'.Aliment Pharmacol Ther 2001; 15: 143-149.

[80] Borody TJ, Pang G, Wettstein AR, Clancy R, Herdman K, Surace R, Llorente R, Ng C. Efficacy and safety of rifabutincontaining 'rescue therapy' for resistant *Helicobacter pylori* infection. Aliment Pharmacol Ther 2006; 23: 481-488.

[81] Kwon DH, Lee M, Kim JJ, Kim JG, El-Zaatari FA, Osato MS, Graham DY. Furazolidone- and nitrofurantoin-resistant *Helicobacter pylori*: prevalence and role of genes involved in metronidazole resistance. Antimicrob Agents Chemother 2001; 45:306-308.

[82] Heep M, Kist M, Strobel S, Beck D, Lehn N. Secondary resistance among 554 isolates of *Helicobacter pylori* after failure of therapy. Eur J Clin Microbiol Infect Dis 2000; 19: 538-541.

[83] Xiao SD, Liu WZ, Hu PJ, Ouyang Q, Wang JL, Zhou LY, Cheng NN. A multicentre study on eradication of *Helicobacter pylori* using four 1-week triple therapies in China. Aliment Pharmacol Ther 2001;15: 81-86.

[84] Qasim A, Sebastian S, Thornton O, Dobson M, McLoughlin R, Buckley M, O'Connor H, O'Morain C. Rifabutin- and furazolidone- based *Helicobacter pylori* eradication therapies after failure of standard first- and second-line eradication attempts in dyspepsia patients. Aliment Pharmacol Ther 2005; 21: 91-96.

[85] Cammarota G, Martino A, Pirozzi G, Cianci R, Branca G, Nista EC, Cazzato A, Cannizzaro O, Miele L, Grieco A, Gasbarrini A, Gasbarrini G. High effi cacy of 1-week doxycycline- and amoxicillin- based quadruple regimen in a culture-guided, third-line treatment approach for *Helicobacter pylori* infection. AlimentPharmacol Ther 2004; 19: 789-795.

[86] Pipkin, GA, Dixon JS, Williamson R, Wood JR.Clarithromycin dual therapy regimens for eradication of *Helicobacter pylori*. Helicobacter, 1997; 159-171.

[87] Megraud F. Resistance of *Helicobacter pylori* to antibiotics: the main limitation of current proton-pump inhibitor triple therapy. Eur J Gastroenterol Hepatol 1999; 11 (2) S35–37.

[88] Vaira D, Ali A, Gatta L, O'Morain C. Treatment of *Helicobacter pylori*. Curr Opin Gastroent 1999;14 (1) S71–78.

[89] Lind T, Megraud F, Unge P,. The MACH2 Study: role of omeprazole in eradication of *Helicobacter pylori* with 1-week triple therapies. Gastroenterology 1999;116: 248–253.

[90] Wang J, Tauchi Y, Deguchi Y, Morimotov K, Tabata Y, Ikada Y. Positively charged gelatin microspheres as gastric mucoadhesive drug delivery system for eradication of *H. pylori*,. Drug Delivery 2003 ; 7(4) : 237– 243.

[91] Blaser MJ, Kirschner D. Dynamics of *Helicobacter pylori* colonization in relation to the host response. Proc Natl Acad Sci USA 1999; 96: 8359–8364.

[92] Dubois A, Berg DE, Incecik ET, Fiala N,. Host specificity of *Helicobacter pylori* strains and host responses in experimentally challenged nonhuman primates. Gastroenterology 1999; 116: 90–96.

[93] Fox JG, Perkins S, Yan L,. Local immune response in *Helicobacter pylori* infected cats and identi. cation of *H. pylori* in saliva, gastric fluid and faeces. Immunology 1996;88: 400–406.

[94] Wotherspoon AC, Doglioni C, Diss TC. Regression of primary low grade B cell gastric lymphoma of mucosa-associated lymphoid tissue after eradication of *Helicobacter pylori*. Lancet 1993; 342: 575–577.

[95] Smythies, LE., Novak, MJ., Waites, KB., Lindsey, JR., Morrow, CD., Smith, PD. Poliovirus replicons encoding the B subunit of *Helicobacter pylori* urease protect mice against *H. pylori* infection. Vaccine 2005; 23: 901–909.

[96] Hoffelner, H., Haas, R. Recombinant bacterial ghosts: versatile targeting vehicles and promising vaccine candidates. Int J Med Microbiol 2004; 294:303–311.

[97] Panthel, K, Jechlinger, W, Matis, A, Rohde, M, Szostak, M, Lubitz, W, Haas, R Generation of Helicobacter pylori ghosts by PhiX protein E-mediated inactivation and their evaluation as vaccine candidates. Infect Immun 2003b; 71: 109–116.

[98] Leonard, M, De Boisseson, MR, Hubert, P, Dalencon, F, Dellacherie, E Hydrophobically modified alginate hydrogels as protein carriers with specific controlled release properties. J Control Release, 2004; 98: 395–405.

[99] Dzwonek, A, Mikula, M, Woszczynski, M, Hennig, E, Ostrowski, J. Protective effect of vaccination with DNA of the *H. pylori* genomic library in experimentally infected mice. Cell Mol Biol Lett 2004; 9: 483–495.

[100] Hatzifoti, C, Bajaj-Elliott, M, Dorrell, N, Anyim, M, Prentice, MB, Nye, KE, Wren, B, Morrow, WJ. A plasmid immunization construct encoding urease B of *Helicobacter pylori* induces an antigen-specific antibody response and upregulates the expression of betadefensins and IL-10 in the stomachs of mmunized mice. Vaccine 2004; 22: 2651–2659.

[101] Sommer, F., Wilken, H., Faller, G., Lohoff, M. Systemic Th1 immunization of mice against Helicobacter pylori infection with CpG oligodeoxynucleotides as adjuvants does not protect from infection but enhances gastritis. Infect Immun 2004;72: 1029–1035.

[102] Garland, SM. Imiquimod. Curr Opin Infect Dis 2003; 16: 85–89.

[103] Wang R, Epstein, J, Charoenvit Y, Baraceros FM, Rahardjo N, Hoffman SL. Induction in humans of CD8+ and CD4+ Tcell and antibody responses by sequential immunization with malaria DNA and recombinant protein. J Immunol 2004;172: 5561–5569.

[104] Manoj S, Griebel PJ, Babiuk LA, van Drunen Littel-van den Hurk S. Modulation of immune responses to bovine herpesvirus-1 in cattle by immunization with a DNA vaccine encoding glycoprotein D as a fusion protein with bovine CD154. Immunology 2004;112: 328–338.

[105] Alm RA, Ling L-SL, Moir DT, ae.al. Genomic –sequence comparision of two unrelated isolates of human gastric pathogen Helicobacter pylori. Nature 1999; 397: 176-180.

[106] McClain MS, Shaffer CL, Israel DA, Peek RM Jr, Cover TL. Genome sequence analysis of Helicobacter pylori strains associated with gastric ulceration and gastric cancer BMC Genomics. 2009; 5;10-3

[107] Tomb JF, White O, Kerlavage AR. The complete genome sequence of the gastric pathogen Helicobacter pylori. Nature 1997;, 388:539-547.

[108] Axon, A T R. Treatment of Helicobacter pylori: future therapeutic and prophylactic perspectives. *Gut* 1998;43;70-73.

[109] Tatusov RL., Koonin EV, Lipman.D.J. A genomic perspective on protein families. Science 1997;278:631–637.

[110] Beier, D, Frank R. Molecular characterization of two-component systems of *Helicobacter pylori*. J Bacteriol 2000;182:2068–2076.

[111] Bereswill S, Lichte F, Greiner S, Waidner B, Fassbinder F, Kist N. The ferric uptake regulator (Fur) homologue of *Helicobacter pylori*: functional analysis of the coding gene and controlled production of the recombinant protein in *Escherichia coli*. Med Microbiol Immunol 1999;188:31–40.

[112] Dorrell N, Wren, BW. Helicobacter pylori research from genes to genome biology: a new era in. *Gut 1998;* 42;451-453.

[113] Donald T. Moir 1, Karen J, Roberta S, Gerald F. Vovis1 Genomics and Antimicrobial Drug Discovery. Antimicrob. Agents Chemother 1999;43:3:439–446.

[114] Rajinikanth PS and Mishra B. Floating in situ gelling system for stomach site-specific delivery of clarithromycin to eradicate *H. pylori*. J. Contr. Rel 2008; 4(1), 33-41.

[115] P.S.Rajinikanth, and B.Mishra, Development and in vitro evaluation of floating in situ gelling system of acethydroxamic acid for clearance of *H.pylori*. Drug. Dev. Ind. Pharm 2008;34, 577-584.

[116] Shah S, Qaqish R, Patel V, Amiji M. Evaluation of the factors influencing stomach-specific delivery of antibacterial agents for *Helicobacter pylori* infection. J. Pharm Pharmacol 1999; 51: 667–672.

[117] Yokel RA, Dickey KM, Goldberg AH. Selective adherence of a sucralfate-tetracycline complex to gastric ulcers: implications for the treatment of *Helicobacter pylori*. Biopharm Drug Dispos 1995; 16: 475–479.

[118] Myung-Kwan C, Hongkee S, Hoo-Kyun C. Preparation of mucoadheive microspheres containing antimicrobial agents for eradication of *H.pylori*. Int J Pharm 2005; 297 : 172-179.

[119] Yang L, Eshrafh J, Fassihi R. A new intragastric delivery system for the treatment *of Helicobacter pylori* associated gastric ulcer: in vitro evaluation. J Contr Rel 1999; 57: 215-225.

[120] Umamaheshwari RB, Jain S, Bhadra D, Jain NK. Floating microspheres bearing acetohydroxamic acid for the treatment of Helicobacter pylori. J Pharm. Pharmacol 2003;55 :12: 1607– 1613.

[121] P.S.Rajinikanth, and B.Mishra, Development and evaluation of floating–mucoadhesive microspheres of clarithromycin for eradication of *H.pylori*. Chem. Pharm. Bull 2008;52(12), 45-53.

[122] P.S.Rajinikanth, J.Balasubramaniam and B.Mishra Development and evaluation of a novel floating in situ gelling system of amoxicillin for eradication of *H.pylori*. International Journal of Pharmaceutics 2007; 335, 114-122.

[123] P.S.Rajinikanth and B.Mishra, Preparation and In Vitro Characterization of Gellan based Floating Beads of Acetohydroxamic Acid for Eradication of *H.pylori.*, Acta Pharmaceutica 2007; 57 (1), 413–427.

[124] Umamaheshwari RB Jain S, Tripathi PK, Agrawal GP, Jain NK. Floating-bioadhesive microspheres containing acetohydroxamic acid for clearance of Helicobacter pylori, Drug Deliv 9 :4 :223– 231, 2002.

[125] Umamaheshwari RB, Jain S, Jain JK. Anew approach in gastroretentive drug delivery system using cholestyramine. Drug delivery 2003;1(10):151-160.

[126] Kattayama H, Nishimura T, Ochi S, Tsuruta Y,. Sustained release liquid preparation using sodium alginate for eradication of *Helicobacter pylori*.. Bio Pharm Bull 1999; 55-60.

[127] Park H, Rabinson JR. Mechanism of bioadhesion of poly(acrylic acid) hydrogels. Pharm Res 1987; 4 : 457-464.

[128] Nagahara N, Akiyama Y, Nakao M, Tada M, Kitano M, Ogawa Y. Mucoadhesive microspheres containing amoxicillin for clearance of *Helicobacter pylori*. Antimicrob Agents Chemother 1998;42 : 2492–2494.

[129] Wang J, TabataY, Bi D, Morimoto K. Evaluation of gastric mucoadhesive properties of aminated gelatin microspheres. J Contr Rel 2002; 73 : 223–231.

[130] Umamaheshwar RB, Ramteke S, Jain JK. Anti–*Helicobacter Pylori* Effect of mucoadhesive nanoparticles bearing amoxicillin in experimental gerbils model., AAPS PharmSci Tech 2004;, 5 (2) Article 32.

[131] Radi H, Mansoor A. Stomach anti *H.pylori* therapy I: Preparation and characterization of tetracycline – loaded chitosan microspheres. Int J Pharm 2002; 235 : 87-94.

[132] Zhepeng L, Weiyue L, Quian L, Xuhui Z, Pengyun Z. In vitro and in vivo studies on mucoadgesive microspheres of amoxicillin. J Contr Rel 2002;102 :135-144.

[133] Osaki T, Yamaguchi H, Taguchi H, Fukada M, Kawakami H, Hirano H, Kamiya S. Interleukin-8 induction and adhesion of the coccoid form of *Helicobacter pylori*. J Med Microbiol 2002;51 :4: 295– 299.

[134] Sisto F, Brenciaglia MI, Scaltrito MM, Dubini F. *Helicobacter pylori*: ureA, cagA and vacA expression during conversion to the coccoid form. Int J Antimicrob Agents 2000;15 (4)277–282.

[135] Khin, MM, Hua JS, Ng HC, Wadstrom T, Bow H. Agglutination of Helicobacter pylori coccoids by lectins. World J Gastroenterol 2000;6(2)202– 209.

3

Helicobacter pylori Infection and Gastric Cancer — Is Eradication Enough to Prevent Gastric Cancer

Aleksandra Sokic-Milutinovic, Dragan Popovic,
Tamara Alempijevic, Sanja Dragasevic,
Snezana Lukic and Aleksandra Pavlovic-Markovic

1. Introduction

Helicobacter pylori (H. pylori) is a gram negative, microaerophilic spiral bacterium with a clear role in the pathogenesis of gastric and duodenal ulcer, low grade B cell gastric lymphoma (MALT lymphoma) and gastric cancer. The bacterium was successfully cultivated by Warren and Marshall in 1982. Their discovery led to completely different therapeutic approach to patients with peptic ulcer disease and gastric MALT lymphoma. Despite initial skepticism concerning *H. pylori* role in gastric carcinogenesis, in 1991 two epidemiological studies [1,2] confirmed previously published reports suggesting higher incidence of gastric cancer in *H. pylori* infected individuals [3-5]. Furthermore, cohort studies in California, Hawaii and Great Britain confirmed increased risk for gastric cancer in *H. pylori* infected individuals. As a result of accumulated scientific evidence *Helicobacter pylori* was marked as human carcinogen by International Agency for Research on Cancer in 1994. Gastric cancer is the third most common cancer among males and fifth most common among females. The incidence of gastric cancer is declining in developed countries, but the global burden is rising due to cases occurring in developing countries. The five-year survival for advanced stage gastric cancer is below 20% even in developed countries [6].

Different outcomes of *Helicobacter pylori* infection are to be expected depending on distinct patterns of gastritis that were identified and described in detail. Namely, antrum-predominant gastritis leads to duodenal ulcer formation while chronic corpus predominant and multifocal atrophic gastritis lead to increased risk for gastric cancer formation [7-9].

The outcome of *Helicobacter pylori* infection depends on characteristics of the microorganism, characteristics of the host and environmental factors.

2. *Helicobacter pylori* virulence factors

Helicobacter pylori virulence depends on different factors enabling it to colonize gastric mucosa and induce tissue damage. Epidemiological studies revealed so far six distinct *H. pylori* strains (hpEurope, hpEastAsia, hpAsia2, hpAfrica 1, hpAfrica2 and hpNEAfrica) that are related to geographic regions and correlate well with the incidence of gastric cancer [10].

H. pylori is a highly heterogeneous bacterium [11,12]. Several *H. pylori* virulence factors are thought to contribute to gastric cancer development and this review will focus on cytotoxin-associated gene A and CagA protein (CagA), vacuolating cytotoxin (VacA) and outer inflammatory protein (OipA) (Figure 1) with a brief comment on possible role of duodenal ulcer–promoting gene (dupA).

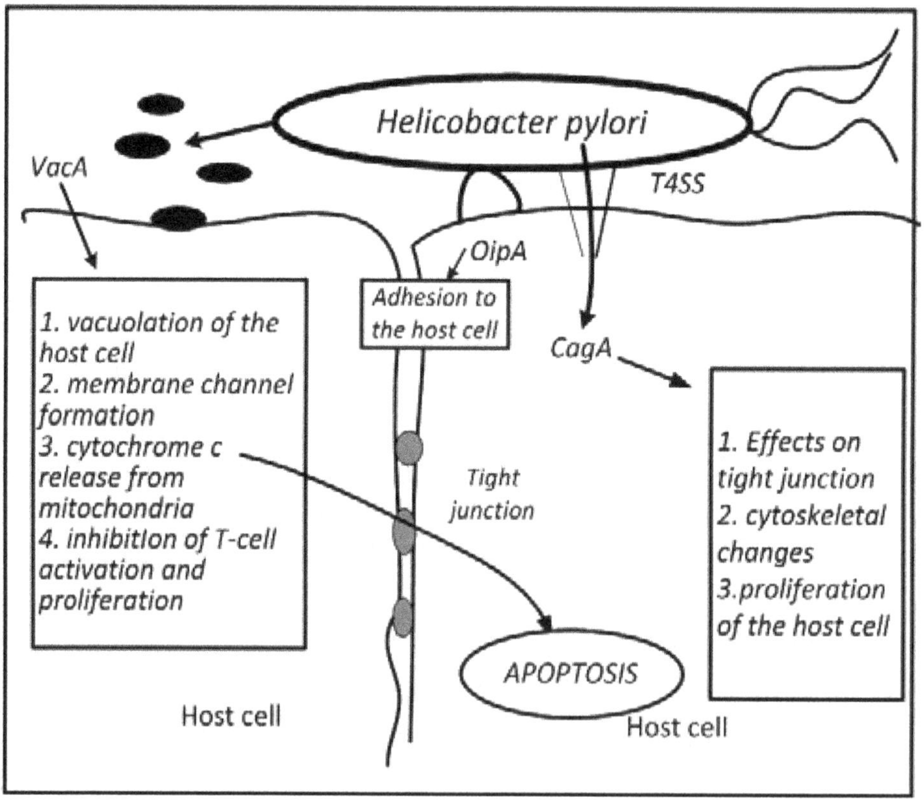

Figure 1. Mechanism of *Helicobacter pylori* induced host cell injury

2.1. *cagA*

There are two types of clinical *H. pylori* isolate: CagA-producing (*cagA* positive) strains and CagA-nonproducing (*cagA* negative) strains. Results of studies obtained on animal model revealed that gastric cancer developed only in animals infected with *cagA* positive *H. pylori* strains or when CagA protein was artificially introduced into the host [13,14] and authors concluded that CagA protein was important factor in gastric carcinogenesis. Further investigations revealed that *cagA* gene polymorphisms could at least partly explain why only some *cagA* positive individuals develop gastric cancer. Namely, there are different number of repeat sequences located on 3` region of the cagA gene in different *H. pylori* strains. It is now well known that sequences of these repeat regions differ significantly between strains isolated in East Asia and Western strains [15]. Each repeat region of the CagA protein contains Glu-Pro-Ile-Tyr-Ala (EPIYA) motifs. The first repeat region is termed EPIYA-A and EPIYA-B and second repeat region EPIYA-C or EPIYA-D segments [11]. Western type CagA has EPIYA ABC, ABCC or ABCCC, while East Asian CagA has EPIYA ABD segments [11].

CagA protein is composed of a disordered C-terminal region that contains the EPIYA motifs and a structured N-terminal region with several conserved regions. When the bacterium contacts the host cell CagA is injected into the host cell via the *cag* pathogenicity island (*cag*PAI)-encoded type IV secretion system (T4SS). Upon injection, CagA is linked to the inner leaflet of the cell membrane probably via an electrostatic interaction with phosphatidylserine [16]. When injected into the cytoplasm via the T4SS, CagA can be phosphorylated by the host and alter host cell signaling in both phosphorylation-dependent and phosphorylation-independent manner. CagA is phosphorylated on EPIYA motifs [17]. Induction of heme oxygenase 1, which exhibits anti-inflammatory and antioxidant effects, reduced CagA phosphorylation during *H. pylori* infection of gastric epithelial cells *in vitro*. However, there is data suggesting that the bacterium developed a strategy to diminish heme oxygenase 1 gene expression in gastric epithelial cells [18].

Recently it was demonstrated that another protein component of T4SS termed CagL induces hypergastrinemia, which is a major risk factor for the development of gastric adenocarcinoma [17].

2.2. *vacA*

VacA induces vacuolation of the host cell, membrane-channel formation, cytochrome *c* release from mitochondria leading to apoptosis, induces autophagy and alters host immune response [17,20,21]. VacA also inhibits T-cell activation and proliferation [22]. All *H. pylori* strains have a functional *vacA* gene. There is a variation in the vacuolating activity among different *H. pylori* strains [23] related to differences in the *vacA* gene structure at the signal (s1 and s2) region, middle region (m1 and m2) and intermediate (i1 and i2) region. Combination of subtype of these three regions influences the levels of VacA activity and is related to risks for different gastrointestinal diseases.

The most cytotoxic are s1/m1 strains, followed by s1/m2 strains, whereas s2/m2 strains have no cytotoxic activity and s2/m1 strains are rare [24]. Individuals infected with s1 or m1 *H. pylori* strains have an increased risk of peptic ulcer or gastric cancer compared with individuals infected with s2 or m2 strains [11]. In East Asia most *H. pylori* strains are s1 type that led to conclusion (based on epidemiological data) that in East Asia presence of m1 region leads to increased risk for gastric cancer [11] and its typing is the best marker for gastric cancer risk out of all *vacA* regions.

Intermediate region of *vacA* is identified between s and m regions few years ago. All s1/m1 strains belong to the type i1, and all s2/m2 strains are type i2. Strains tha contain s1/m2 can be type i1 or i2. Strains with i1 region are more pathogenic. In some populations typing of i-region is superior in predicting gastric cancer risk than typing of s region, while in other populations it has no predictive value [25].

The deletion (d) region—was identified between the i-region and the m region [26]. The d region is divided into d1 and d2. The study of Western strains demonstrated that d1 was a risk factor for gastric mucosal atrophy; however, almost all East Asian strains are classified as s1/i1/d1 [11].

2.3. oipA

Outer membrane proteins (OMPs) are coded by different genes in *Helicobacter pylori* genome. One of the OMPs that can function as adhesin is OipA, which was identified in 2000 [11].

OipA is a protein that induces proinflammatory response and its activity leads to increase in mucosal interleukin-8 (IL8) levels. OipA is involved in the attachment of *H. pylori* to gastric epithelial cells *in vitro* [27]. Results from animal studies demonstrated that OipA alone plays a role in the development of gastric cancer [13].

The production of CagA, VacA and OipA is linked and the majority of *H. pylori* strains produce either all of these proteins or none of them. Almost all East Asian strains of *H. pylori* are classified as CagA-producing, VacA-producing (*vacA* s1), and OipA-producing strains and are highly pathogenic. In addition, CagA, VacA and OipA are all thought to be involved in the development of both gastric cancer and duodenal ulcer [11].

2.4. *dupA*

Duodenal ulcer–promoting gene *dupA* was described in 2005. It is localized in the plasticity zone and it is involved in T4SS formation. Initial report suggested it to be the first disease-specific *H. pylori* virulence factor that induced duodenal ulcer formation and had a suppressive action on gastric cancer (DupA) [28]. After this report multiple studies failed to demonstrate correlation between *dupA* gene and specific gastroduodenal disease [10,29,30]. This gene is,however, highly polymorphic, and that could explain the conflicting data obtained in different studies [17].

2.5. Geographic differences in gastric cancer incidence related to *Helicobacter pylori* strains

Multilocus sequence typing (MLST) of the housekeeping genes revealed six *H. pylori* strains (hpEurope, hpEastAsia, hpAsia2, hpAfrica 1, hpAfrica2 and hpNEAfrica) that are related to geographic regions and correlate well with the incidence of gastric cancer.

Sequence differences among the examined housekeeping genes of the six major genotypes probably have no influence on the disease outcome but serve as a marker for other virulence factors related to the disease outcome (i.e *cagA* and *vacA*) [10]. In 2003, Falush et al analyzed 370 *H. pylori* isolates and assigned the strains to four main clusters: hpEurope, hpEastAsia, hpAfrica1 and hpAfrica2 due to their obvious geographical associations [31]. HpEurope is common in Europe and countries colonized by Europeans and most isolates from East Asia belong to hpEastAsia. HpAfrica2 is very distinct and has only been isolated in South Africa. Four years later Linz et al expanded the analysis using 769 *H. pylori* isolates and assigned the isolates to six distinct groups, adding to previously descried clusters (hpEurope, hpEastAsia, hpAfrica1 and hpAfrica2) two new clusters termed hpAsia 2 and hpNEAfrica. Cluster hpAsia2 was isolated in South and Southeast Asia. Cluster hpNEAfrica is predominant among isolates from Northeast Africa [12].

Populations with high rates of gastric cancer correspond with regions presenting hpEastAsia strains. In contrast, incidence of gastric cancer is very low in Africa, where most strains are hpNEAfrica, hpAfrica1 or hpAfrica2, and in South Asia, where most strains are hpAsia2. The differences in *H. pylori* isolates in different populations are considered to be an explanation of the both African and Asian enigma. Namely, populations with high incidences of *Helicobacter pylori* infection in East Asian countries have high incidences of gastric cancer, as opposed to low incidence of gastric cancer in other highly infected populations in Africa (African enigma) and South Asia (Asian enigma) [10].

3. Host factors

Host characteristics and immune response to *Helicobacter pylori* infection also play a role in gastric carcinogenesis. Different gene polymorphisms that affect host immune response and extent of cell proliferation are described and linked to gastric carcinogenesis together with gene polymorphisms for growth factors and growth factor receptors. Majority of these polymorphisms are single nucleotide polymorphisms (SNP). In recent years, host genetic polymorphisms involved in inflammatory response, carcinogen metabolism, antioxidant protection, mucosal protection and cell proliferation regulation have been widely studied as potential biomarkers to predict gastric cancer risk.

4. Cytokine gene polymorphisms

Cytokines modulate inflammatory response to *Helicobacter pylori* infection and indirectly the risk for gastric cancer. Gene polymorphisms for interleukin-1 beta and its receptor antagonist, tumor necrosis factor alpha, interleukin-8 and interleukin-10 were extensively studied and reported as relevant in determining gastric cancer risk.

4.1. Interleukin-1

Interleukin-1 beta (IL-1β) is a potent inhibitor of gastric acid secretion. Reduced gastric acid secretion on the other hand promotes development of *H. pylori* induced pangastritis, gastric mucosa atrophy and subsequently, in a subset of individuals, gastric cancer development. El-Omar et al described in 2000 polymorphisms in the pro-inflammatory *IL-1B* gene (encoding IL-1β) and *IL-IRN* (encoding IL-1β receptor antagonist) associated with elevated risk for hypochlorhydria and gastric cancer in the persons with *H. pylori* infection [32] (El-Omar). Presence of *IL-1B*-31C or -511T and *IL-IRN**2/*2 polymorphisms is associated with a 2-3-fold increase in risk for intestinal and diffuse non-cardia gastric cancer among *H. pylori*-infected persons [33]. These genetic polymorphisms modulate gastric cancer risk by increasing expression of pro-inflammatory cytokine IL-1β. It was later established that these polymorphisms interact synergistically with bacterial virulence factors (*cagA* positive, *vacA* s1 and *vacA* m1). Gastric cancer risk is highest among those with both host and bacterial high-risk genotypes [34].

Results of meta-analysis provided by Persson et al. based on available data from epidemiological studies showed strongest association of IL1RN2 polymorphism with increased risk for gastric cancer [35] in non-Asian populations for both intestinal and diffuse cancers. The *IL1RN22* genotype has been reported to cause high circulating IL-1receptor antagonist and IL-1β levels resulting in a severe and prolonged inflammatory response. IL1B-511T carriers were found to have an increased risk of gastric cancer in non-Asian populations. Possible explanation is that stronger inflammatory reaction may increase the risk of cancer through damage to gastric cells and bacterial overgrowth and accumulation of toxic byproducts [32]. These findings are supported by results of some [36,37], but not all previously published meta-analysis [38]. Surprisingly, according to Persson et al *IL-1B*-31C polymorphism was associated with a reduced overall risk for gastric cancer in Asian populations [35].

4.2. Tumor necrosis factor alpha

Tumor necrosis factor alpha (TNF-α) is another proinflammatory cytokine produced in gastric mucosa in response to *H. pylori* infection. Polymorphisms in *TNF-A* gene, especially presence of the high producing A allele of *TNF-A* at position 308 (G→A) is considered to be associated with increased risk for non-cardia gastric cancer [6]. This finding is supported by majority [39-41], but not all of available meta-analysis [35].

4.3. Interleukin 10

Interleukin 10 is an anti-inflammatory cytokine that down-regulates *IL-1B, TNF-A,* and interferon-γ gene expression. Previously published studies suggested that individuals carrying the *IL-10* ATA haplotype associated with low IL-10 production (-592, -819, -1082) have an increased risk for non-cardia gastric cancer [33]. Nevertheless meta-analysis failed to confirm these observations except for *IL10*-1082G where the effect of polymorphism depends on ethnicity of the host. It seems that this polymorphism increases gastric cancer risk in Asians, but has no significant effect in non-Asian populations [39].

4.4. Interleukin 8

IL-8 is a CXC family cytokine that is a potent chemoattractant for neutrophils and lymphocytes affecting proliferation, migration, and tumor angiogenesis. However, not all studies have replicated the positive associations between pro-inflammatory cytokines polymorphisms and gastric cancer risk [42]. A polymorphisms in *IL-8* (-251 T→A) is associated with increased production of IL-8 in *H. pylori* infected gastric mucosa and with precancerous gastric abnormalities in Caucasians and gastric cancer in Asian populations [43]. Nevertheless, studies in Asian populations [44,45] have failed to confirm relevance of this polymorphism and meta-analysis supported this finding [35], but this can be attributable to small sample size in these studies and limited number of the high quality studies available for the meta-analysis.

4.5. Presence of multiple high-risk cytokine gene polymorphisms

Possession of multiple high-risk host polymorphisms is associated with increased risk for gastric cancer. Presence of 3-4 of the polymorphisms (*IL-B1*-511*T, *IL-IRN**2/*2, *TNF-A*-308*A and *IL-10* ATA/ATA) confers a 27-fold increase in risk of non-cardia gastric cancer [33].

5. Polymorphisms in innate immune response genes

H. pylori attaches to gastric epithelium via receptors. Thus, polymorphisms in the innate immune response genes, which interact with these receptors, could influence outcome of infection and potentially the risk of gastric cancer.

5.1. Toll like receptor 4 (TLR4)

TLR4 is a cell-surface signaling receptor involved in the recognition and host response to *Helicobacter pylori*. Toll-like receptor 4 gene codes for a lipopolysaccharide (LPS) receptor molecule involved in innate immune recognition of microbe pathogen-associated molecular patterns. The *TLR4*+896A>G polymorphism linked with impaired reactivity to bacterial lipopolysaccharide may play a role in gastric carcinogenesis [44] and is associtaed with hypochlorhydria and upper gastrointestinal cancer. *TLR4* 896 polymorphisms results in changed conformation of the extra cellular domain of the TLR4 receptor and carriers are unable to adequately respond to LPS challenge. The defective signaling through TLR4 leads to an exaggerated inflammatory response with severe tissue destruction that causes gastric atrophy and severe hypochlorhydria. Two independent case-control studies have demonstrated that *TLR4*+896G carriers have eightfold increase in odds ratio for hypochlorhydria and gastric atrophy, and over two-fold increase for gastric cancer [44,45]

6. Cell proliferation-related gene polymorphisms

Meta-analysis by Gao et al identified 23 polymorphisms significantly related to gastric cancer in at least one published study suggesting the importance of polymorphisms in genes implicated in cell proliferation in development of gastric cancer. The overall effect of these polymorphisms is probably modest but should not be neglected [46].

6.1. Cell cycle and apoptosis regulators

Cell cycle and apoptosis regulators are directly involved in the initiation of malignant proliferation of the cell. Polymorphisms of functional regulators of *TP53, TP53BP2* (tumor protein P53 binding protein 2) and *MDM2* (gene encoding Mouse double minute 2 homolog, an important negative regulator of the p53 tumor suppressor) were found to be related to the development of gastric cancer. *TP3* gene encodes a multi-purpose protein (P53) that takes part in regulating the cell cycle, carrying out programmed cell death, initiating DNA repair, and regulating the transcription of a large number of genes that cells use for various biological purposes. Given its many essential functions, P53 is frequently found inactivated in tumor cells. Results of meta-analysis confirm that association of *TP3* gene polymorphisms vary by population and type of gastric cancer. The *TP3* Arg allele carriers of Asian origin have an increased risk for gastric cancer, while same polymorphism seems to have protective effects in Caucasians [43]. Possible explanation is difference in environmental factors that act together with either apoptotic or DNA repairing mechanisms. Data obtained for other two polymorphisms in cell-cycle related genes that were extensively studied are inconsistent, both for *Lmyc* (nuclear oncogen) EcoRI polymorphism and *p21* (gene encoding P21/ cyclin-dependent kinase inhibitor 1) polymorphism (Arg31Ser), probably due to relatively small sample sizes and underestimated importance of environmental factors and their interplay with host genetics.

PPAR-γ (peroxisome proliferator-activated receptors γ) is a member of the nuclear hormone receptor family that plays an important role in cell differentiation and regulation of metabolism. A potential interplay between *PPAR-γ* Pro12Ala polymorphism and *H. pylori* infection was observed in the development of gastric cancer [47,48].

6.2. Growth factors and growth factor receptors

Polymorphisms determining higher level of growth factors and related receptors, which are important for tissue repair, were associated with reduced risk of gastric cancer. Such associations were observed for gene encoding epidermal growth factor (EGF) *EGF* 5′ UTR 61G>A, [49], polymorphisms for transforming growth factor beta (TGFB) i.e. *TGFB1* -509C>T, *TGFBR2*-875G>A [50] and gene encoding insulin-like growth factor-binding protein 3 *IGFBP3* -202A>C and Gly32Ala [51,52].

7. Environmental factors

Environmental regulation of virulence factors could be an interesting concept explaining why not all infected individuals develop severe complications of disease despite infection with pathogenic *Helicobacter pylori* strains.

Recent study demonstrated that high salt diet could influence *H. pylori* protein expression [53].

7.1. Diet

In 2007 World Cancer Research Fund declared that high intake of vegetables and fruit probably decrease risk of gastric cancer, and that high intakes of salt and salty food probably increase risk of gastric cancer [54]. The proposed underlying mechanism for the inverse association of gastric cancer risk with vegetable and fruit/rich diet is related to the presence of antioxidants. Salt on the other hand acts directly on the stomach lining, destroying the mucosal barrier, causes gastritis and increased epithelial cell proliferation [55]. A synergistic interaction between diet and *Helicobacter pylori* infection with risk of gastric cancer has been proposed [56]. Recent study demonstrated that high salt diet could influence *Helicobacter pylori* protein expression leading to increased risk of gastric cancer [53]. Salt responsive increase in *cagA* expression attributable to increased CagA transcription was described that could lead to increased risk of gastric cancer.

7.2. Smoking

Tobacco smoking is the risk factor associated with the largest number of cancer cases worldwide and the causal link with stomach cancer is recognized [54]. A recent meta-analysis found significant positive associations of smoking with risk of both cardia and non-cardia gastric cancer among the majority of studies, overall increasing risk by 62% for male and 20% for female current smokers [57]. It is possible that tobacco smoke carcinogens affect gastric cancer risk directly through contact with the stomach mucosa or indirectly through the blood flow [54]. In a large population-based study in Europe (EPIC), 17.6% of gastric cancer cases were attributed to smoking [56]. The cancer risk in past smokers can remain up to 14 years after cessation of smoking [57,58]. The effect of smoking on gastric cancer is dose-dependent and additive in the presence of other risk factors [59,60]. However, passive smoking does not seem to increase the risk [61].

7.3. Non-steroidal anti-inflammatory drugs

Protective effect of regular use of non-steroidal anti-inflammatory drugs (NSAIDs) and particularly aspirin on risk of gastric cancer was repeatedly reported in observational studies and then results of meta-analysis [62] confirmed these finding. According to Algra et al regular NSAID users have up to 20% reduced risk of gastric cardia adenocarcinoma and up to 36% reduced risk of distal gastric adenocarcinoma [62]. NSAIDs suppress the production of cyclooxygenase enzymes. Data on clinical efficacy of NSAIDs in prevention of gastric cancer first suggested that aspirin reduces risk for both proximal and distal gastric cancer [63]. Recent results from population-based intervention trial by Wong et al revealed that celecoxib treatment or *Helicobacter pylori* eradication alone had beneficial effects on the regression of advanced gastric lesions. Nevertheless no favourable effects were seen for *H. pylori* eradication followed by celecoxib treatment [64]. Meta-analysis by Tian et al suggests significant protective effects of NSAIDs against gastric cancer [65].

7.4. Socioeconomic status

Lower socioeconomic status is associated with at least two-fold greater risk of gastric cancer irrespective of the country incidence of gastric cancer [54]. Possible explanation is related to increased likelihood of transmission and re-infection with *H. pylori* (large family, poor sanitation, less frequent use of antibiotics). Also, low socioeconomic status is related to a diet lower in fresh fruits and vegetables.

8. Importance of *Helicobacter pylori* eradication in prevention of gastric cancer development-current knowledge and evidence

Helicobacter pylori infection is mainly associated with distal forms and intestinal-type gastric carcinoma [7-9]. Namely, there are two distinct sites of gastric adenocarcinoma: proximal (cardia) and distal (non-cardia), with different epidemiological and clinical characteristics. Main risk factors for cardia gastric cancer are obesity, gastro-oesophageal reflux disease and Barrett's oesophagus [66] and its incidence is increasing over last decades. On the contrary, main risk factors for development of distal gastric cancer are *H.pylori*, low socioeconomic status, smoking, salty and smoked food intake, low consumption of fruits and vegetables and a family history of gastric cancer. Clear decline in incidence of distal gastric cancer is observed in the last decades [67].

Histologically gastric cancer is, according to Lauren classification, divided into two subtypes: intestinal and diffuse type. The intestinal type is related to corpus-predominant gastritis with intestinal metaplasia and is closely related to long-lasting *H.pylori* infection, whereas the diffuse originates from superficial pangastritis without atrophy [7-9].

Intestinal type gastric adenocarcinoma results from a prolonged precancerous process. The link between gastric intestinal metaplasia and cancer was proposed by pathologists in Java and Sumatra in 1938. This idea was over time only occasionally revisited by scientists until in 1975 Correa et al proposed a model of gastric carcinogenesis. This model postulated that intestinal type of gastric cancer was a result of progressive changes in the gastric mucosa [68]. Authors updated their model in 1988 and 1992. In Correa cascade the following consecutive steps are now recognized: normal gastric mucosa, superficial (non-atrophic) gastritis, multifocal atrophic gastritis (MAG), complete (small intestine type) intestinal metaplasia followed by intestinal metaplasia of the incomplete (colonic) type, low-grade dysplasia, high-grade dysplasia and invasive adenocarcinoma. [7-9, 68]. Loss of normal glandular tissue is the first specific recognizable step in the precancerous cascade. However, the changes of the precancerous lesions over time remain an issue difficult to assess leading to the fact that the point of no return, although of critical importance for timely eradication, still remains unidentified.

Five randomized controlled trials (RCT) reported effects of *H.pylori* infection eradication on invasive gastric cancer or premalignant histological lesions of gastric mucosa. [69-75]

Study by Wong et al. was designed as RCT conducted in a high-risk gastric cancer region in China that evaluated gastric cancer incidence as a primary outcome [69]. Authors identified healthy individuals with *H. pylori* infection and treated them either with eradication therapy or placebo. During a follow-up period of 7.5 years authors failed to demonstrate overall decrease in gastric cancer incidence. The study concluded that incidence of gastric cancer development in the general population was similar between subjects receiving *H. pylori* treatment and placebo. The study, however, suggested the possible protective role of *H. pylori* eradication in participants without precancerous lesions, including gastric atrophy, intestinal metaplasia, or dysplasia.

Other above cited trials were not designed to assess gastric cancer as a primary outcome [70, 71] or had low numbers of gastric cancer cases [69, 72] to provide an informative assessment of the effects of eradication on cancer occurrence. Nevertheless, recently an important study was published by Ma et al [74] with the long-term follow-up results of a randomized trial in which 2258 *H. pylori* seropositive adults from a general population in China were randomly assigned to three interventions (*H. pylori* eradication, garlic supplements, supplemental vitamins) or control groups. After 15 years there were 34 new gastric cancers in *H. pylori* eradication group and 52 in the corresponding control group (relative risk of 0.61, 95 % confidence interval 0.38-0.96) that clearly demonstrated benefit of eradication therapy in gastric cancer prevention.

This year Lee et al [76] evaluated the benefit of mass eradication of *H. pylori* infection started in Taiwanese population with high incidence of *H. pylori* infection. Individuals who were aged 30 years and older were tested for the presence of *H. pylori* infection and those positive underwent endoscopic screening and subsequent eradication therapy. Authors demonstrated the success of eradication in 78.7%. Gastric atrophy incidence decreased in over 77% after successful eradication of *H. pylori* with no significant change in intestinal metaplasia. Gastric cancer incidence during the chemoprevention period was reduced by 25%. Based on these findings authors suggest that ultimate benefit in reducing gastric cancer incidence and its mortality should be validated by a further long-term follow-up.

Over a decade ago Uemura et al. [77] first reported that *H. pylori* eradication could reduce the subsequent development of metachronous gastric cancer after endoscopic resection of early gastric carcinoma. Namely, 132 *H. pylori* serology-positive patients who underwent endoscopic resection were assigned to the *H. pylori*-treatment group or the no treatment group according to the patients' preference. Regular endoscopic follow-up for up to 4 years found no metachronous cancer in *H. pylori*-treated patients compared to 9% in the no treatment group.

Some years later, Fukase et al. [75] reported the results of a trial in which more than five hundred patients in Japan who had previously undergone endoscopic resection for treatment of early gastric cancer were randomized to either *H. pylori* eradication or usual care. They demonstrated statistically significant 65 % reduction in the risk of metachronous gastric carcinoma compared with the control group.

The evidence from more recent trial reports [74-76], taken together with the epidemiological and experimental evidence for the carcinogenic activity of chronic *H. pylori* infection, provides support for a protective effect of *H. pylori* eradication in gastric cancer.

9. Conclusion

H. pylori infection contributes 5.5% to global cancer burden and is the single most important cause of infection-associated cancer globally [6]. It is therefore reasonable to consider eradication therapy as optimal preventive approach in infected individuals. Interrupting transmission of infection is primary prevention, secondary should be eradication therapy and tertiary prevention includes identification of the individuals with early gastric cancer. However data from large study in China that included 1630 healthy carriers of *H. pylori* infection that were given eradication therapy or placebo detected no difference of gastric cancer incidence between these two groups [69]. Benefit would probably be seen in patients where gastric cancer cascade did not cross the point of no return, which would explain results of recently published studies [74,76]. Namely, intestinal-type gastric cancer results from a multistep process of mucosal alterations leading from chronic inflammation (gastritis) to glandular atrophy followed by development of intestinal metaplasia and dysplasia resulting in invasive carcinoma. Clinical studies should aim to identify a 'point of no return', a situation when mucosal alterations are no longer reversible after *H. pylori* eradication and progression to gastric cancer became independent of presence of the bacterium.

Higher risk for gastric cancer might be modulated by an overall pro-inflammatory host genetic profile in the adaptive and innate immune systems genes (e.g. *IL-1B, TNFA, IL-10, IL-8,* and *TLR4*) [77]. This pro-inflammatory profile might drive the immune response to *H. pylori* infection to a severe chronic inflammatory phenotype, reduced gastric acid secretion, bacterial overgrowth, and oxidative stress to the gastric mucosa.

Therefore timely eradication of *H pylori* infection especially in individuals with proinflammatory genetic profile could prevent development and in long term possibly decrease incidence of gastric cancer.

Author details

Aleksandra Sokic-Milutinovic[1,2], Dragan Popovic[1,2], Tamara Alempijevic[1,2], Sanja Dragasevic[2], Snezana Lukic[1,2] and Aleksandra Pavlovic-Markovic[1,2]

1 School of Medicine, University of Belgrade, Belgrade, Serbia

2 Clinic for Gastroenterology and Hepatology, Clinical center of Serbia, Belgrade, Serbia

References

[1] Talley NJ, Zinsmeister AR, Weaver A, DiMagno EP, Carpenter HA, Perez-Perez GI, Blaser MJ. Gastric adenocarcinoma and *Helicobacter pylori* infection. J Natl Cancer Inst 1991;83(23):1734-1739

[2] Parsonnet J, Friedman GD, Vandersteen DP, Chang Y, Vogelman JH, Orentreich N, Sibley RK. *Helicobacter pylori* infection and the risk of gastric carcinoma.N Engl J Med 1991;325(16):1127-1131.

[3] Scott N, Lansdown M, Diament R, Rathbone B, Murday V, Wyatt JI, McMahon M, Dixon MF, Quirke P. Helicobacter gastritis and intestinal metaplasia in a gastric cancer family. Lancet 1990;335(8691):728.

[4] Marwick C. Helicobacter: new name, new hypothesis involving type of gastric cancer. JAMA 1990;264(21):2724-2727.

[5] Caruso ML, Fucci L. Histological identification of *Helicobacter pylori* in early and advanced gastric cancer.J Clin Gastroenterol 1990;12(5):601-602.

[6] Mbulaiteye SM, Hisada M, El-Omar EM *Helicobacter pylori* associated global gastric cancer burden. Front Biosci (Landmark Ed). 2009;14:1490-1504.

[7] Correa P. A human model of gastric carcinogenesis. Cancer Res 1988; 48: 3554–3360.

[8] Correa P. Human gastric carcinogenesis: a multistep and multifactorial process – First American Cancer Society Award lecture on cancer epidemiology and prevention. Cancer Res 1992; 52: 6735–6740.

[9] Correa P, Piazzuelo MB. The gastric precancerous cascade. J Dig Dis 2012;13:2-9.

[10] Yamaoka Y, Kato M, Asaka M. Geographic differences in gastric cancer incidence can be explained by differences between *Helicobacter pylori* strains. Intern Med. 2008;47(12):1077-1083

[11] Yamaoka Y. Mechanisms of disease: *Helicobacter pylori* virulence factors. Nat Rev Gastroenterol Hepatol. 2010;7(11):629-641.

[12] Linz B, Balloux F, Moodley Y, Manica A, Liu H, Roumagnac P, Falush D, Stamer C, Prugnolle F, van der Merwe SW, Yamaoka Y, Graham DY, Perez-Trallero E, Wadstrom T, Suerbaum S, Achtman M.An African origin for the intimate association between humans and *Helicobacter pylori*. Nature 2007;445:915–918

[13] Franco AT, Johnston E, Krishna U, Yamaoka Y, Israel DA, Nagy TA, Wroblewski LE, Piazuelo MB, Correa P, Peek RM Jr. Regulation of gastric carcinogenesis by *Helicobacter pylori* virulence factors. Cancer Res 2008;68:379–387

[14] Ohnishi N, Yuasa H, Tanaka S, Sawa H, Miura M, Matsui A, Higashi H, Musashi M, Iwabuchi K, Suzuki M, Yamada G, Azuma T, Hatakeyama M.Transgenic expression of *Helicobacter pylori* CagA induces gastrointestinal and hematopoietic neoplasms in mouse. Proc Natl Acad Sci USA 2008;105:1003–1008.

[15] Yamaoka Y, Osato MS, Sepulveda AR, Gutierrez O, Figura N, Kim JG, Kodama T, Kashima K, Graham DY. Molecular epidemiology of *Helicobacter pylori*: separation of *H. pylori* from East Asian and non-Asian countries. Epidemiol Infect 2000;124:91–96.

[16] Hayashi T, Senda M, Morohashi H, Higashi H, Horio M, Kashiba Y, *et al.* Tertiary structure-function analysis reveals the pathogenic signaling potentiation mechanism of *Helicobacter pylori* oncogenic effector CagA. Cell Host Microbe 2012;12:20–33.

[17] Cid TP, Fernández MC, Benito Martínez S, Jones NL. Pathogenesis of *Helicobacter pylori* Infection. Helicobacter 2013;18 Suppl 1:12-17

[18] Gobert AP, Verriere T, de Sablet T, Peek RM Jr, Chaturvedi R, Wilson KT. Haem oxygenase-1 inhibits phosphorylation of the *Helicobacter pylori* oncoprotein CagA in gastric epithelial cells. Cell Microbiol 2013;15:145–156.

[19] Wiedemann T, Hofbaur S, Tegtmeyer N, Huber S, Sewald N, Wessler S, Backert S, Rieder G. *Helicobacter pylori* CagL dependent induction of gastrin expression via a novel alphavbeta5-integrin-integrin linked kinase signalling complex. Gut 2012;61:986–996.

[20] Atherton JC. The pathogenesis of *Helicobacter pylori*-induced gastro-duodenal diseases. Annu Rev Pathol Mech Dis 2006;1:63–96.

[21] Cover TL, Blanke SR. *Helicobacter pylori* VacA, a paradigm for toxin multifunctionality. Nat Rev Microbiol 2005;3:320–332

[22] Gebert B, Fischer W, Weiss E, Hoffmann R, Haas R. *Helicobacter pylori* vacuolating cytotoxin inhibits T lymphocyte activation. Science. 2003;301:1099–1102.

[23] Cover TL, Blaser MJ. Purification and characterization of the vacuolating toxin from *Helicobacter pylori*. J Biol Chem. 1992;267:10570–10575.

[24] Atherton JC, Cao P, Peek RM Jr, Tummuru MK, Blaser MJ, Cover TL. Mosaicism in vacuolating cytotoxin alleles of *Helicobacter pylori*Association of specific *vacA* types with cytotoxin production and peptic ulceration.

[25] Ogiwara H, Graham DY, Yamaoka Y. *vacA* i-region subtyping. Gastroenterology. 2008;134:1267.

[26] Ogiwara H, Sugimoto M, Ohno T, Vilaichone RK, Mahachai V, Graham DY, Yamaoka Y.Role of deletion located between the intermediate and middle regions of the *Helicobacter pylori vacA* gene in cases of gastroduodenal diseases. J Clin Microbiol. 2009;47:3493–3500.

[27] Yamaoka Y, Kita M, Kodama T, Imamura S, Ohno T, Sawai N, Ishimaru A, Imanishi J, Graham DY. *Helicobacter pylori* infection in mice: Role of outer membrane proteins in colonization and inflammation. Gastroenterology. 2002;123:1992–2004.

[28] Lu H, Hsu PI, Graham DY, Yamaoka Y. Duodenal ulcer promoting gene of *Helicobacter pylori*. Gastroenterology. 2005;128:833–848.

[29] Douraghi M, Mohammadi M, Oghalaie A, Abdirad A, Mohagheghi MA, Hosseini ME, Zeraati H, Ghasemi A, Esmaieli M, Mohajerani N. *dupA* as a risk determinant in *Helicobacter pylori* infection. J Med Microbiol. 2008;57:554–562.

[30] Nguyen LT, Uchida T, Tsukamoto Y, Kuroda A, Okimoto T, Kodama M, Murakami K, Fujioka T, Moriyama M.*Helicobacter pylori dupA* gene is not associated with clinical outcomes in the Japanese population. Clin Microbiol Infect. 2010;16:1264–1269.

[31] Falush D, Wirth T, Linz B, Pritchard JK, Stephens M, Kidd M, Blaser MJ, Graham DY, Vacher S, Perez-Perez GI, Yamaoka Y, Mégraud F, Otto K, Reichard U, Katzowitsch E, Wang X, Achtman M, Suerbaum S.Traces of human migrations in *Helicobacter pylori* populations. Science 2003;299: 1582-1585.

[32] El-Omar EM, Carrington M, Chow WH, McColl KE, Bream JH, Young HA, Herrera J, Lissowska J, Yuan CC, Rothman N, Lanyon G, Martin M, Fraumeni JF, Jr, Rabkin CS. Interleukin-1 polymorphisms associated with increased risk of gastric cancer. Nature. 2000;404:398–402.

[33] El-Omar EM, Rabkin CS, Gammon MD, Vaughan TL, Risch HA, Schoenberg JB, Stanford JL, Mayne ST, Goedert J, Blot WJ, Fraumeni JF, Jr, Chow WH. Increased risk of noncardia gastric cancer associated with proinflammatory cytokine gene polymorphisms. Gastroenterology 2003;124:1193–201.

[34] Figueiredo C, Machado JC, Pharoah P, Seruca R, Sousa S, Carvalho R, Capelinha AF, Quint W, Caldas C, van Doorn LJ, Carneiro F, Sobrinho-Simoes M. *Helicobacter pylori* and interleukin 1 genotyping: an opportunity to identify high-risk individuals for gastric carcinoma. J Natl Cancer Inst 2002;94:1680–7

[35] Persson C, Canedo P, Machado JC, El-Omar EM, Forman D. Polymorphisms in Inflammatory Response Genes and Their Association With Gastric Cancer: A HuGE Systematic Review and Meta-Analyses. Am J Epidemiol. 2011 February 1; 173(3): 259–270.

[36] Wang P, Xia HH, Zhang JY, Dai LP, Xu XQ, Wang KJ.Association of interleukin-1 gene polymorphisms with gastric cancer: a meta-analysis. Int J Cancer 2007;120(3): 552–562.

[37] Camargo MC, Mera R, Correa P, Peek RM Jr, Fontham ET, Goodman KJ, Piazuelo MB, Sicinschi L, Zabaleta J, Schneider BG.Interleukin-1β and interleukin-1 receptor antagonist gene polymorphisms and gastric cancer: a meta-analysis. Cancer Epidemiol Biomarkers Prev 2006;15(9):1674–1687

[38] Kamangar F, Cheng C, Abnet CC, Rabkin CS.Interleukin-1B polymorphisms and gastric cancer risk—a meta-analysis. Cancer Epidemiol Biomarkers Prev 2006;15(10): 1920–1928.

[39] Loh M, Koh KX, Yeo BH, Song CM, Chia KS, Zhu F, Yeoh KG, Hill J, Iacopetta B, Soong R.Meta-analysis of genetic polymorphisms and gastric cancer risk: variability in associations according to race. Eur J Cancer 2009;45(14):2562–2568.

[40] Gorouhi F, Islami F, Bahrami H, Kamangar F.Tumour-necrosis factor-A polymorphisms and gastric cancer risk: a meta-analysis. Br J Cancer 2008;98(8):1443–1451.

[41] Zhang J, Dou C, Song Y, et al. Polymorphisms of tumor necrosis factor-alpha are associated with increased susceptibility to gastric cancer: a meta-analysis. J Hum Genet 2008;53(6):479–489.

[42] Kamangar F, Abnet CC, Hutchinson AA, Newschaffer CJ, Helzlsouer K, Shugart YY, Pietinen P, Dawsey SM, Albanes D, Virtamo J, Taylor PR. Polymorphisms in inflammation-related genes and risk of gastric cancer (Finland) Cancer Causes Control 2006;17:117–25.

[43] Canedo P, Castanheira-Vale AJ, Lunet N, Pereira F, Figueiredo C, Gioia-Patricola L, Canzian F, Moreira H, Suriano G, Barros H, Carneiro F, Seruca R, Machado JC. The interleukin-8-251*T/*A polymorphism is not associated with risk for gastric carcinoma development in a Portuguese population. Eur J Cancer Prev 2008;17:28–32.

[44] Hold GL, Rabkin CS, Chow WH, Smith MG, Gammon MD, Risch HA, Vaughan TL, McColl KE, Lissowska J, Zatonski W, Schoenberg JB, Blot WJ, Mowat NA, Fraumeni JF, Jr, El-Omar EM. A functional polymorphism of toll-like receptor 4 gene increases risk of gastric carcinoma and its precursors. Gastroenterology 2007;132:905–12.

[45] Arbour NC, Lorenz E, Schutte BC, Zabner J, Kline JN, Jones M, Frees K, Watt JL, Schwartz DA. TLR4 mutations are associated with endotoxin hyporesponsiveness in humans. Nat Genet2000; 25: 187-191

[46] Gao L, Nieters A, Brenner H. Cell proliferation-related genetic polymorphisms and gastric cancer risk: systematic review and meta-analysis. Eur J Hum Genet. 2009;17:1658-67.

[47] Liao SY, Zeng ZR, Leung WK, Zhou SZ, Chen B, Sung JJ, Hu PJ.Peroxisome proliferator-activated receptor-gamma Pro12Ala polymorphism, *Helicobacter pylori* infection and non-cardia gastric carcinoma in Chinese. Aliment Pharmacol Ther. 2006;23:289–294.

[48] Prasad KN, Saxena A, Ghoshal UC, Bhagat MR, Krishnani N. Analysis of Pro12Ala PPAR gamma polymorphism and *Helicobacter pylori* infection in gastric adenocarcinoma and peptic ulcer disease. Ann Oncol 2008;19:1299–1303

[49] Hamai Y, Matsumura S, Matsusaki K, K, Kitadai Y, Yoshida K, Yamaguchi Y, Imai K, Nakachi K, Toge T, Yasui W. A single nucleotide polymorphism in the 50 untranslated region of the EGF gene is associated with occurrence and malignant progression of gastric cancer. Pathobiology 2005;72: 133 – 138.

[50] Jin G, Wang L, Chen W, Hu Z, Zhou Y, Tan Y, Wang J, Hua Z, Ding W, Shen J, Zhang Z, Wang X, Xu Y, Shen H. Variant alleles of TGFB1 and TGFBR2 are associated with a decreased risk of gastric cancer in a Chinese population.Int J Cancer 2007;120: 1330 – 1335.

[51] Zhang ZW, Newcomb PV, Moorghen M Zhang ZW, Newcomb PV, Moorghen M, Gupta J, Feakins R, Savage P, Hollowood A, Alderson D, Holly JM.Insulin-like growth factor binding protein-3: relationship to the development of gastric pre-ma-

lignancy and gastric adenocarcinoma (United Kingdom). Cancer Causes Control 2004;15:211 – 218.

[52] Chen W, Wang L, Ke Jin G, Tan Y, Zhou Y, Hu Z, Ma H, Wang J, Hua Z, Ding W, Shen J, Xu Y, Shen H. The role of IGFBP3 functional polymorphisms in the risk of gastric cancer in a high-risk Chinese population.Eur J Cancer Prev 2008;17: 82 – 87.

[53] Loh JT, Friedman DB, Piazuelo MB, Bravo LE, Wilson KT, Peek RM Jr,Correa P, Cover TL. Analysis of *Helicobacter pylori cag*A promoter elements required for salt-induced upregulation of CagA expression. Infect Immun 2012;80:3094–106.

[54] Blanca Piazuelo M, Epplein M, Correa P. Gastric cancer: An infectious disease. Infect Dis Clin North Am 2010; 24(4): 853–869

[55] Fox JG, Dangler CA, Taylor NS, King A, Koh TJ, Wang TC. High-salt diet induces gastric epithelial hyperplasia and parietal cell loss, and enhances *Helicobacter pylori* colonization in C57BL/6 mice. Cancer Res 1999;59(19):4823–8.

[56] Yamaguchi N, Kakizoe T. Synergistic interaction between *Helicobacter pylori* gastritis and diet in gastric cancer. Lancet Oncol 2001;2(2):88–94.

[57] Ladeiras-Lopes R, Pereira AK, Nogueira A, Pinheiro-Torres T, Pinto I, Santos-Pereira R, Lunet N. Smoking and gastric cancer: systematic review and meta-analysis of cohort studies. Cancer Causes Control 2008; 19:689 – 701.

[58] Koizumi Y, Tsubono Y, Nakaya N, Kuriyama S, Shibuya D, Matsuoka H, Tsuji I. Cigarette smoking and the risk of gastric cancer: a pooled analysis of two prospective studies in Japan. Int J Cancer 2004; 112: 1049 – 1055.

[59] Sjodahl K, Lu Y, Nilsen TI, Ye W, Hveem K, Vatten L, Lagergren J. Smoking and alcohol dinking in relation to risk of gastric cancer: a population-based,prospective cohort study. Int J Cancer 2007; 120: 128 – 132.

[60] Moy KA, Fan Y, Wang R, Gao YT, Yu MC, Yuan JM. Alcohol and tobacco use in relation to gastric cancer: a prospective study of men in Shanghai,China. Cancer Epidemiol Biomarkers Prev 2010; 19: 2287 – 2297.

[61] Duan L, Wu AH, Sullivan-Halley J, Berstein L. Passive smoking and risk of oesophageal and gastric adenocarcinomas. Br J Cancer 2009;100: 1483 – 1485

[62] Algra AM, Rothwell PM. Effects of regular aspirin on long-term cancer incidence and metastasis: a systematic comparison of evidence from observational studies versus randomised trials. Lancet Oncol 2012;13(5):518-27.

[63] Bosetti C, Rosato V, Gallus S, Cuzick J, La Vecchia C. Aspirin and cancer risk: a quantitative review to 2011. Ann Oncol 2012;23(6):1403-15.

[64] Wong BC, Zhang L, Ma JL, Pan KF, Li JY, Shen L, Liu WD, Feng GS, Zhang XD, Li J, Lu AP, Xia HH, Lam S, You WC. Effects of selective COX-2 inhibitor and *Helicobacterpylori* eradication on precancerous gastric lesions. Gut 2012;61(6):812-8.

[65] Tian W, Zhao Y, Liu S, Li X. Meta-analysis on the relationship between nonsteroidal anti-inflammatory drug use and gastric cancer. Eur J Cancer Prev. 2010 ;19(4):288-98

[66] Conteduca V, Sansonno D, Ingravallo G, Marangi S, Russi S, Lauletta G, Dammacco F. Barrett's esophagus and esophageal cancer: an overview. Int J Oncol 2012; 41:414–424.

[67] Fuccio L, Eusebi LH, Bazzoli F. Gastric cancer, *Helicobacterpylori* infection and other risk factors. World J Gastrointest Oncol 2010; 2:342–347.

[68] Correa P, Haenszel W, Cuello C, Tannenbaum S, Archer M. A model for gastric cancer epidemiology. Lancet 1975; 2: 58–60.

[69] Wong BC, Lam SK, Wong WM, Chen JS, Zheng TT, Feng RE, Lai KC, Hu WH, Yuen ST, Leung SY, Fong DY, Ho J, Ching CK. *Helicobacterpylori* eradication to prevent gastric cancer in a high-risk region of China: a randomized controlled trial. JAMA 2004;291:187–194.

[70] Leung WK, Lin SR, Ching JY, To KF, Ng EK, Chan FK, Lau JY, Sung JJ. Factors predicting progression of gastric intestinal metaplasia: results of a randomised trial on *Helicobacterpylori* eradication.Gut 2004;53(9):1244–1249

[71] Correa P, Fontham ET, Bravo JC, Bravo LE, Ruiz B, Zarama G, Realpe JL, Malcom GT, Li D, Johnson WD, Mera R. Chemoprevention of gastric dysplasia: randomized trial of antioxidant supplements and anti-*Helicobacterpylori* therapy. J Natl Cancer Inst 2000;6;92:1881–1888.

[72] Mera R, Fontham ET, Bravo LE, Bravo JC, Piazuelo MB, Camargo MC, Correa P. Long term follow up of patients treated for *Helicobacterpylori* infection. Gut 2005;54(11):1536–1540.

[73] You WC, Brown LM, Zhang L, Li JY, Jin ML, Chang YS, Ma JL, Pan KF, Liu WD, Hu Y, Crystal-Mansour S, Pee D, Blot WJ, Fraumeni JF Jr, Xu GW, Gail MH. Randomized double-blind factorial trial of three treatments to reduce the prevalence of precancerous gastric lesions. J Natl Cancer Inst 2006; 98:974-983.

[74] Ma JL, Zhang L, Brown LM, Li JY, Shen L, Pan KF, Liu WD, Hu Y, Han ZX, Crystal-Mansour S, Pee D, Blot WJ, Fraumeni JF Jr, You WC, Gail MH. Fifteen-year effects of *Helicobacterpylori*, garlic, and vitamin treatments on gastric cancer incidence and mortality. J Natl Cancer Inst 2012;104:488-492.

[75] Fukase K, Kato M, Kikuchi S, Inoue K, Uemura N, Okamoto S, Terao S, Amagai K, Hayashi S, Asaka M; Japan Gast Study Group.Effect of eradication of *Helicobacterpylori* on incidence of metachronous gastric carcinoma after endoscopic resection of early gastric cancer: an open-label, randomised controlled trial. Lancet 2008;372:392-397.

[76] Lee YC, Chen TH, Chiu HM, Shun CT, Chiang H, Liu TY, Wu MS, Lin JT. The benefit of mass eradication of *Helicobacterpylori* infection: a community-based study of gastric cancer prevention. Gut 2013;62:676-82

[77] El-Omar EM. Role of host genes in sporadic gastric cancer. Best Pract Res Clin Gastroenterol. 2006;20:675–86.

4

Floating Drug Delivery Systems for Eradication of *Helicobacter pylori* in Treatment of Peptic Ulcer Disease

Yousef Javadzadeh and Sanaz Hamedeyazdan

1. Introduction

Peptic ulcer (gastric or duodenal ulcer) is one of the most common disorders affecting the gastrointestinal system. The lifetime cumulative incidence of peptic ulcer disease is more than 10% of adult population in western countries (Ofman et al., 2000). The pathophysiology of peptic ulcer disease is an imbalance between mucosal defense factors (bicarbonate, mucin, prostaglandin, nitric oxide and other peptides and growth factors) and injurious factors (acid and pepsin). The management and prevention of these acid-related disorder are possible either by decreasing the level of gastric acidity or by enhancing mucosal protection (Brunton et al., 2008). Various factors, including genetic, diet, pharmacologic and psychologic might contribute to peptic ulcers (Wyatt, 1989). *Helicobacter pylori* (*H. pylori*) is a prominent etiologic factor influencing peptic ulcer disease (Hauser et al., 2005). Regarding the fact that *H. pylori* play a dominant role in the majority of peptic ulcers, prevention of relapse is focused on eradication of this organism from the stomach.

Nowadays it is believed that, *H. pylori* and non-steroidal anti-inflammatory drugs (NSAID) are the two major contributing factors causing peptic ulcer disease (Graham, 1996). *H. pylori* is found in approximately 100% of chronic active antral gastritis cases; 90% to 95% of duodenal ulcer patients and 50% to 80% of gastric ulcer patients (Kluwer, 2004). Owing to the fact that chronic infection with *H. pylori* weakens the natural defenses of the lining of the stomach against the ulcerating action of acid, medications that neutralize stomach acid, antacids, and medications that decrease the secretion of acid in the stomach such as H_2-blockers and proton pump inhibitors (PPIs) have been used effectively for many years to treat ulcers. Obviously, antacids, H_2-blockers and PPIs not only would have no effect on *H. pylori* eradication from the stomach, but also the ulcers are frequently returned promptly after these medications are discontinued. Accordingly, eradication of *H. pylori* also is important in the treatment of the pylori-related ulcers which could be achieved through the commonly used antibiotics.

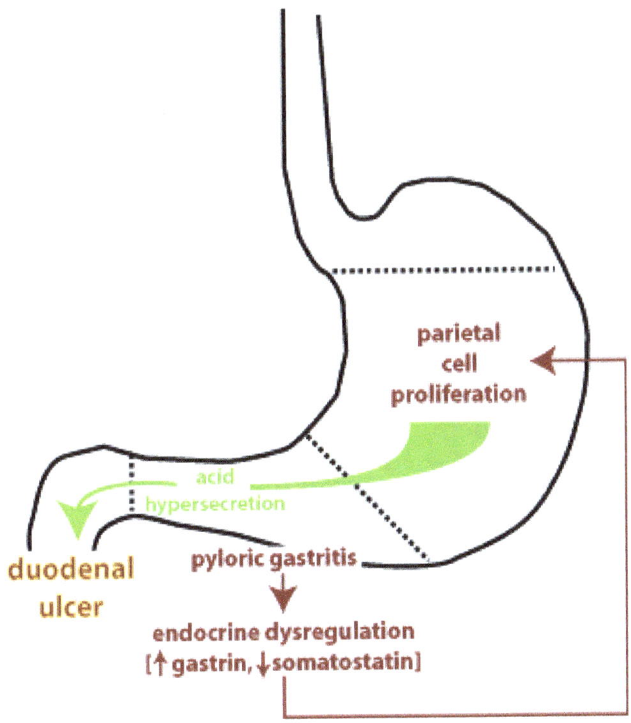

Figure 1. *H. pylori* in peptic ulcers.

Not surprisingly, the wide range of effective medicinal agents available today is one of the greatest scientific achievements. Regardless of the effectiveness and safety of the medicines embedded in dosage forms, the pharmaceutical concept of the latter is growing to be ever more eminent in the management of different diseases. The oral dosage forms of the medications available for *H. pylori* eradication, typically, possess several physiological restrictions such as non-uniform drug absorption profiles, incomplete drug release and shorter residence time of the dosage form in the stomach (MotlekarYouan, 2006; Adibkia et al., 2011; GisbertCalvet, 2011). Rate of the transition for a dosage form through the gastrointestinal (GI) tract is highly affected by the physiological properties of the GI tract as well as the formulation properties (Bardonnet et al., 2006a; Khobragade et al., 2009). Hence, suitable pharmaceutical dosage forms in *H. pylori* eradication is also an important basic principle of the drug delivery system dominating these constraints and offering a proper delivery strategy that would function independent of the digestive state, clinical condition, or GI motility of the individual. Since the bioavailability of drugs often depends on the GI transit rate of the dosage form, it appears necessary to establish an appropriate sustained release system for drug delivery (Hu et al., 2010; JavadzadehHamedeyazdan, 2012).

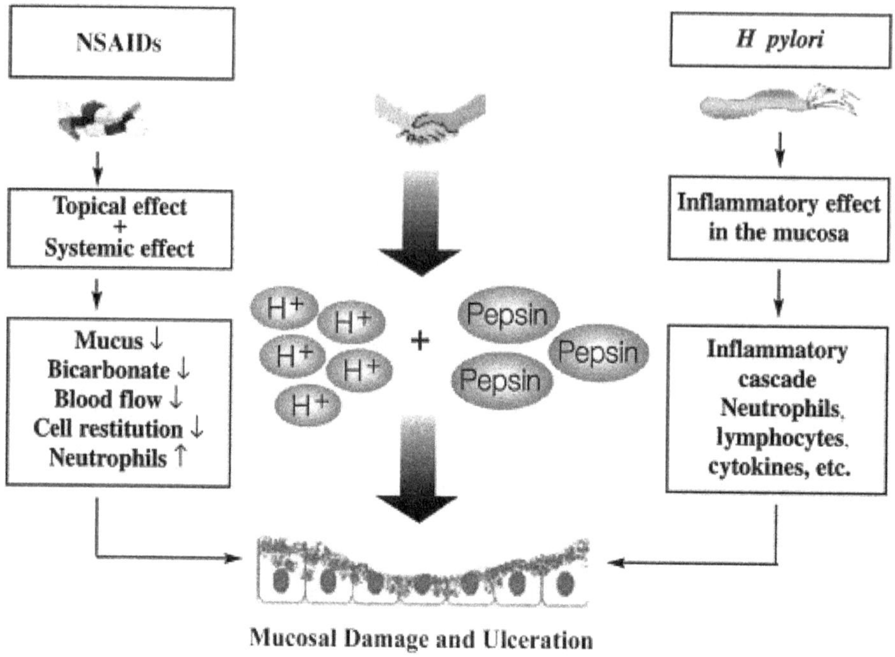

Figure 2. Major factors causing mucosal damage and ulceration (Peura, 2004).

2. Prolongation of GI retention

Scientific and technological advancements have been made in the research and development of different types of drug delivery systems. Keeping up with the rapid development in designing novel drug delivery systems, it is advisable to explore the existing delivery concept and new intra gastric delivery systems which would be expected to overcome the current medication limitations of the treatment of *H. pylori* associated peptic ulcer. It is obvious that formulating dosage forms that retained in the stomach for a prolonged and predictable period of time seem to be advantageous in *H. pylori* eradication.

The most feasible method for achieving a prolonged and predictable drug delivery in the GI tract is to control the gastric residence time by gastro retentive and sustained release dosage forms that have some beneficial in safety and efficacy over normal release systems. This method of application is especially helpful in delivery of sparingly soluble and insoluble drugs used in *H. pylori* eradication. It is acknowledged that, as the solubility of a drug decreases, the time available for drug dissolution becomes less adequate and so the transit time becomes an important factor affecting drug absorption in drugs with lower solubility. Other drug candidates suitable for gastroretentive drug delivery systems include those drugs that are locally active in the stomach, drugs with narrow absorption window in GI tract, drugs that are unstable in the intestinal or colonic environment, drugs that act locally in the proximal part of GI tract or disturb normal colonic microbes like antibiotics and also drugs that exhibit low solubility at high pH values. Concerning the pharmacotherapy of the stomach through local drug release of gastroretentive dosage forms, bringing about high levels of drug concentrations at the gastric mucosa (eradication of *H. pylori* from the submucosal tissue of the stomach), and treating stomach and duodenal ulcers, gastritis and oesophagitis, the risk of gastric carcinoma would be drastically reduced. In contrast, there are drugs that do not fit in gastroretentive drug delivery systems; Drugs that have very limited acid solubility, drugs that suffer instability in the gastric environment, and drugs intended for selective release in the colon should follow other techniques of drug delivery to reach for their intended site of action. Hence, gastroretentive dosage forms despite providing rather constant drug concentrations in the bloodstream for longer periods of time do not fulfill this benefit with several groups of drugs (Javadzadeh-Hamedeyazdan, 2012; Pahwa et al., 2012b).

One of the advantages of the sustained release dosage forms is that medication is administered less often than other dosage forms reducing fluctuations of drug concentration in the bloodstream. As a result, the patient is not repeatedly subjected to different levels of drug which are less or more than adequate. Nor does the blood chemistry undergo frequent chemical imbalances, which might be risky to the patient's health. Additionally, through gastroretentive dosage forms not only the bioavailability and therapeutic efficacy of drugs are improved but also it may allow for a possible reduction in the dose because of the steady therapeutic levels of drugs. Drugs that have poor solubility in higher pH, absorption windows in stomach, requiring local delivery in stomach could be delivered ideally to the site of action by the gastroretentive formulations. On the other hand, drugs that cause irritation to gastric mucosa and the ones meet first-pass metabolism or have stability problems in gastric fluids are not appropriate for these kinds of drug delivery systems (JavadzadehHamedeyazdan, 2012; Pahwa et al., 2012a; Pawar et al., 2012).

In brief, gastric retention is a means to enable a delivery strategy that will function irrespective of the digestive state, clinical condition, or GI motility of the individuals with longer drug residence time in the stomach being advantageous in superior drug bioavailabilities and also in certifying local action of some drugs in the upper part of the GI tract, that are used in *H. pylori* eradication (Bardonnet et al., 2006b; Nama et al., 2008; Badhan et al., 2009; Shah et al., 2009; AdebisiConway, 2013).

3. *H. pylori* associated peptic ulcer

3.1. Acidic condition of stomach

The human stomach can produce and secrete about 2.2 to 3 L of gastric acid per day with basal secretion levels being typically highest in the evening. Normally no bacteria or viruses can survive in this medium that is composed of digestive enzymes and concentrated hydrochloric acid. Consequently, stomach has been regarded as a sterile ingestion organ for its hostile and acidic environment that could be considered as a barrier for invasion of various microorganisms. However, this notion has been totally changed since *H. pylori* as a major cause of peptic ulcer disease and gastritis in human was firstly isolated by Marshall and Warren in 1983 (Yang et al., 1999). *H. pylori*, a spiral-shaped gram-negative rod, is classified as *Campylobacter pyloridis* due to its similar histological and growth properties to the *Campylobacter* species. Based on the unique morphological and biochemical characteristics, *Campylobacter pyloridis* was regrouped into a new genus *Helicobacter* (Brooks et al., 2004).

3.2. Pathogenesis of *H. pylori*

H. pylori is associated with antral gastritis, peptic ulcer disease (gastric and duodenal ulcer disease) and gastric carcinoma, however, it initially induces chronic gastritis to develop peptic ulcer rather than directly causing the ulcer disease (Wyatt, 1989). Ever since, *H. pylori* grows optimally at a pH of 6-7, it would not grow at the pH of the gastric lumen. Gastric mucus is relatively impermeable to acid and has a strong buffering capacity so deep mucus layer near the epithelial surface where the pH is about physiologic of 7.4 is an appropriate place for *H. pylori* growth. The bacterium produces a protease modifying the gastric mucus to reduce the ability of acid to diffuse through the mucus. In addition, *H. pylori* also has potent urease activity, which yields production of ammonia and further buffering of acid, which may directly damage the cells, too (Brooks, Butel et al., 2004; Abe et al., 2011). Although, the mechanisms by which *H. pylori* causes mucosal inflammation and damage, are not well known but they may involve both bacterial and host factors. Compared to other infectious diseases, the *H. pylori* associated morbidity is relatively high, which is about 10% for peptic ulcer disease and 0.5% for gastric adenocarcinoma (Kusters, 2001). Once *H. pylori* eradication has been achieved, re-infection rates are less than 0.5% per year, and ulcer recurrence rates are dramatically reduced (Kluwer, 2004). Since, there is not any clear hypothesis about spread of *H. pylori*, prevention is rather difficult issue. Then in treatment of peptic ulcer disease, clinicians are logically focusing on the eradication of *H. pylori* (Ables et al., 2007; Yamaoka, 2010).

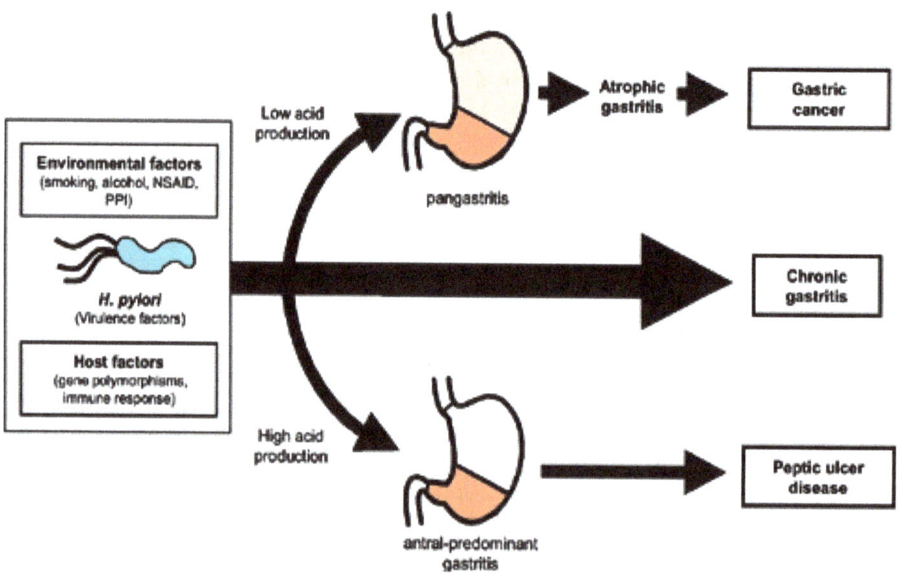

Figure 3. Pathogenesis of *H. pylori* (Kusters et al., 2006).

3.3. Treatments for *H. pylori* associated peptic ulcer disease

Basically, the goals for peptic ulcer treatments have been defined as: alleviation of symptoms, healing of the ulceration, prevention of recurrence of ulcer. Primarily, before the bacterium was found, it was believed that stomach ulcers occur when excess acid damaged the gastric mucosa so the treatment was based on reduction or neutralization of that acid (Gisbert et al., 2010; GisbertPajares, 2010). Patients were treated with long-term suppressive therapy by giving acid-blocking medications, for instance, H_2-blockers and, more recently, proton pump inhibitors (BreuerGraham, 1999). This kind of treatment could certainly relieve ulcer-related symptoms, heal gastric mucosal inflammation and even heal the ulcer. Unfortunately, it has a high recurrence rate just owing to the lack of basic treatment of the infection and eradication of the bacterium, *H. pylori* (Brunton, Parker et al., 2008). The identification of *H. pylori*, and understanding of *H. pylori* associated peptic ulcer disease have greatly changed therapeutic regiments covering peptic ulcer disease. Eradication of *H. pylori* is now recognized to be the correct approach in the treatment of the disease (Yang, Eshraghi et al., 1999; Chuah et al., 2011). The treatment of peptic ulcer with antibiotics is recognized as the choice treatment for patients (Beales, 2001). Savings of costs and time are the major benefits of this protocol to therapy with acid reducing medications. The same drug and dosage regimens could be applied to the treatment for both gastric and duodenal ulcer as there are no important differences between these two ulcer diseases (DzieniszewskiJarosz, 2006). Antibiotics and agents used to eradicate *H. pylori*, attack three main areas, i.e. the bacterium cell wall, the ribosome and nuclear DNA. For instance, metronidazole, a nitroimidazole antiprotozoal drug that also has potent antibacterial activity against anaerobes, including bacteroides and clostridium species, can disrupt the bacterial DNA helix preventing replication and interrupting gene expression, bismuth salt may disrupt bacterial cell wall or membrane (Malfertheiner, 1996).

3.3.1. Combination therapy

Although *H. pylori* is sensitive to many antibiotics *in vitro*, this sensitivity is not correlated with eradication of the organism *in vivo* (Drumm, 1990). Recurrence of the infection is common after treatment of *H. pylori* by bismuth alone or monotherapy antibiotic (Rauws et al., 1988; Oderda et al., 1989; Chang et al., 2009). It has been postulated that the failure of antibiotic monotherapy to clear *H. pylori in vivo* may be due to the lack of efficacy of the antibiotics in the acid environment of the stomach (Drumm, 1990). Other possible reason of failure could be the area that *H. pylori* colonized and resistance to bacteria. As a result of failure of single antibiotic therapies, combination regiments are suggested to increase the rate of *H. pylori* eradication. Nonetheless, many regimens for *H. pylori* eradication have been proposed, the ideal regimen in this setting should achieve a cure rate of >80% (Brunton, Parker et al., 2008).

3.3.2. Triple combination therapy

Triple combination therapy, using two antibacterial antibiotics and a proton pump inhibitor, had achieved a high eradication rate and seems to be the most effective regimens for *H. pylori* eradication (AxonMoayyedi, 1996; Ishizone et al., 2007). Proton pump inhibitors promote eradication of *H. pylori* through several mechanisms: direct antimicrobial properties (minor);

raising intra-gastric pH and lowering the minimal inhibitory concentrations of antibiotics against *H. pylori.* One of the principal treatment regimens consists of a 10–14 day regimen of "triple therapy": a proton pump inhibitor (standard dose, b.i.d.), clarithromycin, (500 mg, b.i.d.) and amoxicillin (1 g, b.i.d.). For patients who have allergy to penicillin, metronidazole, 500 mg twice daily, should be substituted for amoxicillin. Moreover, after completion of triple therapy, the proton pump inhibitor has been recommended to be continued once daily for a total of 4–6 weeks to ensure complete ulcer healing (Katzung, 2006). Other triple therapies that are being mentioned in other reference includes combinations of bismuth salts and various antibiotics (Rauws, Langenberg et al., 1988).

3.3.3. *Quadruple combination therapy*

In the case of *H. pylori* eradication quadruple therapy has been offered for 14 days: Proton pump inhibitor twice a day, metronidazole 500 mg three times daily, bismuth subsalicylate 525 mg, tetracycline 500 mg four times daily or H_2-receptor antagonist twice a day, bismuth subsalicylate 525 mg, metronidazole 250 mg, tetracycline 500 mg four times daily (Brunton, Parker et al., 2008). Antibiotics from systemic circulation have to traverse the epithelial layer (Malfertheiner, 1996; Hsu et al., 2011). Seeing as, in systemic administration of drugs the gastric emptying makes the effective local concentrations of drugs difficult to maintain, the effects of drug is not local and is through its systemic absorption, the frequent doses of oral antibiotics are required leading to higher drug dosages, lower patient compliance, and adverse drug effects.

3.4. Drug delivery systems for *H. pylori* eradication

3.4.1. *Importance of drug delivery systems in treatment of diseases*

It is judicious to be reminiscent of the GI tract being a primary site for the absorption of drugs with a variety of limitations making the *in vivo* performance of drug delivery systems uncertain. Despite tremendous advancement in drug delivery, the oral rout still remains the preferred route for the administration of therapeutic agents in consequence of the low cost of therapy, and ease of administration, as well as patient compliance. However, oral dosage forms hold several physiological restrictions like non-uniform absorption profiles, incomplete drug release and shorter residence time of the dosage form in the stomach (Adibkia, Hamedeyazdan et al., 2011). Undoubtedly, rate of drug transition through the gastrointestinal (GI) tract is highly controlled by the physiological properties of the GI tract as well as the formulation properties. Since, bioavailability of drugs in this route of administration often depends on the GI transit rate of the dosage form it is of value to distinguish between an appropriate drug delivery system for an especial objective in treatment of diseases. Acquiring a clear notion of why certain medications are prone to problems in reaching the desired efficiency and bioavailability, to dominate the relative constraints offering successful medication therapy recalling some fundamental characteristics of the stomach would be of note.

3.4.2. Stomach and drug delivery systems

As far as we know, the stomach is a muscular, hollow, dilated part of the alimentary canal which functions as an important organ of the human body located between the esophagus and the small intestine. Surface epithelium of stomach retains its integrity throughout the course of its lifetime, even though it is constantly exposed to a high concentration of hydrochloric acid and powerful enzymes. This self protection mechanism is due to the fact that the specialized goblet cells located in the stomach and continuously secrete a large amount of mucus that remains closely applied to the surface epithelium (Chein, 1992). In general, stomach is an important site of enzyme production with small surface area, offering an imperfect site of absorption (Chein, 1992). The main function of stomach is to store food temporarily, grind it, and then release it slowly in to the duodenum. The process of gastric emptying occurs both during fasting and fed states; however, the pattern of motility differs markedly in the two states. Fasted state is characterized by an inter-digestive series of electrical events which cycle both through the stomach and small intestine every 2–3 h which is called the inter-digestive myoelectric cycle or migrating myoelectric complex (Fell, 1996). In the fed state, the gastric emptying rate is slowed since the feeding results in a lag time prior to the onset of gastric emptying, depending upon the physiological state of the subject and the design of pharmaceutical formulation, the emptying process can last from a few minutes to 12 h. Alterations in gastric emptying occurs due to factors such as age, race, sex, and disease states, as they may seriously affect the release of a drug from the drug delivery system (SinghKim, 2000).

The complex and highly variable nature of gastric emptying process making the *in vivo* performance of conventional drug delivery systems uncertain draw researchers' attention to find a clue and dominate these constraints and present suitable drug delivery strategies that would serve independent of the digestive state, clinical condition, or GI motility of the individual. Conventional oral dosage forms provide a specific drug concentration in the systemic circulation without offering any control over the rate of drug delivery, whilst controlled-release drug delivery systems provide drug release at a predetermined, predictable, and controlled rate of drug release (Hwang et al., 1998). Nevertheless, in some cases the insufficient residency of drugs in the vicinity of absorption site for the life time of drug delivery restricts the use of controlled-release drug delivery systems. The inadequate drug residence in the vicinity of absorption site might arise from differences in GI transit time of drugs in individuals, and physical properties of the object ingested as well as the physiological conditions of the alimentary canal. Correspondingly, medications with sustained drug release forms have some benefits over normal release systems in safety and efficacy in reducing the frequency of drug dosage, together with the diminished incidence of adverse drug reactions. Hence, if medications used in *H. pylori* eradication therapy are used in terms of sustained release dosage forms some advantages are fulfilled seeing as the medications are administered less often than other dosage forms, fluctuations of drug concentration in the blood would be reduced, and the patient is not repeatedly subjected to amounts of the drug which are less or more than adequate, nor the blood chemistry experience frequent chemical imbalances, which might be detrimental to the patient's health (Klausner et al., 2003; Javadzadeh et al., 2007; Tang et al., 2007; Javadzadeh et al., 2009; Javadzadeh et al., 2012). Several methods have been developed for extension of GI transit time via enhancing the residence time of drug delivery systems in the stomach.

3.4.3. Floating drug delivery systems

One of the approaches followed to extend the residency of medications in the stomach is floating dosage forms with lower density than the gastric fluids to be capable of floating on the gastric juice in the stomach (SinghKim, 2000; Adibkia, Hamedeyazdan et al., 2011). According to the mechanism of buoyancy, two evidently different technologies are applied in development of floating dosage forms, effervescent and non-effervescent systems. In general, the principle rule is indelible in all approaches and that is to float on gastric juice with a specific density of less than 1.004 g/cm of the gastric juice in the stomach.

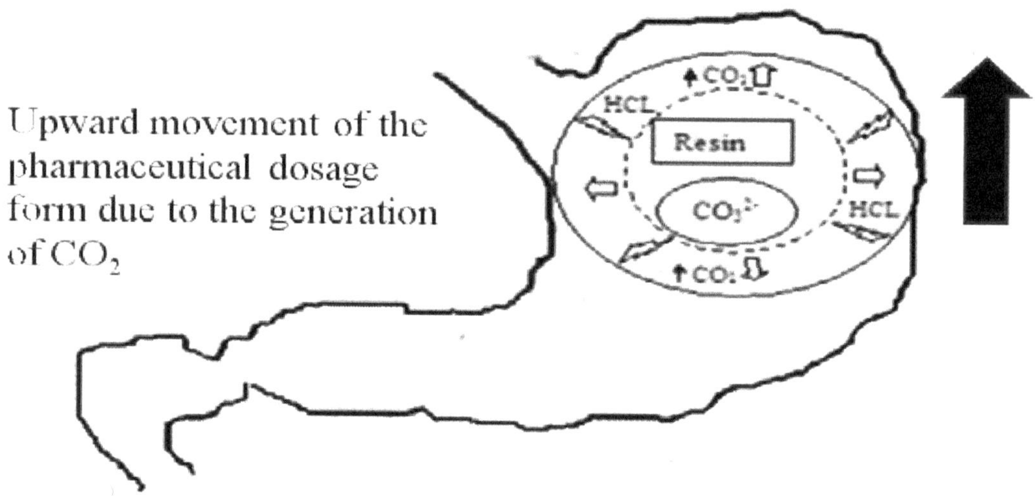

Figure 4. Effervescent floating drug delivery system in the stomach

Besides, multi-particulates of floating dosage forms consisting of small discrete units in which the active substance is offered as a number of small independent subunits are less reliant on gastric emptying, bringing about less inter and intra-subject variability in GI transit time. Moreover, they are also well distributed and less likely to cause local irritation. Nowadays, much emphasis is being laid on the development of multi particulate dosage forms rather than single unit systems due to potential benefits of them such as increased bioavailability, reduced risk of systemic toxicity, reduced risk of local irritation as well as predictable gastric emptying (MohamadDashevsky, 2007; GuptaPathak, 2008).

A number of factors that affect gastric emptying of a dosage form, such as density, size, and shape of dosage form, concomitant intake of food and drugs such as anticholinergic agents (e.g., atropine, propantheline), opiates (e.g., codeine), prokinetic agents (e.g., metoclopramide, cisapride), and biological factors like gender, posture, age, body mass index, and disease states (e.g., diabetes, Crohn's disease) could be controlled by these floating dosage forms providing a more convenient medication therapy (SinghKim, 2000).

These systems are also appropriate for drugs which are locally active to the gastric mucosa in the stomach, such as administration of metronidazole (MZ) as an antibiotic for *H. pylori* eradication in the treatment of peptic ulcer disease (Murata et al., 2000; Rajinikanth et al., 2007; RajinikanthMishra, 2007; RajinikanthMishra, 2008). Treatment of *H. pylori* infection by topical administration of antimicrobial agents has been reported. In order to avoid the side effects of standard triple therapy, Satoh used a technique of instilling a combination of bismuth subnitrate, amoxicillin and metronidazole into the stomach via a naso-gastric tube for 1 hour. He found that topical therapy was highly successful with high eradication rate of *H. pylori* and none-ulcer dyspepsia as well. Although this local administration successfully avoids some of the side effects of standard triple therapy, it is inconvenient and still complicated to patient when compared to oral dosage delivery system (Satoh, 1996). Elsewhere, the hydrodynamically balanced delivery system of Clarithromycin was developed which, after oral administration had the ability of prolonged gastric residence time with the desired *in vitro* release profile for the localized action in the stomach, in the treatment of *H. pylori* mediated peptic ulcer. In this study, wet granulation technique was applied for preparing of floating tablets of Clarithromycin. The proportion of sodium bicarbonate was varied to get the least possible lag time, also the polymer part varied to get the desired release. The formulation that developed using 66.2% Clarithromycin, 12% HPMC K4M polymer, 8% sodium bicarbonate gave floating lag time less than 3 min with a floating time of 12 h, and an *in vitro* release profile very near to the desired release. *In vivo* radiographic studies also suggested that the tablet had increased gastric residence time for the effective localized action of the antibiotic (Clarithromycin) in the treatment of *H. pylori* mediated peptic ulcer. The mechanism of release of Clarithromycin from the floating tablets was anomalous diffusion transport and followed by zero order kinetics (Nama, Gonugunta et al., 2008). In another study by Pornsak Sriamornsak, oil-entrapped calcium pectinate gel floating beads were prepared using selected oils that were floated immediately and remained floating for 24 hours. They concluded that this lasting intra-gastric buoyancy of a controlled release dosage form may also provide a suitable manner to deliver drugs that are locally active to the gastric mucosa in the stomach and, hence, achieve a site-specific therapeutic action (e.g., antibiotic administration for *H. pylori* eradication in the treatment of peptic ulcer disease (Sriamornsak et al., 2004). Then again, in another study Sriamornsak et al. evaluated the effects of some variables on release behavior of metronidazole from floating emulsion gel beads of calcium pectinate. They detected a notable prolongation drug release profile by coating the beads with Eudragit or by hardening with glutaraldehyde, whereas no clear effect on drug release was obtained using PEG10000, glyceryl monostearate and Eudragit as additives in the formulations (Sriamornsak, Thirawong et al., 2004; Sriamornsak et al., 2005).

Considering the fact that prolongation of the local availability of the antibacterial agents show positive effects of increasing in the effectiveness of *H. pylori* treatment ensuring a high drug concentration in the gastric mucosa, we had tried to formulate metronidazole in floating pharmaceutical dosage forms to encounter higher concentrations of the antibacterial agent in the gastric mucosa and clarify the mechanism of the release obtaining a general kinetic model for drug release profiles. In our previously published papers, we had reported the use of two different mechanisms in preparation of metronidazole floating matrix tablets including: A low density producing agent (gas generating agent/porous agent) and hydrocolloid-forming polymer(s) (Asnaashari et al., 2011). Carbonate acted as the gas generating agent when it came into contact with an acidic environment of the stomach under fed condition which got entrapped inside the system, producing bubbles, decreasing the density of the formulation. Preparing a low-density system using calcium silicate a characteristically porous structure with many pores and a large pore volume which forms a porous buoyant system (Jain et al., 2005). The hydrocolloids such as HPMC, carbopol, psyllium in the metronidazole formulations were hydrated and formed a colloid gel barrier that controled the rate of drug release, around its surface with thickness growing by time and increasing of volume due to hydration that in a bulk density less than 1 g/cm3 remaining buoyant on the gastric fluid. The established suitable release metronidazole floating matrix tablets could ensure a more localized drug concentration which might be useful for *H. pylori* eradication. In other survey, we had prepared alginate beads of metronidazole employing gas generating and porous agents followed by physicochemical evaluations for the prepared formulations (Javadzadeh et al., 2010). Alginates due to their high biocompatibility and nontoxic nature in oral administration that also demonstrate protective effect on the mucous membranes of the upper GI tract are a remarkable natural polymers found in brown algae that have been studied for a variety of biomedical applications. Sodium-Alginate beads (Na-Alg) have been developed in recent years as a unique vehicle for drug delivery. Alginates, which are naturally substances, are found in brown algae and can be considered as block polymers, which mainly consist of mannuronic acid (M), guluronic acid (G) and mannuronic-guluronic (MG) blocks. Alginate is known to be nontoxic when taken orally and also have protective effect on the mucous membranes of the upper gastrointestinal tract. The alginate beads with the structure of spherical gels are taken shape through dropwise addition of aqueous alginate solution to the aqueous solution containing calcium ions and/or other di and polyvalent cations (10). The pH dependent reswelling property of dried alginate beads let them to be administrated as controlled release system in gastrointestinal tract. The drug release from pharmaceutical dosage forms is a major determinant in their biological effect, thus evaluation of drug release kinetic is of paramount importance in the field. The findings of our study revealed high compatibility of the alginate beads in achieving a suitable floating pharmaceutical dosage forms which could control metronidazole release from the beads with a definite kinetic of drug release. Identifying drug release kinetics of a drug which is an important variable in obtaining one or two physically meaningful parameters in relating the drug release parameter with important parameters such as *in vivo* drug bioavailability is of substantial value in pharmaceutical manufacturing.

Hence, developing an efficient floating dosage form is reliant to a better understanding of the relation among the physiological properties of the GI tract, formulation variables and the performance of these floating systems *in vivo* and clinical stages, leading to a superior floating drug delivery system in special cases like *H. pylori* eradication.

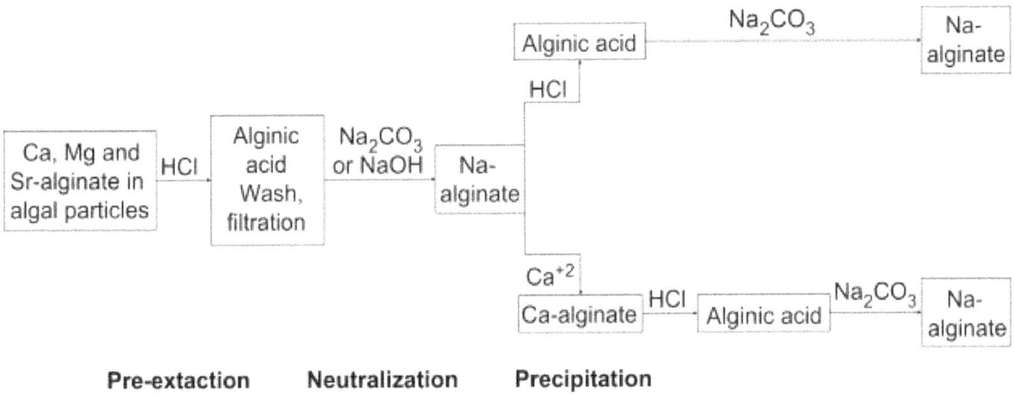

Figure 5. Alginates in floating drug delivery systems

4. Conclusion

Overall, developing an efficient floating dosage form for *H. pylori* eradication could be established by the combination of two buoyancy mechanisms, gas generating systems with swellable polymers, being advantages in view point of obtaining an appropriate floating lag time and duration of buoyancy which guarantees the optimum efficiency of the pharmaceutical dosage form. Nonetheless, further investigations may focus on the compatibility of the mentioned concepts in the interplay of the pharmacokinetic and pharmacodynamic parameters *in vivo* and also in clinical aspect to provide the effectiveness of the floating drug delivery systems in *H. pylori* eradication therapies.

Author details

Yousef Javadzadeh and Sanaz Hamedeyazdan

Biotechnology Research center, Tabriz University of Medical Sciences, Iran

References

[1] Abe, T., Kodama, M., Murakami, K., Matsunari, O., Mizukami, K., Inoue, K., Uchida, M., Okimoto, T., Fujioka, T., Uchida, T., Moriyama, M. & Yamaoka, Y. (2011). Impact of Helicobacter pylori CagA diversity on gastric mucosal damage: an immunohistochemical study of East-Asian-type CagA. *J. Gastroenterol. Hepatol.*, Vol.26, No.4, pp. 688-693.

[2] Ables, A.Z., Simon, I. & Melton, E.R. (2007). Update on Helicobacter pylori treatment. *Am. Fam. Physician.*, Vol.75, No.3, pp. 351-358.

[3] Adebisi, A.O. & Conway, B.R. (2013). Preparation and characterisation of gastroretentive alginate beads for targeting H. pylori. *J Microencapsul*, pp.

[4] Adibkia, K., Hamedeyazdan, S. & Javadzadeh, Y. (2011). Drug release kinetics and physicochemical characteristics of floating drug delivery systems. *Expert Opin. Drug Deliv.*, Vol.8, No.7, pp. 891-903.

[5] Asnaashari, S., Khoei, N.S., Zarrintan, M.H., Adibkia, K. & Javadzadeh, Y. (2011). Preparation and evaluation of novel metronidazole sustained release and floating matrix tablets. *Pharm. Dev. Technol.*, Vol.16, No.4, pp. 400-407.

[6] Axon, A.T. & Moayyedi, P. (1996). Eradication of Helicobacter pylori: omeprazole in combination with antibiotics. *Scand. J. Gastroenterol. Suppl.*, Vol.215, pp. 82-89.

[7] Badhan, A.C., Mashru, R.C., Shah, P.P., Thakkar, A.R. & Dobaria, N.B. (2009). Development and evaluation of sustained release gastroretentive minimatrices for effective treatment of H. pylori infection. *AAPS PharmSciTech*, Vol.10, No.2, pp. 459-467.

[8] Bardonnet, P.L., Faivre, V., Pugh, W.J., Piffaretti, J.C. & Falson, F. (2006a). Gastroretentive dosage forms: overview and special case of Helicobacter pylori. *J. Control. Release*, Vol.111, No.1-2, pp. 1-18.

[9] Bardonnet, P.L., Faivre, V., Pugh, W.J., Piffaretti, J.C. & Falson, F. (2006b). Gastroretentive dosage forms: overview and special case of Helicobacter pylori. *J Control Release*, Vol.111, No.1-2, pp. 1-18.

[10] Beales, I.L. (2001). Efficacy of Helicobacter pylori eradication therapies: a single centre observational study. *BMC Gastroenterol.*, Vol.1, pp. 7.

[11] Breuer, T. & Graham, D.Y. (1999). Costs of diagnosis and treatment of Helicobacter pylori infection: when does choosing the treatment regimen based on susceptibility testing become cost effective? *Am. J. Gastroenterol.*, Vol.94, No.3, pp. 725-729.

[12] Brooks, G., Butel, J., Morse, S., Melnick, J., Jawetz, E. & Adelberg, E. (2004). *Jawetz, Melnick, & Adelberg's Medical Microbiology*. United States of America, McGraw-Hill Professional.

[13] Brunton, L., Parker, K., Blumenthal, D. & Buxton, L. (2008). *Goodman & Gilman's Manual of Pharmacology and Therapeutics*. United States of America, McGraw-Hill Companies.

[14] Chang, W.L., Sheu, B.S., Cheng, H.C., Yang, Y.J., Yang, H.B. & Wu, J.J. (2009). Resistance to metronidazole, clarithromycin and levofloxacin of Helicobacter pylori before and after clarithromycin-based therapy in Taiwan. *J. Gastroenterol. Hepatol.*, Vol.24, No.7, pp. 1230-1235.

[15] Chein, Y.W. (1992). *Novel Drug Delivery System*. New York, Marcel Dekker, Inc.

[16] Chuah, S.K., Tsay, F.W., Hsu, P.I. & Wu, D.C. (2011). A new look at anti-Helicobacter pylori therapy. *World J. Gastroentero.*, Vol.17, No.35, pp. 3971-3975.

[17] Drumm, B. (1990). Helicobacter pylori. *Arch. Dis. Child.*, Vol.65, No.11, pp. 1278-1282.

[18] Dzieniszewski, J. & Jarosz, M. (2006). Guidelines in the medical treatment of Helicobacter pylori infection. *J. Physiol. Pharmacol.*, Vol.57 Suppl 3, pp. 143-154.

[19] Fell, J.T. (1996). Targeting of drugs and delivery systems to specific sites in the gastrointestinal tract. *J. Anat.*, Vol.189 (Pt 3), pp. 517-519.

[20] Gisbert, J.P. & Calvet, X. (2011). Review article: the effectiveness of standard triple therapy for Helicobacter pylori has not changed over the last decade, but it is not good enough. *Aliment. Pharm. Ther.*, Vol.34, No.11-12, pp. 1255-1268.

[21] Gisbert, J.P., Calvet, X., O'Connor, A., Megraud, F. & O'Morain, C.A. (2010). Sequential therapy for Helicobacter pylori eradication: a critical review. *J. Clin. Gastroenterol.*, Vol.44, No.5, pp. 313-325.

[22] Gisbert, J.P. & Pajares, J.M. (2010). Treatment of Helicobacter pylori infection: the past and the future. *Eur. J. Intern. Med.*, Vol.21, No.5, pp. 357-359.

[23] Graham, D.Y. (1996). Nonsteroidal anti-inflammatory drugs, Helicobacter pylori, and ulcers: where we stand. *Am. J. Gastroenterol.*, Vol.91, No.10, pp. 2080-2086.

[24] Gupta, R. & Pathak, K. (2008). Optimization studies on floating multiparticulate gastroretentive drug delivery system of famotidine. *Drug Dev. Ind. Pharm.*, Vol.34, No. 11, pp. 1201-1208.

[25] Hauser, K., Longo, B. & Jameson, F. (2005). *Harrison's Principles of Internal Medicine.* United States of America, McGraw-Hill companies.

[26] Hsu, P.I., Wu, D.C., Wu, J.Y. & Graham, D.Y. (2011). Modified sequential Helicobacter pylori therapy: proton pump inhibitor and amoxicillin for 14 days with clarithromycin and metronidazole added as a quadruple (hybrid) therapy for the final 7 days. *Helicobacter*, Vol.16, No.2, pp. 139-145.

[27] Hu, L.D., Xing, Q.B., Shang, C., Liu, W., Liu, C., Luo, Z.L. & Xu, H.X. (2010). Preparation of rosiglitazone maleate sustained-release floating microspheres for improved bioavailability. *Pharmazie*, Vol.65, No.7, pp. 477-480.

[28] Hwang, S.J., Park, H. & Park, K. (1998). Gastric retentive drug-delivery systems. *Crit Rev Ther Drug Carrier Syst*, Vol.15, No.3, pp. 243-284.

[29] Ishizone, S., Maruta, F., Suzuki, K., Miyagawa, S., Takeuchi, M., Kanaya, K., Oana, K., Hayama, M., Kawakami, Y. & Ota, H. (2007). *In vivo* bactericidal activities of Japanese rice-fluid against H. pylori in a Mongolian gerbil model. *Int. J. Med. Sci.*, Vol.4, No.4, pp. 203-208.

[30] Jain, S.K., Awasthi, A.M., Jain, N.K. & Agrawal, G.P. (2005). Calcium silicate based microspheres of repaglinide for gastroretentive floating drug delivery: preparation and *in vitro* characterization. *J. Control. Release,* Vol.107, No.2, pp. 300-309.

[31] Javadzadeh, Y., Asnaashari, S. & Hamedeyazdan, S. (2012). Recrystallization of Drugs: Significance on Pharmaceutical Processing Recrystallization. K. Sztwiertnia. Croatia, InTech.

[32] Javadzadeh, Y. & Hamedeyazdan, S. (2012). Novel Drug Delivery Systems for Modulation of Gastrointestinal Transit Time Recent Advances in Novel Drug Carrier Systems. A. D. Sezer. Croatia, InTech: 393-418.

[33] Javadzadeh, Y., Hamedeyazdan, S., Adibkia, K., Kiafar, F., Zarrintan, M.H. & Barzegar-Jalali, M. (2010). Evaluation of drug release kinetics and physico-chemical characteristics of metronidazole floating beads based on calcium silicate and gas-forming agents. *Pharm. Dev. Technol.,* Vol.15, No.4, pp. 329-338.

[34] Javadzadeh, Y., Jafari-Navimipour, B. & Nokhodchi, A. (2007). Liquisolid technique for dissolution rate enhancement of a high dose water-insoluble drug (carbamazepine). *Int J Pharm,* Vol.341, No.1-2, pp. 26-34.

[35] Javadzadeh, Y., Mohammadi, A., Khoei, N.S. & Nokhodchi, A. (2009). Improvement of physicomechanical properties of carbamazepine by recrystallization at different pH values. *Acta Pharm,* Vol.59, No.2, pp. 187-197.

[36] Katzung, B. (2006). *Basic and Clinical Pharmacology.* San Francisco, mc graw hill pressed.

[37] Khobragade, D.S., Parshuramkar, P.R., Ujjainkar, A.P., Mahendra, A.M., Phapal, S.M. & Patil, A.T. (2009). Conception and evaluation of sustained release polymeric matrix beads for enhanced gastric retention. *Curr. Drug. Deliv.,* Vol.6, No.3, pp. 249-254.

[38] Klausner, E.A., Lavy, E., Friedman, M. & Hoffman, A. (2003). Expandable gastroretentive dosage forms. *J. Control. Release,* Vol.90, No.2, pp. 143-162.

[39] Kluwer, W. (2004). *Drug Facts and Comparisons.* St. Louis, USA., Facts and Comparisons.

[40] Kusters, J.G. (2001). Recent developments in Helicobacter pylori vaccination. *Scand. J. Gastroenterol. Suppl.,* No.234, pp. 15-21.

[41] Kusters, J.G., van Vliet, A.H. & Kuipers, E.J. (2006). Pathogenesis of Helicobacter pylori infection. *Clin Microbiol Rev,* Vol.19, No.3, pp. 449-490.

[42] Malfertheiner, P. (1996). Management of Helicobacter pylori-positive peptic ulcer disease. *Scand. J. Gastroenterol. Suppl.,* Vol.215, pp. 69.

[43] Mohamad, A. & Dashevsky, A. (2007). *In vitro* and *in vivo* performance of a multiparticulate pulsatile drug delivery system. *Drug Dev. Ind. Pharm.,* Vol.33, No.2, pp. 113-119.

[44] Motlekar, N.A. & Youan, B.B. (2006). The quest for non-invasive delivery of bioactive macromolecules: a focus on heparins. *J. Control. Release*, Vol.113, No.2, pp. 91-101.

[45] Murata, Y., Sasaki, N., Miyamoto, E. & Kawashima, S. (2000). Use of floating alginate gel beads for stomach-specific drug delivery. *Eur. J. Pharm. Biopharm.*, Vol.50, No.2, pp. 221-226.

[46] Nama, M., Gonugunta, C.S. & Reddy Veerareddy, P. (2008). Formulation and evaluation of gastroretentive dosage forms of Clarithromycin. *AAPS PharmSciTech*, Vol.9, No.1, pp. 231-237.

[47] Oderda, G., Dell'Olio, D., Morra, I. & Ansaldi, N. (1989). Campylobacter pylori gastritis: long term results of treatment with amoxycillin. *Arch. Dis. Child.*, Vol.64, No.3, pp. 326-329.

[48] Ofman, J.J., Etchason, J., Alexander, W., Stevens, B.R., Herrin, J., Cangialose, C., Ballard, D.J., Bratzler, D., Elward, K.S., FitzGerald, D., Culpepper-Morgan, J. & Marshall, B. (2000). The quality of care for Medicare patients with peptic ulcer disease. *Am. J. Gastroenterol.*, Vol.95, No.1, pp. 106-113.

[49] Pahwa, R., Saini, N., Kumar, V. & Kohli, K. (2012a). Chitosan-based gastroretentive floating drug delivery technology: an updated review. *Expert Opin Drug Deliv*, Vol.9, No.5, pp. 525-539.

[50] Pahwa, R., Singh, M., Kumar, V. & Kohli, K. (2012b). Recent advances and patent perspectives in gastroretentive technology. *Recent Pat Drug Deliv Formul*, Vol.6, No.3, pp. 278-290.

[51] Pawar, V.K., Kansal, S., Asthana, S. & Chourasia, M.K. (2012). Industrial perspective of gastroretentive drug delivery systems: physicochemical, biopharmaceutical, technological and regulatory consideration. *Expert Opin Drug Deliv*, Vol.9, No.5, pp. 551-565.

[52] Peura, D.A. (2004). Prevention of nonsteroidal anti-inflammatory drug-associated gastrointestinal symptoms and ulcer complications. *Am J Med*, Vol.117 Suppl 5A, pp. 63S-71S.

[53] Rajinikanth, P.S., Balasubramaniam, J. & Mishra, B. (2007). Development and evaluation of a novel floating in situ gelling system of amoxicillin for eradication of Helicobacter pylori. *Int. J. Pharm.*, Vol.335, No.1-2, pp. 114-122.

[54] Rajinikanth, P.S. & Mishra, B. (2007). Preparation and in vitro characterization of gellan based floating beads of acetohydroxamic acid for eradication of H. pylori. *Acta Pharm.*, Vol.57, No.4, pp. 413-427.

[55] Rajinikanth, P.S. & Mishra, B. (2008). Floating in situ gelling system for stomach site-specific delivery of clarithromycin to eradicate H. pylori. *J. Control. Release*, Vol.125, No.1, pp. 33-41.

[56] Rauws, E.A., Langenberg, W., Houthoff, H.J., Zanen, H.C. & Tytgat, G.N. (1988). Campylobacter pyloridis-associated chronic active antral gastritis. A prospective study of its prevalence and the effects of antibacterial and antiulcer treatment. *Gastroenterology*, Vol.94, No.1, pp. 33-40.

[57] Satoh, K. (1996). Treatment of Helicobacter pylori infection by topical administration of antimicrobial agents. *Scand. J. Gastroenterol. Suppl.*, Vol.214, pp. 56; discussion 57-60.

[58] Shah, S.H., Patel, J.K. & Patel, N.V. (2009). Gastroretentive floating drug delivery systems with potential herbal drugs for Helicobacter pylori eradication: a review. *Zhong Xi Yi Jie He Xue Bao*, Vol.7, No.10, pp. 976-982.

[59] Singh, B.N. & Kim, K.H. (2000). Floating drug delivery systems: an approach to oral controlled drug delivery via gastric retention. *J. Control. Release*, Vol.63, No.3, pp. 235-259.

[60] Sriamornsak, P., Thirawong, N. & Puttipipatkhachorn, S. (2004). Morphology and buoyancy of oil-entrapped calcium pectinate gel beads. *AAPS J.*, Vol.6, No.3, pp. e24 (21-27).

[61] Sriamornsak, P., Thirawong, N. & Puttipipatkhachorn, S. (2005). Emulsion gel beads of calcium pectinate capable of floating on the gastric fluid: effect of some additives, hardening agent or coating on release behavior of metronidazole. *Eur. J. Pharm. Sci.*, Vol.24, No.4, pp. 363-373.

[62] Tang, Y.D., Venkatraman, S.S., Boey, F.Y. & Wang, L.W. (2007). Sustained release of hydrophobic and hydrophilic drugs from a floating dosage form. *Int. J. Pharm.*, Vol. 336, No.1, pp. 159-165.

[63] Wyatt, J.I. (1989). The role of Campylobacter pylori in the pathogenesis of peptic ulcer disease. *Scand. J. Gastroenterol. Suppl.*, Vol.157, pp. 7-11; discussion 21-12.

[64] Yamaoka, Y. (2010). Mechanisms of disease: Helicobacter pylori virulence factors. *Nat. Rev. Gastroenterol. Hepatol.*, Vol.7, No.11, pp. 629-641.

[65] Yang, L., Eshraghi, J. & Fassihi, R. (1999). A new intragastric delivery system for the treatment of Helicobacter pylori associated gastric ulcer: *in vitro* evaluation. *J. Control. Release*, Vol.57, No.3, pp. 215-222.

5

Can Drinking Water Serve as a Potential Reservoir of *Helicobacter pylori*? Evidence for Water Contamination by *Helicobacter pylori*

Malgorzata Plonka, Aneta Targosz and
Tomasz Brzozowski

1. Introduction

This review was designed to highlight the available evidence that suggests drinking water and possible survival in water as a probable transmission mode for *H. pylori*.

Although the natural niche for *H. pylori* is the human stomach, for widespread infection to occur the organism may need to survive in the external environment [1]. Documented evidence relating to the survival of *H.pylori* outside the gastric niche is extremely limited. However, there are no established culture methods for the detection of viable *H. pylori* in the environment, in particular drinking water supplies, preventing the development of true epidemiological and risk assessments [2]. A number of drinking water studies have identified *H. pylori* in water pre- and post-chlorination [3]. Baker and colleague [4] found that *H. pylori* were more resistant to low levels of free chlorine than E. coli or C. jejuni. Moreno and colleagues [5] have shown that *H. pylori* could survive disinfection procedures that are normally used in drinking water treatment when bacterium *H. pylori* was found in the viable but not-culturable (VBNC) state. However, they did find that culture of *H. pylori* was lost after 5 min in water despite free chlorine levels of 0.96 mg/2l of water. Children born into high-income families supplied with municipal water are considered 12 times more likely to become colonized with *H. pylori* than those supplied from community wells. This suggests that municipal water is a possible risk factor in the transmission and acquisition of *H. pylori*. It is plausible to suggest that breaks in municipal pipes allow for infiltration of contaminated surface water [6].

2. *Helicobacter pylori* — sources and pathways of transmission

2.1. A Brief history

It has been over a century since Walery Jaworski at Cracow University detected a spiral bacteria named *Vibrio rugula,* in the sediment after gastric washing from patients with gastric cancer and over a quarter of century since Marshall and Warren drew attention to the spiral bacteria, *H. pylori* as a pathogen in various gastric diseases. The Nobel Prize was awarded to Marshall and Warren in 2005 for the discovery of *H. pylori* within the gastric mucosa and its role in gastritis and peptic ulcer disease [7].

H. pylori infecting almost half of the world's population, has become the cause of one of the most common infections. It is a pathogen of constant interest among researchers still looking for the answers to many questions. One of them is the question: "How are *H. pylori* transmitted and what is its source?"

The answer to this question hangs within the realm of conjecture, because - so far - no dominant route of infection by *H. pylori* has been defined. The following routes of transmission are currently taken into consideration: oral - oral transmission, fecal - oral transmission, iatrogenic transmission and vector-borne transmission (Fig. 1). The most likely way in which the *H. pylori* infection is spread has been found to be by passing from person to person by oral- oral or fecal - oral transmission [8, 9]. All the scientists involved in research on the etiology of *H. pylori* infection are unanimous about the fact that this bacterium has to get invaded into the stomach through the mouth - this is a non-invasive micro-organism, and therefore cannot colonize the gastric mucosa in any other way.

2.2. Oral-oral transmission

Data for the confirmation of oral - oral transmission is based on various observations that are related to, among others, research on infection within the family. Research showed that if one person in the family was found to be infected with *H. pylori,* the probability of infecting the other family members was significantly higher [10, 11]. By studying the frequency of infected couples, Italian and German epidemiologists have shown the relationship between the prevalence of infection among uninfected spouses and the length of time in which they live with an infected partner [12, 13]. German studies [14, 15] have also demonstrated particularly strong dependence of the cross-infection between mother and child, with emphasis on the key role of the mother in this form of transmission. Evidence for the dominance of the oral- oral and fecal - oral transmissions was also provided by research conducted in closed institutions such as care facilities for the mentally and physically handicapped, nursing homes, preschools/ kindergartens and orphanages. Research conducted by Lambert and others [16], carried out on adult residents of a home for mentally and physically handicapped persons in Australia, reported a higher prevalence rate of *H. pylori* infection in the population of the institution, than in the general population, as well as the relationship between the prevalence of infection and the length of stay in such a care facility. Similar conclusions were reached by Dutch and Japanese researchers [17, 18]. Indeed, a higher degree of *H. pylori* infection was also detected

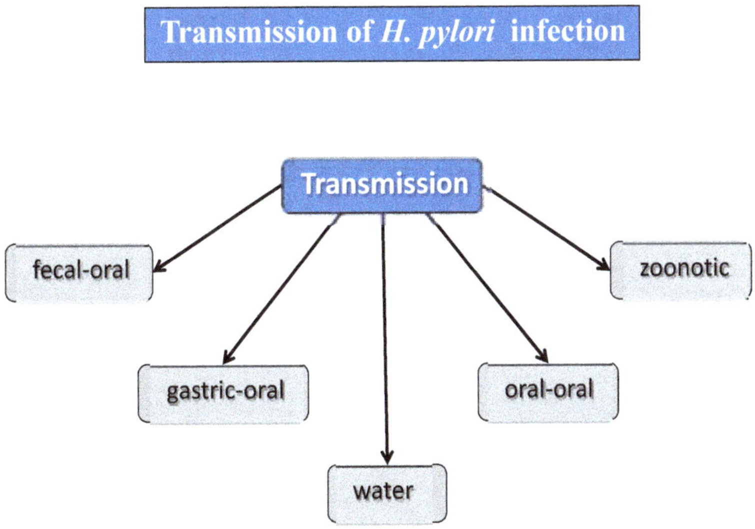

Lee A et al., 1999, Brown LM et al., 2000 Konturek PC et al. 2009

Figure 1. The different mode of transmission of *H.pylori* in humans.

in closed institutions: in England [19, 20], Russia [21], and France [22]. The oral - oral route of transmission is confirmed by the presence of bacteria in the saliva, the dental plate and dental pockets. Evidence that the bacterium *H. pylori* can be transmitted by saliva come from studies conducted by Mègraund`s [23], Pytko - Polonczyk et al [24] and Parsonnet et al [25]. Mègraund in the cited work [23] also reported an increased risk of transmission associated with the chewing of food by mothers in West Africa before the feeding it to their children. The transmission of bacteria through vomiting up the stomach contents into the mouth was confirmed in clinical trials by Parsonnet et al [25] who bred *H. pylori* from all samples collected from 16 vomiting seropositive asymptomatic patients.

2.3. Fecal -oral transmission

An important argument for transmission of *H. pylori* by the fecal - oral route was the isolation and growth of the bacteria from human faeces by Thomas et al [26]. Another proponent of the spreading of the *H. pylori* infection by the fecal - oral route is a David Graham, who demonstrated the transmission's similarity to other bacterial gastrointestinal infections transmitted in this way, in particular hepatitis A (HAV) [27].

An important factor in the acquisition of *H. pylori* infection by the fecal - oral route may be the contamination of water with faeces (Fig. 2). The active, spiral form of *H. pylori* can survive in river water for at least a week, and coccoid of the bacteria can survive for a year or more. Klein et al [28] also demonstrated that *H. pylori* can survive in water, and then penetrate into particular parts and organs of the gastrointestinal tract through the contaminated water. They found that the water resources in Lima (Peru) may be responsible for the bacterium *H. pylori* infection, especially if it is stored in tanks or extracted from urban scenes.

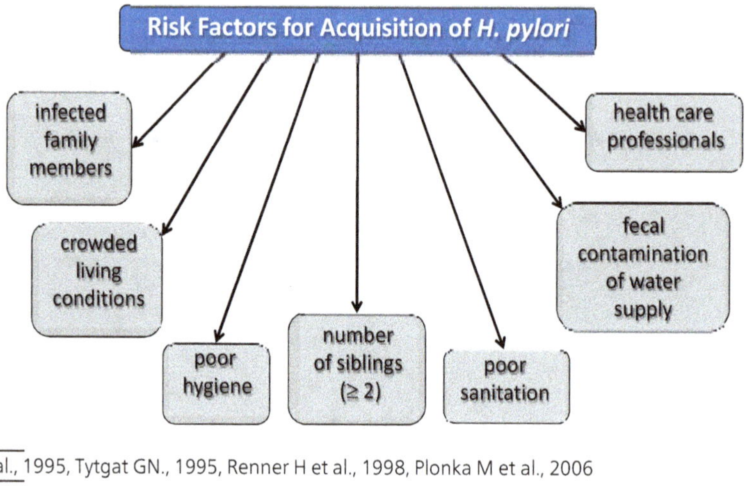

Figure 2. Major epidemiologic risk factors for acquisition of *H.pylori* in humans.

2.4. Iatrogenic and vector-borne transmission

In view of the widespread use of the gastroscopy as a means for diagnosing the upper gastrointestinal tract disorders, the iatrogenic transmission of *H. pylori* could be a potential risk factor for infecting patients undergoing colonoscopies. Tytgat [29] proposed that the major cause of this phenomenon is the complex structure of gastroscope and the difficulties involved in its disinfection. It should be noted, however, that the risk of bug infection in this way is negligible. Lin et al [30, 31] believe that the medical staff performing endoscopic examinations are at greater risk of becoming infected with *H. pylori*, as opposed to dentists and dental nurses whose level of risk is negligible. This suggests that infected gastric mucosa may play a more important role in the spread of infection than infected saliva. Although the principal reservoir for *H. pylori* infection seems to be a human being, there may be other reservoirs of *H. pylori*, such as livestock. Handt et al [32] isolated *H. pylori* from cats and implied that this so called "pet transmission" may have public health implications. However, there is no convincing epidemiological data of *H. pylori* infection in cats, which is why the current risk of infection from cats is considered to be rather small. Other animal organisms that were found to be colonized with *H. pylori* are monkeys [33]. The monkey to human mode of transmission of *H. pylori* could be, however, unlikely due to limited human contact with monkeys. However, a much more likely vector in the transmission of *H. pylori* is a housefly. It was Grubel et al [34, 35] who found that houseflies infected with *H.pylori* in the laboratory may be a reservoir of living bacteria, found both in the gut and on the hairs covering the fly's body. The probability that flies can carry *H. pylori* from infected faeces to food or human mucosal surfaces is indirectly confirmed by numerous epidemiological studies conducted in countries with particularly difficult sanitary conditions such as Colombia, Peru and Japan (Fig. 3). However, there is no direct evidence that the flies which have been in contact, under natural conditions, with faeces infected by *H. pylori* are the source of infection or that this microorganism can be transferred from contaminated flies to food in an amount sufficient enough to infect humans [36]. Goodman et al [37] have found interesting results on the risk of *H. pylori* infection in children from the Colombian Andes, who played with sheep (Fig. 3). A study by Dore et al [38] revealed a significantly higher prevalence of *H. pylori* infection among Sardinian sheep herders, but not among members of their families. Papiez et al [39] and Plonka et al [40] detected an increased risk of *H. pylori* infection in both Polish sheepherders from the Tatra Mountains, as well as entire families in that region. Despite the significance of issue at hand, the epidemiology of the *H. pylori* infection still remains obscure. Studies often present conflicting results, especially when it comes to sources and modes of transmission of infection and associated risk factors. In world literature, authors of various studies emphasize the high volatility of risk, depending on environmental and geographical factors. They also emphasize the lack of a sufficient number of epidemiological studies in the countries of Central and Eastern Europe, including Poland.

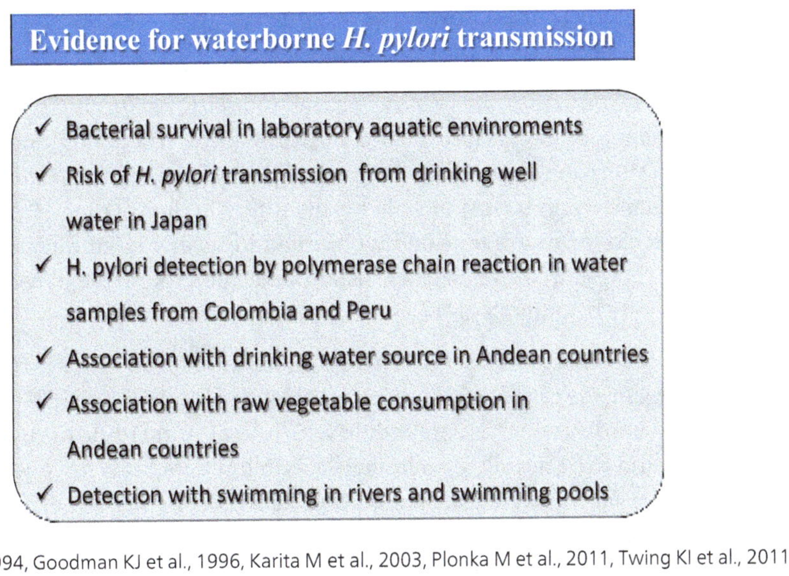

Figure 3. Literature evidence that water may serve as a potential source and reservoir of *H.pylori*.

2.5. Water serves as a potential reservoir of *H. pylori*

The breakthrough discovery that water can be a source and route of the *H. pylori* infection resulted in a flurry of research. The fact that water can be a source of *H. pylori* infection was reported in a study, conducted in the Colombian Andes, by Goodman and others [37]. They found that drinking water from streams, bathing and swimming in streams and pools significantly increases the risk of infection in children in Colombia (Fig. 3). Similar conclusions were reached by Klein et al [28] on the basis of the abovementioned studies conducted in Lima. However, Teh et al [41] of Taiwan and Hopkins et al [42] in Chile found no increased risk in subjects who acquired their drinking water from rivers, and even in those that swam near the polluted beaches in local rivers, irrigation canals or lakes. The problem of *H.pylori* contamination of water resources requires further studies with a proper way of assessment of bacteria in water environment.

3. Methods for the detection of waterborne *H. pylori*

The following methods are used in order to detect the presence of *H. pylori* in water samples taken from a variety of intakes:

1. Culturable methods – that utilize the specialized media bacterial growth, and
2. The methods of molecular assessment of *H. pylori* using the polymerase chain reaction (PCR).

3.1. Culturable methods in the culturing of *H. pylori*

H. pylori is a Gram-negative bacterium, measuring 2 to 4 μm in length and 0.5 to 1 μm in width. Culturing *H. pylori* from areas outside the human stomach has been difficult because of a morphological change in the bacterium and overgrowth by competing microorganisms. *H. pylori* rapidly transforms into a coccoid form which is in a viable but nonculturable (VNBC) state. The VBNC state could be responsible for the difficulty in isolating *H. pylori* from water samples [43]. Coccoid forms are repeatedly observed in several environments, but since it is not known if they represent cell death or a resistant state, their role in the transmission pathway of *H. pylori*, especially by animals and food, is still controversial [44, 45].

We found only a few studies that report successful isolation of *H. pylori* from environmental water samples [46]. In one case, the bacterium was isolated from a municipal wastewater canal on the US-Mexico border, which is compatible with a fecal – oral route of contamination [47]. This canal was found to be heavily contaminated with untreated raw sewage in an area know to have a high *H. pylori* prevalence. The authors used a combination of non standardized immunomagnetically separation (IMS) and culturing techniques. Following separation the bead-*H. pylori* conjugates were streaked onto Columbia blood agar plates and incubated for 3 to 5 days in microaerophilic condition at 37°C, the small, gray colonies were selected and stained with Gram stain to verify morphology. Colonies with Gram-negative rods or coccoid forms were tested by three diagnostic techniques: a rapid urea test, of cytochrome oxidase test and catalase test. In order to fully confirm detection of *H. pylori* one should remember that besides to be positive in all the three mentioned tests, *H. pylori* is a Gram-negative bacterium. A total of 37 out of 132 isolates from culture were selected as putative *H. pylori* and then 23 out of 37 isolates were confirmed to be *H. pylori* by 16S rRNA PCR (Fig. 4).

In the second case, *H. pylori was* isolated from a seawater sample [48]. Colonies were only obtained in residues on 200 μm filters but not in residues on 0.64 and 0.22 μm filters. *H. pylori* could only be isolated from fractionated seawater samples, containing large zooplankton organisms; without zooplankton, *H. pylori* cells could not be recovered from any other fractions by growth-dependent detection protocols [48, 49]. This suggests that bacterium *H. pylori* requires an organic or proteins matrix to remain culturable. This should be further investigated and other studies attempting to isolate *H. pylori* from water sources using similar approaches are needed.

In another study [50] drinking water samples (n= 600) were collected from ground-drilled water supplied by water and sanitation agencies in different localities within the Lahore metropolitan area, Pakistan, and were used within six hours for culturing of *H. pylori*. Water Samples with isolated bacteria was cultured on modified *H. pylori* medium and detected by biochemical tests. The culture-based method sometimes may lead to false negative results due to contamination of microbial species present in the environment that contain the combination of antibiotic resistant genes. In order to remove this discrepancy the grown bacterial cultures were rechecked on another *H. pylori* agar plate followed by urease and catalase tests and was also checked under a microscope to minimize the probability of mixed microbial growth. It was found that 225 out of 600 drinking water samples (37.5%) were positive for *H. pylori* on the *H. pylori* agar medium. The samples that were positive for *H. pylori* were selected on the basis of the formation of a discrete red color zone around the bacterial colony during incubation in 5% CO_2 at 37°C for 3-5 days. And then PCR analysis showed that 90 out of 225 *H. pylori* positive drinking water samples were confirmed 139 bp gene segment of 16S rRNA *H. pylori* strains from water in the Lahore metropolitan area were studied to find the presence of virulence genes and also to correlate with the global genetic structure and evolution of *H. pylori*. The presence of *H. pylori* in drinking water samples of Lahore metropolitan city was approximately 40%, which is an alarming situation. The presence of a high percentage of *H. pylori* contamination in different water sources may be due to low socioeconomic factors such as a lack of public health education, poverty, overcrowding, poor sanitation and unsafe water supplies (Fig. 2). The results for the presence of *H. pylori* in the test samples are in agreement with the results of other studies [51]. The epidemiological survey also suggests that water is the potential source for the transmission of *H. pylori* infection [52] suggesting that water is one of the vectors required for prevalence and transmission of *H. pylori*.

Survival studies in water samples demonstrate that *H. pylori* can be cultured for a limited period of time in a temperature dependent manner [53, 54]. Elevated temperature results in loss of cultivability [55]. The presence of *H. pylori* associated with biofilm from wells, rivers and water distribution systems has been reported recently [56, 57]. Biofilms are slimy films of bacteria, other microbes and organic materials that cover underwater surfaces, particularly inside plumbing. This makes them rather inaccessible and provides a matrix difficult to be reached by disinfectants. The detachment of biofims is the principal form of contamination of treated water [58, 59]. Aside from these studies, positive culture of *H pylori* from drinking water has not been successful, despite efforts to produce a culture-specific media sensitive and selective enough to isolate and grow this organism. A simple plating medium for the detection of *H. pylori* in the environment was investigated independently by Stoodley et al [59], however, the culturable methods employed were unsuccessful in the culturing of *H. pylori*.

3.2. The methods of molecular assessment of *H. pylori*

3.2.1. Fluorescent in situ hybridization (FISH)

Fluorescent in situ hybridization (FISH) with rRNA oligonucleotide probes has been used for detection and identification of VBNC forms of bacteria [62]. In addition to PCR, FISH was validated as a quick and sensitive method for detection of *H. pylori* in environmental samples [63].

In the United States, actively respiring *H. pylori* from surface and well water has been detected using fluorescent antibody - tetrazolium reduction (FACTC) microscopy [64] and confirmed using species-specific PCR [65]. Sen et al. [66] investigated the development of internal controls for PCR assays by spiking drinking water with 100 cells of *H. pylori* and demonstrated similar cycle thresholds to those of recombinant *Escherichia coli* during chlorine disinfection. In addition to PCR, FISH was validated as a quick and sensitive method for detection of *H. pylori* in environmental samples [63]. These findings suggest the presence of *H. pylori* in the natural environment and a possible waterborne route of transmission.

3.2.2. The determination of gene expression by PCR method in the biological material collected from humans and from water sources

This method allows the identification of DNA which is specific for *H. pylori* in biological material: gastric juice, saliva, feces and as shown, this method could be useful to detect the presence of *H. pylori* in water. The application of this technique to test for *H. pylori* has allowed the cloning and sequencing of important genes involved in colonization and pathogenesis, and for the development of simple patterns to determine a sequence of *H. pylori*-specific genes. It also allows for the detection of the protein CagA and VacA which are encoded by the pathogenic genes of cagA and vacA found in particular strains of *H. pylori* bacteria that cause serious gastric disorders including chronic gastritis, peptic gastric and duodenal diseases and /or even gastric cancer.

Despite the numerous research findings identifying *H. pylori* in water, it is important to consider the fact that the use of PCR and other molecular methods for the detection of pathogens in environmental samples has limitations. This is principally due to the inability of PCR to differentiate between naked DNA from dead and living cells. Consequently, to scientifically interpret data regarding the epidemiology of *H. pylori*, cultured bacteria from appropriate water sources are necessary (Fig. 4).

H. pylori rapidly transforms into VBNC state which is induced by low nutrient and hyperosmotic conditions [67 - 69]. Such stressed conditions are commonly found in water and the watery environment. Nayak and Rose [70] demonstrated that quantitative polymerase chain reaction (qPCR) could determine *H. pylori* concentrations in water. In this study real time qPCR was shown to be a specific, sensitive and rapid method to quantify *H. pylori* in sewage. Prior to these studies a two-stage *in vitro* method for detection of *H. pylori* in spiked water and fecal samples.

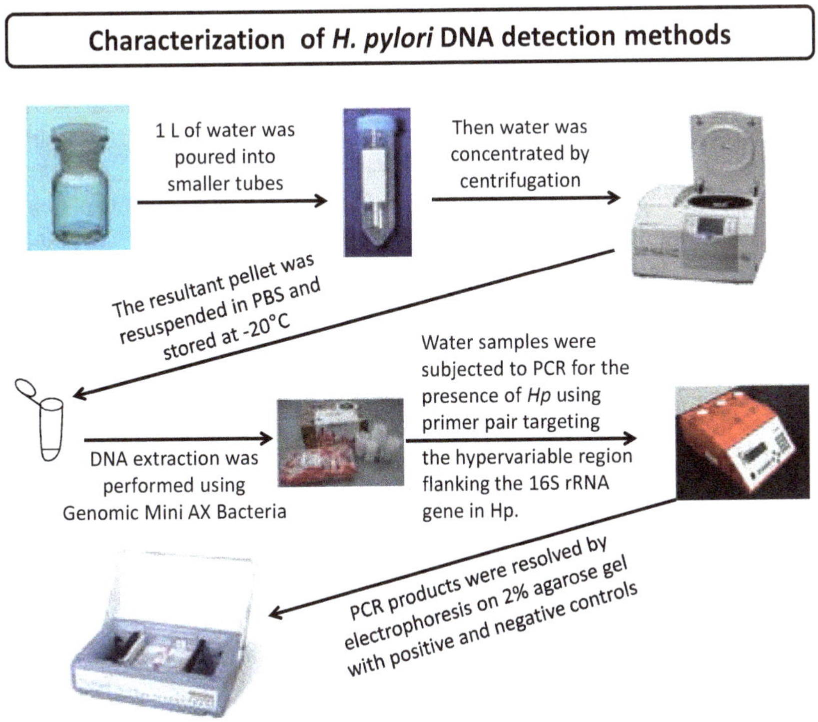

Figure 4. *H.pylori* detection by the assessment of *H.pylori* DNA and 16S rRNA by PCR technique. Proposed steps of detection of *H.pylori* in municipal water.

Janzon et al [71] developed tested and optimized two complementary *H. pylori* specific real-time PCR assays for quantification of *H. pylori* DNA in water. The minimum detection level of the assays including collection procedures and DNA extraction was shown to be approximately 250 *H. pylori* genomes per water sample. They analyzed samples of drinking and environmental water ($n = 75$) and natural water biofilms ($n = 21$) from a high-endemic area in Bangladesh. They could not identify *H. pylori* DNA in any of the samples, even though other pathogenic bacteria have been found previously in the same water samples by using the same methodology. A series of control experiments were performed to ensure that the negative results were not falsely caused by PCR inhibition, nonspecific assays, degradation of template DNA, or low detection sensitivity. Their results suggest that it is unlikely that the predominant transmission route of *H. pylori* in this area is waterborne.

3.2.2.1. H. pylori DNA is not detected in environmental and wastewater samples

Since *H. pylori* DNA was not detected in the household waters, the presence of *H. pylori* DNA in different environmental water sources in Dhaka was evaluated. A total of 15 water samples from ponds and lakes and 6 wastewater samples were collected in the larger Dhaka area between November 2005 and March 2006. The sample volumes ranged between 150 ml and 1,000 ml. Also, these samples were all negative for the presence of *H. pylori* DNA.

3.2.2.2. Determination of inhibitors in samples subjected for PCR.

To evaluate the possibility that the absence of *H. pylori* DNA in the water samples was caused by substances inhibiting the PCR process, two *H. pylori* strains, Hel513 and Hel703, were incubated at approximately 107 bacteria per ml in water samples from three drinking water sources and one pond in Dhaka and in PBS as a control and sampled after 1 and 21 days. The detection rates of less than 100% compared to the level for the control incubated in PBS indicated that PCR inhibitors were present in one of the drinking water sources and in the pond water. However, ten-fold dilution of the purified DNA was shown to remove the effect of the PCR inhibitors.

To further determine the presence of inhibitory factors in the field study water and biofilm samples from Dhaka, the real-time PCR analysis was repeated on all field samples but spiked with 1,000 genomes of *H. pylori* strain J99 in each PCR. Detection rates lower than 30% were found in 41% of the drinking water samples. However, 10-fold dilution of the DNA was shown to remove the inhibitory effect in 90% of samples, but still without positive results. These analyses showed that levels of *H. pylori* DNA were below 250 genome copies in 38% of the samples and below at least 2,500 genome copies in another 52% of the samples. Similar results were found in biofilm and environmental water samples. Interestingly, fewer than 10% of the wastewater samples showed presence of inhibitors, presumably because these were extracted using the Qiagen stool kit, which removes PCR inhibitors but decreases the DNA yield.

3.2.2.3. H. pylori DNA and RNA stability during long-term incubation in tap water and seawater

Possible degradation of *H. pylori* DNA in water was studied using two different *H. pylori* strains, Hel513 and Hel703. Because of the possible confounding effect of inhibitors in the water in Dhaka, water was taken from Gothenburg, Sweden, for this experiment. Morphology, culturability, *hpaA* and *glmM* gene numbers, and RNA integrity were analyzed at different time points. A majority of the initially spiral-shaped *H. pylori* bacteria converted into the coccoid shape within 24 h, and on day 7, no spiral-shaped bacteria were detected and no viable bacteria were recovered. Real-time PCR assays revealed that the copy numbers of both *H. pylori* genes were constant in tap water for up to 35 days, followed by small decreases at 100 days, whereas copy numbers in seawater decreased up to 50-fold after 100 days. However, gel electrophoresis of total RNA showed that RNA was degraded in tap water within 7 days, with no visible 23S or 16S fragments.

4. Evidence that biofilms in water distribution systems may harbor *H. pylori*

It is well known that waterborne bacteria can attach to surfaces by aggregating in a hydrated exopolymer known as a biofilm [72, 73]. The association of bacteria, particularly pathogens, with biofilm communities within a water distribution system may offer vulnerable and susceptible bacteria protection from disinfection and protozoan predation [74]. In fact microorganisms in drinking water are predominantly associated with biofilms rather than in the planktonic state [72, 73, 75]. There is evidence that biofilms in water distribution systems may harbor *H. pylori* [76-78]. In addition a study undertaken in Western Africa, utilizing 16S rDNA sequences, has shown evidence that *H. pylori* can be detected in natural biofilms [79]. A more recent study by Watson and colleagues [80] showed a close link between *Helicobacter* DNA in showerhead biofilm used in domestic households.

4.1. Cultivability of *H. pylori* in water and water-associated biofilms and implications for transmission

Adams et al. [81] have shown that in pure culture *H. pylori* cells remain cultivable longer at 15°C than at 20°C, but in their study it was not possible to recover cultivable *H. pylori* from water samples and biofilms. However, considering the shape of the cells detected by PNA-FISH (peptide nucleic acid fluorescence in situ hybridization) and considering that cultivable cells are spiral shaped, while coccoid cells are VBNC and therefore likely to be non-cultivable, the expectation is that there should be more cultivable *H. pylori* cells at 20°C. It is assumed demonstrating that the behavior of this pathogen in heterotrophic biofilms might be completely different than its behavior in pure culture. Additionally, the PNA probe used in this work targets sites on the 16S rRNA molecule, and it is known that the RNA content of a cell can be indicative of viability which suggests that the cells detected were still viable [82]. It has been shown that the concentration of all *H. pylori* cells in the biofilms formed in this work is either higher than or very similar to the concentrations found when pure-culture biofilms were formed [83]. In addition, the detection of *H. pylori* embedded in biofilms suggests that there is a close association with other bacteria present in the biofilms. These two factors, together with the persistence of a bright PNA-FISH signal, which is indicative of a high rRNA content, suggest that the heterotrophic bacteria present in the biofilms formed in this study were not a negative influence on *H. pylori* but only induced its transformation to the more robust coccoid morphology [84-86].

4.2. The existence of *H. pylori* in the drinking water

The evidence based medicine regarding *H. pylori* transmission is not convincing, making it difficult to avoid the notion that the burden/inconvenience accounts for this bacterial infection. The microbiological and epidemiological studies confirmed that in certain conditions the intake of water contaminated with *H. pylori* might be considered as potential source of human infection with this bug. The water could be considered as a reservoir of *H. pylori* [87].

In the U.S. the problem of drinking water pollution is handled by the Environmental Protection Agency (EPA). On the basis of a survey which was carried out, the Agency has developed and issued a list of microbiological contaminants of water, which are likely to significantly affect the public health of consumers of drinking water. The list includes three species of bacteria: *Aeromonas, Mycobacterium avium* and *H. pylori.*

The water contamination of bacteria was documented specially in suburban areas because the number of systems for discharging sewage to sewage treatment plants is inadequate. The reason of these bacterial contaminations is not fully understood but some mechanisms were already proposed. Moreover, many farms and households either have their own small wastewater treatment plants, which do not always function properly, or in worse cases, waste is disposed of by releasing pollutants into nearby rivers, streams or roadside ditches. Some farms have leaky septic tanks often built near wells from which they derive all their household water.

Recent advances in the role of the particular ionic concentrations and the possible correlation between the presence or absence of contamination of water samples tested for *H. pylori* may be an important contribution for tracing the presence of this microorganism in environmental conditions and attempting to define the role of microelements regarding the inhibition or stimulation of *H. pylori* proliferation in water environment.

Determining the concentrations of the suggested ions and the possible correlation between the presence and absence of contamination of water samples tested for *H. pylori* may be an important contribution for tracing the development of this organism in environmental conditions and to attempt to define the role of microelements on the inhibition or stimulation of *H. pylori* proliferation.

4.2.1. *Sample preparation*

The samples were collected, cooled and stored in polyethylene containers prior to analyses. Before quantitative elemental analysis, if appropriate the samples were filtered and diluted adequately to fit the analytical signal to the linear range of calibration curve.

4.2.2. *Quantitative determination of metals*

Quantitative determinations of sodium and potassium were made using flame photometry method in air acetylene flame in standard conditions (Perkin Elmer AAS spectrometer Model 3110, USA).

Determinations of Fe, Mg and Zn were performed by means of atomic absorption spectrometry, flame technique (air acetylene flame) using Perkin Elmer AAS spectrometer Model 3110, USA. In both methods, analyses were preceded by thorough optimization of measurement conditions (flame characteristic, burner position, and nebulizer performance). Spectral conditions are given in Table 1.

Element	Method	Lamp type	Wavelength (nm)	Slit (nm)
K	AES		766.5	0.7
Na	AES		589.0	0.2
Fe	F AAS	HCL	248.3	0.2
Mg	F AAS	HCL	285.2	0.7
Zn	F AAS	HCL	213.9	0.7

Table 1. Spectral conditions of elements determination.

All measurements were made using the calibration curve technique. In case of Mg measurements, the samples characterized by high Na concentration were quantified using the method of standard additions calibration. Measurements were made in triplicate.

4.2.3. The methods of molecular assessment of H. pylori

We have collected 150 water samples from different municipal water distribution systems (n=49), rivers (n=48), water reservoirs (n=39) and drinking water tanks and wells (n=14) and they were analyzed between June and December 2012. Samples of 1000 ml water were poured into smaller tubes water and were processed to remove organic matter by centrifugation at 121xg for 5 min. The supernatant was concentrated by centrifugation at 7740xg for 15 min. The resultant pellet was dissolve in 1 ml of PBS, followed by centrifugation at 10 000Xg for 5 min. Finally the pellet was stored at -20°C. Total DNA from concentrated samples for PCR was purified using Genomic Mini or Genomic Mini AX Bacteria (A & A Biotechnology, Gdynia, Poland). DNA was stored at -20°C. All PCR amplifications were performed using the GoTaq DNA Polymerase (Promega, WI, USA) in Thermo cycler T3 (Biometra, Gottingen, Germany).

A negative control with sterile water and positive control with *H. pylori* 43504 DNA were included.

PCR with primers specific for *Helicobacter spp.* and *H. pylori* (Table 2) were used to screen samples for potential presence of *H. pylori.*

First, samples were analyzed for *Helicobacter* species with phosphoglucosamine mutase gene and 23S rRNA *Helicobacter spp.* and then were further tested with primer specific for 16S rRNA hyper variable flanking region of *H. pylori.*

For DNA visualization, electrophoresis or PCR products was performed through 2% agarose gel containing ethidium bromide and gels were photographed under UV light. A 100 bp and 50 bp ladder were used as a molecular weight marker.

Primer	Target site	Sequence (5'→3')	Ref*
GlmM-forward	phosphoglucosamine mutase gene	AGG CTT TTA GGG GTG TTA GGG GTT T	[85]
GlmM-reverse		AAG CTT ACT TTC TAA CAC TAA CGC	
Cluster2	16S rRNA hyper variable flanking region of *H. pylori*	GGC GTT ATC AAC AGA ATG GC	[86]
B1J99		CTC AGT TCG GAT TGT AGG CTG C	
HelGen-forward	23S rRNA *Helicobacter spp.*	AAC GGG GCT AAG ATA GAC	[87]
HelGen-reverse		TCT CAT CTA CCT GTG TCG	

*References

Table 2. PCR primer used in this study.

5. Conclusions that arise in relation to the presented results

On the basis of a chemometric analysis that involved the use of multidimensional data analysis known as multivariate data analysis it was possible to distinguish water samples containing DNA *H. pylori* and from samples that did not contain the DNA (Fig. 4). At the same time a correlation was demonstrated between the presence of *H. pylori* DNA in water samples and phosphate, ammonia and iron concentrations.

In analyzing the results of water sampling conducted in the framework of the project "Detection of Helicobacter pylori in drinking water samples. In what way is the water contaminated and what is the source of contamination?" we have reached the conclusion that we cannot yet say with certainty whether water can be considered as a source of *H. pylori* infection. Questions, therefore, arise to which the answers would be helpful in solving the abovementioned problem.

As the results of our study confirmed the presence of the bacteria in tap water only (i.e., after the process of purification/water treatment), but was not found in rivers, reservoirs and in wells where the water is completely untreated, the first question concerns the existence of a link between the amount of bacteria and the degree and process of the water treatment. The link between the amount of bacteria present in tap water and the distance from the point of chlorination can also be taken into consideration (the farther from the treatment, the smaller the concentration of bactericidal chlorine).

On the basis of these results it can be concluded that the presence of *H. pylori* in water is affected by the season. Confirmation of the presence of *H. pylori* in the water samples taken in June, while there was no evidence of it in October, may also result from the fact that each of the water treatment plants in Krakow uses a number of technological processes for water treatment, depending on the quality of the water collected. Accordingly, further examinations should be conducted to ascertain whether the presence of *H. pylori* is actually related to the time of year, or to other factors.

This raises the question - if the bacteria can survive for so long in distilled water, does this mean that the physiologically important endogenous pool of metals is enough for them?

If so we can expect that the metals in the water around them will be important for their survival? On the other hand, there is no doubt about the effects of toxic metals, but these levels are continuously monitored in water - as is the bacterial cell toxicity of heavy metals. And do the levels of acceptable standards for drinking water have anything to do with this.

6. Further research

1. Determination of *H. pylori* interaction with co-occurring elements in water by enriching their culture media with in the laboratory experiment.

2. Understanding the effects of dissolved organic carbon in the survival of bacteria during water treatment.
3. Taking into account the differences in the composition and concentration studied seasonal elements for the possible coexistence of *H. pylori.*

These relationships can be used to develop a better method of treating water in order to minimize the exposure of humans to infection

Acknowledgements

The study was a part of the project of National Center of Science in Poland entitled "Detection of *Helicobacter pylori* in drinking water samples. In what way is the water contaminated and what is the source of contamination?" to Drs. Plonka, Targosz and Brzozowski as principal investigators. This work was supported by grant No 2011/01/B/NZ/01539.

Author details

Malgorzata Plonka[1,2], Aneta Targosz[2] and Tomasz Brzozowski[2*]

*Address all correspondence to: mpbrzozo@cyf-kr.edu.pl

1 University School of Physical Education, Cracow, Poland

2 Department of Physiology Jagiellonian University Medical College, Cracow, Poland

References

[1] Brown LM. Helicobacter pylori: epidemiology and routes of transmission. Epidemiol. Rev. 2000; 22: 283–297.

[2] Percival SL, Thomas JG. Transmission of Helicobacter pylori and the role of water and biofilms. J. Water Health 2009; 7(3): 469-477.

[3] Mazari-Hiriart M, Lopez-Vidal Y, Ponce de Leon S, Castillo-Rojas G, Hernandez-Eugenio C, Rojo F. Bacteria and disinfection byproducts in water from southern Mexico City. Arch. Environ. Health 2003; 58: 233–237.

[4] Baker KH, Hegarty JP, Redmond B, Reed NA, Herson DS. Effect of oxidizing disinfectants (chlorine monochloramine and ozone) on Helicobacter pylori. Appl. Environ. Microbiol. 2002; 68: 981–984.

[5] Moreno Y, Piqueres P, Alonso JL, Jimenez A, Gonzalez A, Ferrus MA. Survival and viability of Helicobacter pylori after inoculation into chlorinated drinking water. Water Res. 2007; 41: 3490–3496.

[6] Frenck RW, Clemens J. Heliocobacter in the developing world. Microbes Infect. 2003; 5: 705–713.

[7] Konturek PC, Konturek SJ, Brzozowski T. Helicobacter pylori infection in gastric cancerogensesis. J Physiol. Pharmacol. 2009; 60(3): 3-21.

[8] Lee A, Fox JG, Otto G, Dick EH, Krakowka S. Transmission of Helicobacter spp. A challenge to the dogma of fecal-oral spread. Epidemiol Infect. 1991; 107(1): 99–109.

[9] Cave DR. How is Helicobacter pylori transmitted? Gastroenterology 1997; 113(6): 9-14.

[10] Malaty HM, Graham DY, Klein PD, Evans DG, Adam E, Evans DJ. Transmission of Helicobacter pylori infection. Studies in families of healthy individuals. Scand. J Gastroenterology 1991; 26: 927–932.

[11] Drum B, Perez-Perez GI, Blaser MJ, Sherman PM. Intrafamilial clustering of Helicobacter pylori infection. N Engl J Med.1990; 322: 359–63.

[12] Brenner H, Rothenbacher D, Bode G, Dieudonne P, Adler G. Active infection with Helicobacter pylori in healthy couples. Epidemiol Infect.1999; 122: 91-95.

[13] Parente F, Maconi G, Sangaletti O, et al. Prevalence of Helicobacter pylori and related gastroduodenal lesions in spouses of Helicobacter pylori positive patients with duodenal ulcer. Gut 1996; 39: 629–33.

[14] Rothenbacher D, Bode G, Berg G, Knayer U, Gonser T, Adler G, Brenner H, Helicobacter pylori among preschool children and their parents: evidence of parent- child transmission. J Infect Dis.1999; 179 (2): 398-402.

[15] Brenner H, Rothenbacher D, Bode G, Adler G. Parental history of gastric or duodenal ulcer and Helicobacter pylori infection among pre-school children: evidence for mother-infant transmission. BMJ 1998; 316: 665.

[16] Lambert JR, Lin SK, Sievert W, Nicholson L, Schembri M, Guest C. High prevalence of Helicobacter pylori antibodies in an institutionalized population: evidence for person-to-person transmission. Am J Gastroenterol. 1995; 90 (12): 2167-71.

[17] Böhmer CJ, Klinkenberg-Knol EC, Kuipers EJ, Niezen-de Boer MC, Schreuder H, Schuckink-Kool F, Meuwissen SG. The prevalence of Helicobacter pylori infection among inhabitants and healthy employees of institutes for the intellectually disabled. Am J Gastroenterol 1997; 92 (6):1000-4.

[18] Kimura A, Matsubasa T, Kinoshita H, Kuriya N, Yamashita Y, Fujisawa T, Terakura H, Shinohara M. Helicobacter pylori seropositivity in patients with severe neurologic impairment. Brain Dev.1999; 21(2):113-7.

[19] Harris AW, Douds A, Meurisse EV, Dennis M, Chambers S, Gould SR. Seroprevalence of Helicobacter pylori in residents of a hospital for people with severe learning difficulties. Eur J Gastroenterol Hepatol. 1995; 7(1):.21-3.

[20] Lewindon PJ, Lau D, Chan A, Tse P, Sullivan PB. Helicobacter pylori in an institution for disabled children in Hong Kong. Dev Med Child Neurol. 1997; 39(10): 682-5.

[21] Malaty HM, Paykov V, Bykova O, Ross A, Graham DP, Anneger JF, Graham DY. Helicobacter pylori and socioeconomic factors in Russia. Helicobacter.1996; 1(2): 82-7.

[22] Vincent P, Gottrand F, Pernes P, Husson MO, Lecomte-Houcke M, Turck D, Leclerc H. High prevalence of Helicobacter pylori infection in cohabiting children. Epidemiology of a cluster, with special emphasis on molecular typing. Gut. 1994; 35(3): 313–316.

[23] Mégraud F. Transmission of Helicobacter pylori: faecal-oral versus oral-oral route. Aliment Pharmacol Ther. 1995; 9(2): 85-91.

[24] Pytko-Polończyk J, Konturek SJ, Karczewska E, Bielański W, Kaczmarczyk A. Oral cavity as permanent reservoir of Helicobacter pylori and potential source of reinfection. J Physiol Pharmacol.1996; 47(1):121–129.

[25] Parsonnet J, Shmuely H, Haggerty T. Fecal and Oral Shedding of Helicobacter pylori From Healthy Infected Adults JAMA. 1999; 282(23): 2240-2245.

[26] Thomas JE, Gibson GR, Darboe MK, Dale A, Weaver LT. Isolation of Helicobacter pylori from human faeces. Lancet 1992; 340(14):1194-5.

[27] Graham DY. Helicobacter pylori: Future Direction in Research Helicobacter pylori. Gastritis and Peptic Ulcer 1990:463-470.

[28] Klein PD, Graham DY, Gaillour A, Opekun AR, Smith EO. Water source as risk factor for Helicobacter pylori infection in Peruvian children. Gastrointestinal Physiology Working Group. Lancet. 1991; 337(22):1503-6.

[29] Tytgat GN. Endoscopic transmission of Helicobacter pylori. Aliment Pharmacol Ther. 1995; 9(2): 105-10.

[30] Lin SK, Lambert JR, Schembri MA, Nicholson L, Johnson IH. The prevalence of Helicobacter pylori in practicing dental staff and dental students. Aust Dent J. 1998; 43(1): 35-9.

[31] Lin SK, Lambert JR, Schembri MA, Nicholson L, Korman MG. Helicobacter pylori prevalence in endoscopy and medical staff. J Gastroenterol Hepatol. 1994; 9(4): 319-24.

[32] Handt LK, Fox JG, Dewhirst FE, Fraser GJ, Paster BJ, Yan LL, Rozmiarek H, Rufo R, Stalis IH. Helicobacter pylori isolated from the domestic cat: public health implications. Infect Immun. 1994; 62(6): 2367-74.

[33] Fox JG. Non-human reservoirs of Helicobacter pylori. Aliment Pharmacol Ther.1995; 9(2):93-103.

[34] Grubel P, Hoffman JS, Chong FK, Burstein NA, Mepani C, Cave DR. Vector potential of houseflies (Musca domestica) for Helicobacter pylori. J Clin Microbiol. 1997; 35(6): 1300-3.

[35] Grubel P, Huang L, Masubuchi N, Stutzenberger FJ, Cave DR. Detection of helicobacter-pylori DNA in houseflies (musca-domestica) on 3 continents. Lancet 1998: 352: 788-789.

[36] Vaira D, Holton J. Vector potential of houseflies (Musca domestica) for Helicobacter pylori. Helicobacter.1998; 3(1):65-6.

[37] Goodman KJ, Correa P, Tenganá Aux HJ, Ramírez H, DeLany JP, Guerrero Pepinosa O, López Quiñones M, Collazos Parra T. Helicobacter pylori infection in the Colombian Andes: a population-based study of transmission pathways. Am J Epidemiol. 1996, 144(3): 290-9.

[38] Dore MP, Bilotta M, Vaira D, Manca A, Massarelli G, Leandro G, Atzei A, Pisanu G, Graham DY, Realdi G. High prevalence of Helicobacter pylori infection in shepherds. Dig Dis Sci. 1999;.44(6):1161-4.

[39] Papiez D, Konturek PC, Bielanski W, Plonka M, Dobrzanska M, Kaminska A, Szczyrk U, Bochenek A, Wierzchos E. Prevalence of Helicobacter pylori infection in Polish shepherds and their families. Dig Liver Dis. 2003; 35(1):10-5.

[40] Plonka M, Bielanski W, Konturek SJ, Targosz A, Sliwowski Z, Dobrzanska M, Kaminska A, Sito E, Konturek PC, Brzozowski T. Helicobacter pylori infection and serum gastrin, ghrelin and leptin in children of Polish shepherds. Dig Liver Dis. 2006; 38(2): 91-7.

[41] Teh BH, Lin JT, Pan WH, Lin SH, Wang LY, Lee TK, Chen CJ. Seroprevalence and associated risk factors of Helicobacter pylori infection in Taiwan. Anticancer Res. 1994; 14, (3B): 1389-92.

[42] Hopkins RJ, Vial PA, Ferreccio C, Ovalle J, Prado P, Sotomayor V, Russell RG. Wasserman SS. Glenn J, Morris J. Seroprevalence of Helicobacter pylori in Chile: Vegetables May Serve as One Route of Transmission. J Infect Dis. 1993; 168(1): 222-226.

[43] She FF, Lin JY, Liu JY, Huang C, Su DH. Virulence of water-induced coccoid Helicobacter pylori and its experimental infection in mice. World Journal of Gastroenterology 2003; 9: 516–520.

[44] Nabwera HM, Logan RP. Epidemiology of Helicobacter pylori: transmission, translocation and extragastric reservoirs. Journal of Physiology and Pharmacology 1999; 50: 711–722.

[45] Velazquez M, Feirtag JM. Helicobacter pylori: characteristics, pathogenicity, detection methods and mode of transmission implicating foods and water. International Journal of Food Microbiology 1999; 53: 95–104.

[46] Vale FF, Vítor JMB.. Transmission pathway of Helicobacter pylori: Does food play a role in rural and urban areas? International Journal of Food Microbiology 2010; 138: 1–12.

[47] Lu Y, Redlinger TE, Avitia R, Galindo A, Goodman K. Isolation and genotyping of Helicobacter pylori from untreatedmunicipal wastewater. Applied and Environmental Microbiology 2002; 68: 1436–1439.

[48] Cellini L, Di CE, Grand R, Di BS, Prenna M., Pasquantonio M, Pane L. Detection of Helicobacter pylori associated with zooplankton. Aquatic Microbial Ecology: International Journal 2005; 40: 115–120.

[49] Cellini L, Del VA, Di CM, Di CE, Favaro M, Donelli G. Detection of free and plankton-associated Helicobacter pylori in seawater. Journal of Applied Microbiology 2004; 97: 285–292.

[50] Samra ZQ, Javaid U, Ghafoor S, Batool A, Dar N, Athar MA. PCR assay targeting virulence genes of Helicobacter pylori isolated from drinking water and clinical samples in Lahore metropolitan, Pakistan. J Water Health 2011; 9(1): 208-16.

[51] Mazari-Hiriart M, Lopez-Vidal Y, Calva JJ. Helieobaeter pylori in water systems for human use in Mexico City. Water Sei. Tech. 2001; 43: 93-98.

[52] Nurgalieva Z. Heiicobacter pylori infection in Kazakhstan: effect of water source and household hygiene. Am. J. Trop. Med. Hyg. 2002; 67: 201-206.

[53] Azevedo NF, Almeida C, Fernandes I, Cerqueira L, Dias S, Keevil CW, Vieira MJ. Survival of gastric and enterohepatic Helicobacter spp. in water: implications for transmission. Applied and Environmental Microbiology 2008; 74: 1805–1811.

[54] Queralt N, Araujo R. Analysis of the survival of H. pylori within a laboratory based aquatic model system using molecular and classical techniques. Microbial Ecology 2007; 54: 771–777.

[55] Shahamat M,Mai U, Paszko-Kolva C, Kessel M, Colwell RR. Use of autoradiography to assess viability of Helicobacter pylori in water. Applied and Environmental Microbiology 1993; 59: 1231–1235.

[56] Percival SL, Thomas JG. Transmission of Helicobacter pylori and the role of water and biofilms. Journal of Water and Health 2009; 7: 469–477.

[57] Giao MS, Azevedo NF, Wilks SA, Vieira MJ, Keevil CW. 2008. Persistence of Helicobacter pylori in heterotrophic drinking-water biofilms. Applied and Environmental Microbiology 74, 5898–5904.

[58] Gouider, M., Bouzid, J., Sayadi, S., Montiel, A. Impact of orthophosphate addition on biofilm development in drinking water distribution systems. Journal of Hazardous Materials 2009; 167: 1198–1202.

[59] Stoodley P, Wilson S, Hall-Stoodley L, Boyle JD, Lappin-Scott HM., Costerton JW. Growth and detachment of cell clusters from mature mixed-species biofilms. Applied and Environmental Microbiology 2001; 67: 5608–5613.

[60] Degnan AJ, Sonzogni WC, Standridge JH. Development of a plating medium for selection of Helieobaeter pylori from water samples. App. Environ. Mierobiol. 2003; 69(5): 2914-2918.

[61] Fernández M, Contreras M, Suárez P, Gueneau P, García-Amado MA. Use of HP selective medium to detect Helicobacter pylori associated with other enteric bacteria in seawater and marine mollusks. Lett Appl Microbiol 2007; 45(2): 213-8.

[62] Rowan NJ. Viable but non-culturable forms of food and waterborne bacteria: quo vadis? Trends Food Sci. Technol. 2004; 15: 462–467.

[63] Moreno Y, Ferrus MA, Alonso JL, Jimenez A, Herandez J. Use of fluorescent in situ hybridization to evidence the presence of Helicobacter pylori in water. Water Res. 2003; 37: 2251–2256.

[64] Hegarty JP, Dowd MT, Baker KH. Occurrence of Helicobacter pylori in surface water in the United States. J. Appl. Microbiol. 1999; 87: 697–701.

[65] Azevedo NF, Pacheco AP, Keevil CW, Vieira MJ. Adhesion of water stressed Helicobacter pylori to abiotic surfaces. J. Appl. Microbiol. 2006; 101: 718–724.

[66] Sen K, Schable NA, Lye DJ. Development of an internal control for evaluation and standardization of a quantitative PCR assay for detection of Helicobacter pylori in drinking water. Appl. Environ. Microbiol. 2007; 73: 7380–7387.

[67] Mizoguchi H, Fujioka T, Nasu M. Evidence for viability of coccoid forms of Helicobacter pylori. J. Gastroenterol. 1999; 34(Suppl.11): 32–36.

[68] Zheng PY, Hua J, Ng HC, Ho B. Unchanged characteristics of Helicobacter pylori during its morphological conversion. Microbios 1999; 98: 51–64.

[69] Moreno Y, Ferrus MA, Alonso JL, Jimenez A, Herandez J. Use of fluorescent in situ hybridization to evidence the presence of Helicobacter pylori in water. Water Res. 2003; 37: 2251–2256.

[70] Nayak AK, Rose JB. Detection of Helicobacter pylori in sewage and water using a new quantitative PCR method with SYBR green. J. Appl. Microbiol. 2007; 103: 1931–1941.

[71] Janzon A, Sjoling A, Lothigius A, Ahmed D, Qadri F, Svennerholm AM. Failure To Detect Helicobacter pylori DNA in Drinking and Environmental Water in Dhaka,

Bangladesh, Using Highly Sensitive Real-Time PCR Assays. Appl. Environ. Microbiol. 2009; 75(10): 3039–3044.

[72] Costerton JW, Stewart PS, Greenberg EP. Bacterial biofilms: a common cause of persistent infections. Science 1999; 284:1318–1322.

[73] Percival SL, Walker J, Hunter PR. Microbiological Aspects of Biofilms and Drinking Water. CRC Press, New York 2000.

[74] Sibille I, Sime-Ngando T, Mathieu L, Block JC. Protozoan bacterivory and Escherichia coli survival in drinking water distribution systems. Appl. Environ. Microbiol. 1998; 64: 197–202.

[75] Percival SL, Chalmers RM, Embrey M, Hunter PR, Sellwood J, Wyn-Jones P. Microbiology of Waterborne Diseases. Elsevier Academic Press 2004, London.

[76] MacKay WG, Gribbon LT, Barer MR, Reid DC. Biofilms in drinking water systems: a possible reservoir for Helicobacter pylori. J. Appl. Microbiol. 1999; 85: 52s–59s.

[77] Andersen LP, Rasmussen L. Helicobacter pylori-coccoid forms and biofilm formation. FEMS Immunol Med Microbiol. 2009; 56 (2): 112-5.

[78] Park SR., MacKay WG, Reid DC. Helicobacter sp. recovered from drinking water biofilm sampled from a water distribution system. Water Res. 2001; 35: 1624–1626.

[79] Bunn JE, MacKay WG, Thomas JE, Reid DC, Weaver LT. Detection of Helicobacter pylori DNA in drinking water biofilms: implications for transmission in early life. Lett. Appl. Microbiol. 2002; 34: 450–454.

[80] Watson CL, Owen RJ, Said B, Lai S, Lee JV, Surman-Lee S, Nichols G. Detection of Helicobacter pylori by PCR but not culture in water and biofilm samples from drinking water distribution systems in England. J. Appl. Microbiol. 2004; 97: 690–698.

[81] Adams BL, Bates TC, Oliver JD. Survival of Helicobacter pylori in a natural freshwater environment. Appl. Environ. Microbiol. 2003; 69: 7462–7466.

[82] Azevedo NF, Vieira MJ, Keevil CW. Establishment of a continuous model system to study Helicobacter pylori survival in potable water biofilms. Water Sci. Technol. 2003; 47:155–160.

[83] Azevedo NF, Pinto AR, Reis NM, Vieira MJ, Keevil CW. Shear stress, temperature, and inoculation concentration influence the adhesion of water-stressed Helicobacter pylori to stainless steel 304 and polypropylene. Appl. Environ. Microbiol. 2006; 72: 2936–2941.

[84] Azevedo NF, Almeida C, Cerqueira L, Dias S, Keevil CW, Vieira MJ. Coccoid form of Helicobacter pylori as a morphological manifestation of cell adaptation to the environment. Appl. Environ. Microbiol. 2007; 73:3423–3427.

[85] Shahamat M, Alavi M, Watts JEM, Gonzalez JM, Sowers KR, Maeder GW, Robb FT. Development of two PCR-based techniques for detecting helical and coccoid forms of Helicobacter pylori. J. Clin. Microbiol. 2004; 3613-3619.

[86] Lu JJ, Perng CI, Shyu RY, Chen CH, Lou Q, Chong SKF, Lee CH. Comparison of five methods for detection of Helicobacter pylori DNA in gastric tissues. J. Clin. Microbiol 1999; 37: 772-774.

[87] Twing KI, Kirchman DL, Campbell BJ. Temporal study of Helicobacter pylori presence in coastal freshwater, estuary and marine waters. Water Research 2011; 45: 1897-1995.

6

Empirical Versus Targeted Treatment of *Helicobacter pylori* Infections in Southern Poland, According to the Results of Local Antimicrobial Resistance Monitoring

Elżbieta Karczewska, Karolina Klesiewicz,
Paweł Nowak, Edward Sito, Iwona Skiba,
Małgorzata Zwolińska–Wcisło, Tomasz Mach and
Alicja Budak

1. Introduction

1.1. General information

Helicobacter pylori (*H. pylori*) is a spiral-shaped, Gram-negative, microaerophilic bacterium inhabiting human gastric mucosa and playing an essential role in dyspepsia, gastritis, gastric ulcer disease and duodenal ulcer disease [1-6]. Moreover, in 1994 the International Agency for Research on Cancer of the World Health Organization (IARC/WHO) concluded that *H. pylori* is a class I carcinogen, involved in gastric cancer and mucosa-associated lymphoid tissue (MALT) lymphoma [2, 7-11]. Furthermore, increasing number of studies showed the association between *H. pylori* infections and pathogenesis of extragastric diseases. The most convincing data appeared in case of iron-deficiency anemia (IDA) of unknown origin and idiopathic thrombocytopenia purpura (ITP) [12]. Eradication of *H. pylori* in IDA patients resulted in normalization of hemoglobin level while in ITP patients lead to a favorable platelet response [13]. Moreover, the findings and ongoing research concerning *H. pylori* infections suggest its association with other diseases such as: heart or vascular diseases (ischemic heart disease, coronary artery disease, cardiac syndrome x), neurological diseases (stroke, Alzheimer's or Parkinson's diseases) as well as obesity, diabetes mellitus, asthma or diseases of oral mucosa [1, 14-18].

H. pylori infection is one of the most common bacterial infections, with the estimated prevalence reaching 50% of the human population worldwide. Nevertheless, the occurrence of *H. pylori* infections correlate with the socioeconomic status and are often reflected in their geographical distribution. The frequency of this infection is markedly higher in the developing countries (80-90%) rather than in the developed countries (<40%) [4]. In Europe the incidence of *H. pylori* varies and can be associated with geographical location and the percentage of compatriots of non-European origin [19]. Current studies show the declining trend in the prevalence of *H. pylori* infections in developed countries such as Denmark or Czech Republic [20, 21], while the frequency of this infection in Asia–Pacific region ranges from 15.5% in Australia, 71.7% in Shanghai China, to 94.3% in Eastern Siberia [6].

The Polish multi-center study performed between 2000 and 2003 revealed that the incidence of *H. pylori* infections was 84% in adult patients [22], whereas our research, conducted in southern Poland between 2009 and 2011, showed that the rate of *H. pylori* infection among adults was 23% [23].

*H. pylor*i has evolved numerous strategies for survival in the gastric niche (especially due to the release of urease, an enzyme, which increases the pH value of the environment around the bacterial cells) [24]. Furthermore, the clinical course of *H. pylori* infection depends from both the bacterial virulence factors and the host susceptibility (e.g. diet, genetic predispositions, degree of the immune response to infection) [3, 7, 25].

It was concluded that untreated *H. pylori* infection led to acid-related disorders of the digestive system. Great majority of individuals colonized by *H. pylori* developed co-existing chronic gastritis, which in subsets of patients could evolve to duodenal or gastric ulcer as well as gastric cancer [7, 8, 26, 27]. Experiments performed in animal models (Mongolian gerbils) confirmed the progressive sequence of lesions from chronic gastritis to gastric cancer by gastric atrophy, intestinal metaplasia, and dysplasia [28]. Figure 1 illustrates the sequential steps of diseases resulting from *H. pylori* infection.

H. pylori infection significantly enhances the risk of development of peptic ulcer disease (up to 15 times) as well as gastric cancer (up to 6 times) [1, 7, 24]. Peptic ulcer disease (PUD) – gastric and/or duodenal ulcer – develops in about 15% of *H. pylori* infected patients, whereas the progression to neoplastic lesions may occur only in a small fraction of patients with *H. pylori* infection. Gastric cancer arises in about 1-5% of patients and MALT cancer in <1% of infected subjects [7, 8, 27, 29].

The information presented above highlights the importance of an effective treatment against *H. pylori*. Furthermore, the increasing resistance of *H. pylori* to antibiotics/chemotherapeutics currently used in empirical therapy justifies the need for continuous surveillance of antibiotic resistance as well as compliance to guidelines of the European Helicobacter Study Group (EHSG) [1].

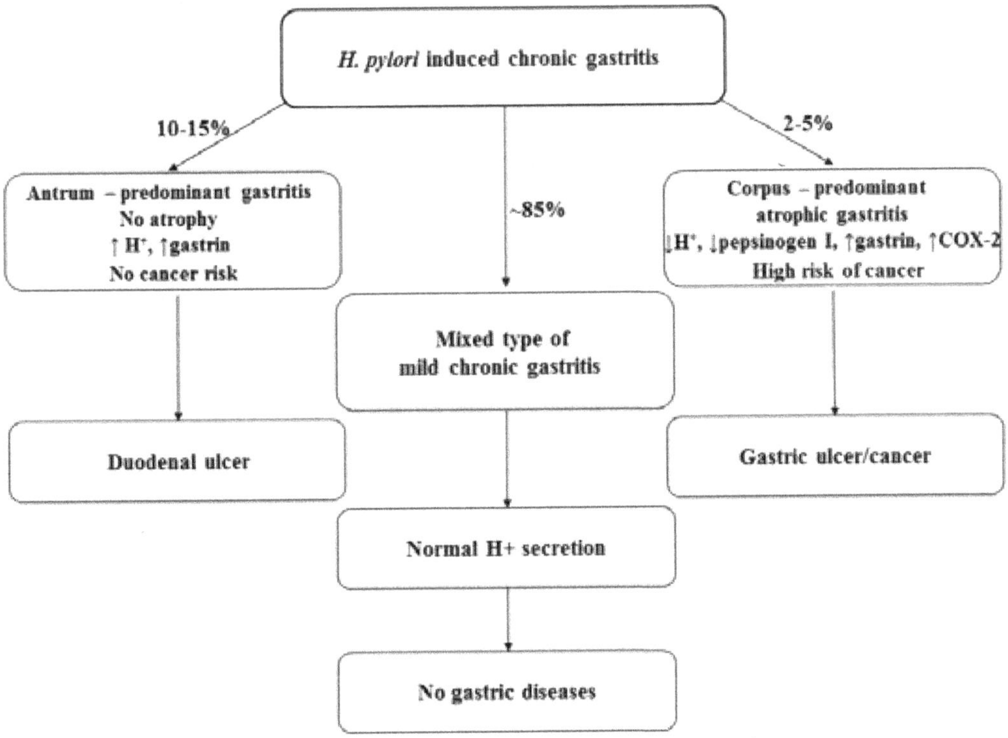

Figure 1. Sequential steps of diseases resulting from *H. pylori* infection *(based on fig. 3 Konturek et. al J Physiol Pharmacol. 2009* [8]).

1.2. Virulence factors (VF)

The pathogenesis of *H. pylori* is determined by wide spectrum of virulence factors, which can be divided into two major groups:

1. VF secreted into the bacterial extracellular environment (e.g. immunogenic protein CagA, vacuolating cytotoxin VacA, secreted enzymes: urease, aliphatic amidase, catalase, oxidase, superoxide dismutase, phospholipases, glycosulfatase and proteolitic enzymes).

2. VF associated with the bacterial surface (e.g. outer membrane proteins, adhesins, flagella, LPS) [24, 25].

CagA. One of the most important *H. pylori* virulence factors is highly immunogenic protein CagA. It is encoded by cytotoxin associated gene (*cag*A gene), which is located on the *cag* pathogenicity island (*cag* PAI) and carried by 56-90% of *H. pylori* strains [8, 24, 29-32]. CagA protein (after translocation into the host cells by the type IV cag secretion system) stimulates epithelial cells to produce the following cytokines: interleukin IL-8 (strong chemotactic factor and activator of inflammatory process on the mucous membrane), IL-6, IL-1β, and tumor necrosis factor α (TNF-α; enhances the inflammatory process) [31, 33, 34] and is also responsible for changes in the host cells such as proliferation, motility, and polarity [25,

35]. Patients infected with *cag*A positive strains usually exhibit a higher inflammatory response and are at a higher risk of developing gastric ulcer disease, atrophic gastritis, or gastric cancer [3, 8, 24, 36, 37].

VacA. Another major *H. pylori* virulence determinant is vacuolating cytotoxin A (VacA). This protein is involved in various mechanisms of programmed cell death (including apoptosis and necrosis) in the target host cells [38]. While VacA encoding gene (*vac*A) occurs in almost all *H. pylori* strains, only approximately 50% of isolates express active protein. Moreover, variations in the *vac*A gene structure considering signal (s) as well as middle (m) region result in differences in vacuolating activity of this cytotoxin [7, 8, 24, 34, 39]. *H. pylori* strains carrying s1/m1 allelic form of *vac*A gene have higher vacuolating activity than isolates with s1/m2 or s2/m1 alleles. Furthermore, polymorphisms among the *vac*A signal region (s1, s1a, s1b, s2) and middle region (m1, m2) are also correlated with the intensity of inflammation process and the severity of gastric epithelial cell injury, respectively. While strains possessing *vac*A s1a genotype cause stronger inflammation process than isolates carrying *vac*A s1b or *vac*A s2 genotype, the strains harboring *vac*A m1 genotype cause more severe gastric epithelial cell injury than the *vac*A m2 strains [34, 40]. Moreover, the infection with *H. pylori* strains possessing *vac*A s1/m1 allele is strongly associated with peptic ulcer disease and gastric cancer [7, 40]. A third polymorphic determinant of vacuolating activity of *vac*A gene was described in mid region and termed the intermediate (i), but its role in the pathogenesis of *H. pylori* infection remains debatable [41].

H. pylori is described as one of the most important risk factors contributing to the development of gastric cancer in more than 50% of cases, while CagA and VacA as major virulence determinants play an important role in this process [2, 7, 8]. Due to the presence/absence of CagA and VacA, *H. pylori* strains were divided into two types: type I (possessing *cag*A gene and expressing vacuolating cytotoxin) and type II (lacking the *cag*A gene and with no expression of vacuolating cytotoxin). Strains belonging to the type I (CagA+, VacA+ phenotype) are more virulent, as their infections are associated with increased risk of peptic ulcer disease and gastric cancer. Strains of the type II (CagA-, VacA- phenotype) are less virulent. Furthermore, an intermediate type of *H. pylori* strain has been described. Isolates belonging to this group have independent expression of CagA and VacA cytotoxins and represent a moderate level of virulence [24, 34, 42].

Urease and aliphatic amidase. Remarkable capacity of *H. pylori* to colonize highly acidic environment of stomach is mostly attributed to the production of urease. This enzyme hydrolyzes urea (to ammonia and carbon dioxide), which results in an increase of pH value in the environment surrounding the bacterium. A similar effect is produced by aliphatic amidase, which also contributes to the pH value of the gastric environment [43]. Furthermore, ammonia which is the product of enzymatic hydrolysis of urea, shows toxicity against epithelial cells [24, 25, 32].

Other pathogenic enzymes.*H. pylori* produces many other groups of enzymes responsible for the pathogenesis. While catalase, oxidase, and superoxide dismutase play a role in protecting the bacterial cells from phagocytosis, phospholipase A2, phospholipases C, and glycosulfatase damage the cells of the mucous membrane [44-48]. Furthermore, *H. pylori* secretes numerous proteolytic enzymes responsible for the gastric mucus degradation [49].

Adhesins. Adherence of *H. pylori* to the host cell receptors triggers cellular changes, which include signal transduction cascades, leading to infiltration of inflammatory cells and to persistence of the organism. *H. pylori* adhesins are proteins, glycoconjugates, or lipids, which are involved in the initial stages of colonization by mediating the interactions between the bacterium and the host cell surface (AlpA, AlpB, BabA, Hsp60, Hsp70, LPS core, LPS O antigen (Lewis X), Nap) [8, 50, 51].

Outer membrane proteins. Outer inflammatory protein (OipA) is an outer membrane inflammatory-related protein significantly associated with the development of duodenal ulcers and gastric cancer. OipA plays an important role in induction of the mucosal cytokines and in gastric mucosal inflammation [7, 8, 36]. The outer membrane proteins contributing to the adherence of *H. pylori* are represented by: SabA, AlpAB [32, 36].

Flagella.*H. pylori* possess up to 6 unipolar flagella composed of two proteins: FlaA and FlaB [24, 52]. Due to the flagella, *H. pylori* is motile and can move within stomach niche between regions of low pH value to regions with higher pH value, which is more hospitable for these bacteria [8, 53]. The motility is also necessary for the successful colonization of the stomach mucosa [52].

LPS. Lipopolysaccharide of *H. pylori* is a unique and a potent immunogen. LPS of *H. pylori* contains O-antigen structures, which resemble human glycosphingolipids due to the presence of common host carbohydrate residues [54]. LPS contains structures like Lewis X and Lewis Y antigens, which are similar to antigens of human blood groups, which occur also in the human gastric epithelium. Due to molecular mimicry, bacteria are able to escape the host immune response. Moreover, the specific structure of *H. pylori* LPS is crucial for the adhesion to epithelial cells and colonization process of the human stomach by *H. pylori* [24, 54, 55].

While in the majority of people *H. pylori* colonization is asymptomatic, long-term carriage significantly increases the risk of development of site-specific diseases [7, 8, 34, 36]. It was also concluded that untreated *H. pylori* infection may lead to serious implications such as gastritis, gastric ulcer disease and gastric cancer, therefore it is crucial to provide effective treatment. Moreover, it was proved that introduction of early effective treatment of *H. pylori* infection in cases of peptic ulcer disease can prevent these patients from developing gastric cancer [1, 26].

1.3. Treatment guidelines

Several recommendations concerning diagnosis and treatment regimen were issued as the infection treatment is often unsuccessful. The first guidelines on diagnostic and therapeutic approaches for the *H. pylori* infection were issued in the United States of America. The second recommendations were introduced by Polish Society of Gastroenterology *Helicobacter pylori* Working Group (PSG-E/HPWG) in 1996. The next guidelines of the PSG-E/HPWG on diagnostic and therapeutic approaches for the *H. pylori* infection were issued in 2000, 2004 and 2008 [22, 56, 57]. The European Helicobacter Study Group (EHSG) took the initiative of introducing recommendations for the clinical management of *H pylori* infection in 1996 in Maastricht and since then four consensus reports have been issued (1997, 2000, 2005, 2012) [1, 5, 58, 59].

Recommendations for the management of *H. pylori* infection are constantly evolving along with the development of knowledge concerning this bacterium and its infections [1]. Current guidelines on the management of *H. pylori* infections were produced by EHSG in 2012 (Maastricht IV/Florence Consensus Report) and should be introduced in the management of this infection in European countries. Despite that fact, the recent Polish recommendations issued in 2008 still support the Third Maastricht Consensus Report (2005). Nevertheless, the new Polish guidelines are under development and will be issued in the near future.

The European Helicobacter Study Group and the Polish Society of Gastroenterology recommend therapeutic regimens, which include three types of drugs: 1) antisecretory (proton pump inhibitors (PPI)), 2) cytoprotectants (drugs containing bismuth salts), and 3) antibiotics/chemotherapeutics (clarithromycin, amoxicillin, metronidazole, tetracycline, levofloxacin, and rifabutin) [1, 22].

The treatment regimens of *H. pylori* infections according to the PSG-E guidelines (2008) [22] are presented in Table 1.

Treatment strategy	**Time of treatment**
The First-Line Treatment (one of the following):	
PPI, amoxicillin (1000 mg) and metronidazole (500 mg) twice a day	
PPI, clarithromycin (500 mg), and metronidazole (500 mg) twice a day	10–14 days
PPI, amoxicillin (500 mg), and clarithromycin (500 mg) twice a day	
The Second-Line Treatment (one of the following):	
PPI, amoxicillin (1000 mg), and metronidazole (500 mg) twice a day and tetracycline (250 mg) three times a day	10–14 days
PPI, amoxicillin (1000 mg), and metronidazole (500 mg) twice a day and bismuth salts (120 mg) four times a day	
The Third-Line Treatment:	
Evaluation of the susceptibility of the strains to the currently used antimicrobial agents: amoxicillin, metronidazole, clarithromycin, and tetracycline	14 days *(prolonged if the previous treatments were shorter)*
Possible introduction of levofloxacin	
Adding a probiotic	

Table 1. Proposed strategy of the first, second and third – line treatment of *H. pylori* infection *(table based on the guidelines of PSG-E Consensus Report, 2008 [22])*

According to the Maastricht IV/Florence Consensus Report guidelines, the treatment regimen should be selected according to the areas of low (<20%) and high (>20%) clarithromycin resistance, to provide the most effective therapy. Figure 2 presents the current EHSG guidelines.

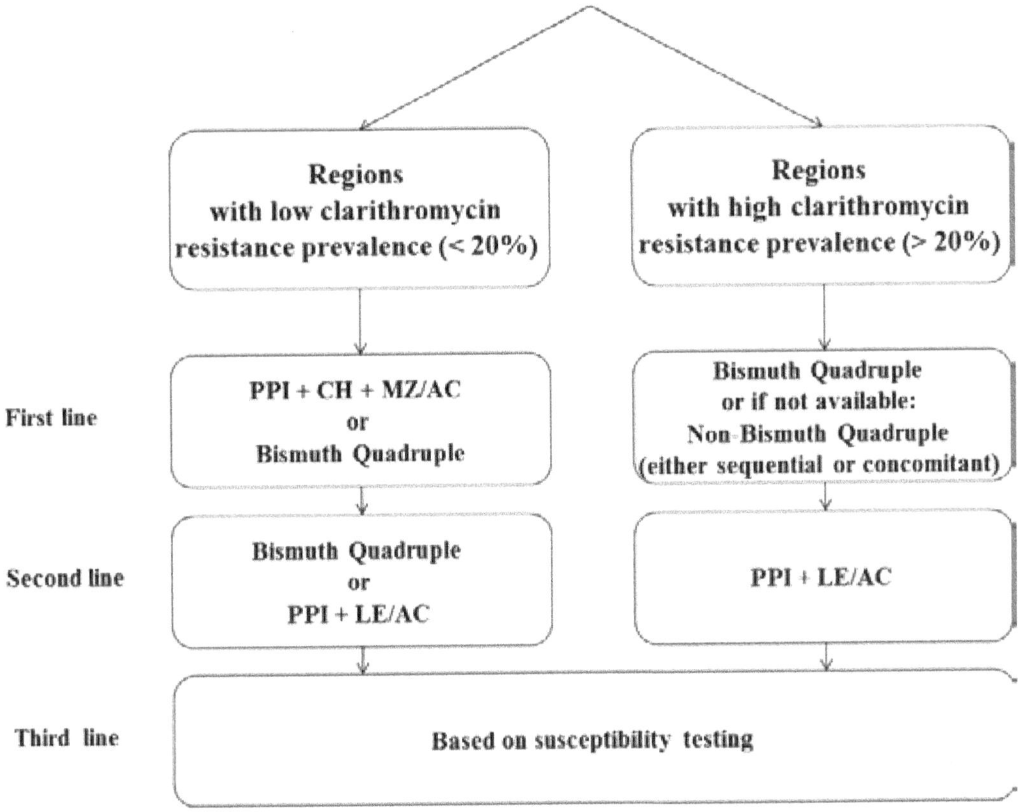

PPI – proton pump inhibitor, **CH** – clarithromycin, **MZ** – metronidazole, **AC** – amoxicillin, **LE** – levofloxacin
Bismuth quadruple therapy: PPI, bismuth, metronidazole, and tetracycline (10 days)
Non-bismuth quadruple sequential therapy: 5-day period with PPI, amoxicillin, followed by 5-day period with PPI, clarithromycin, and metronidazole (or tinidazole)
Non-bismuth quadruple concomitant therapy: clarithromycin, amoxicillin, and metronidazole + PPI (10-14 days)

Figure 2. Treatment schemes of *Helicobacter pylori* infection considering the regions of low and high prevalence of clarithromycin-resistant strains (based on the Maastrich/Florence IV Consensus Report) [1].

In regions with high prevalence of resistance to clarithromycin (>20%), it is recommended to abandon clarithromycin in the empirical treatment of *H. pylori* infections, if the antibiotic susceptibility cannot be tested. As the first line empirical treatment, the bismuth–containing quadruple therapy is recommended. If the bismuth salts are not available in certain countries (e.g. Poland), then non-bismuth quadruple therapies (sequential or concomitant) could be prescribed. Non-bismuth quadruple sequential therapy consists of 5-days of PPI plus amoxicillin, followed by 5-day period with PPI, clarithromycin, and metronidazole (or tinidazole), whereas non-bismuth quadruple concomitant therapy comprises simultaneous use of clarithromycin, amoxicillin, metronidazole, and PPI for 10-14 days. Although both non-bismuth quadruple therapies contain clarithromycin, these regimens could be applied only as targeted therapy based on testing of the bacterial susceptibility to clarithromycin. In regions, where bismuth salts are not available and high clarithromycin resistance occurs, targeted therapy with clarithromycin seems to be the best option.

After failure of the first line treatment, the second line treatment regimen with PPI, levofloxacin, and amoxicillin should be prescribed. It should be emphasized that levofloxacin cannot be used in patients with chronic bronchitis or pneumonia, who may have taken fluoroquinolones, hence it is recommended to perform susceptibility testing to levofloxacin. Moreover, increasing resistance rate to antimicrobial agents should be taken into account [1], for instance in Poland we noted an increasing resistance rate to levofloxacin [23]. Susceptibility testing conducted before treatment, can protect against increasing resistance rate.

If the second line regimen failed, a third line treatment based on antimicrobial susceptibility testing should be introduced. If susceptibility testing is not available, the empirical third line regimen should contain antimicrobials not used previously. Except for the drugs already mentioned, rifabutin is a therapeutic option (its use is limited to mycobacterial infections) [1].

Taking into account the EHSG recommendations, the rationale is to perform susceptibility testing whenever possible to prevent the increase of drug resistance, especially in regions where the resistance to clarithromycin is high.

1.4. Antimicrobial agents and bacterial resistance

Recent data show that combination of standard therapeutic strategies have lost some efficacy. This fact is attributed to increasing antimicrobial resistance of *H. pylori* strains.

Clarithromycin. Among antimicrobial agents used in the treatment of *H. pylori* infections, clarithromycin was considered to be one of the most effective drugs; nonetheless emergence of clarithromycin resistance became the major risk factor of the treatment failure. In susceptible strains, the eradication rates amounted to 87.7%, whereas in resistant strains the rates decreased to 18.3% [5]. One of the most significant factors contributing to clarithromycin resistance is the extensive use of macrolides, particularly in the treatment of upper and lower respiratory tract infections in children [60]. Furthermore, studies conducted between 2001 and 2008 in 18 European countries confirmed the correlation between antibiotic resistance of *H. pylori* strains and outpatient antibiotic consumption in adults. According to this multi-center study, *H. pylori* clarithromycin resistance rates in Europe amounted to 17.5% and were considerably higher in western/central and southern Europe (>20%) than in the northern European countries (<10%) [61]. In Poland, the prevalence of *H. pylori* resistance to clarithromycin was 28% (data published by PSG-E) [22]. Nevertheless, according to our recent study conducted in the years 2006-2008 and 2009-2011, resistance of *H. pylori* strains isolated in southern Poland was also high and amounted to 34% and 22%, respectively [23, 62].

The major mechanism responsible for *H. pylori* clarithromycin resistance is associated with the decrease in the binding of the antibiotic to the ribosome which is caused by the occurrence of the point mutations within the peptidyltransferase-encoding region of 23S rRNA. The most frequently reported point mutation is A-G transition at position 2143 (A2143G), which occurs in 69.8% of *H. pylori* strains resistant to clarithromycin, while the less common mutations are represented by A2142G and A2143C. Furthermore, other mutations, such as A2115G, G2141A,

C2147G, T2190C, C2195T, A2223G, and C2694A, might also be associated with clarithromycin resistance. Molecular assays have a significant impact on improving the availability and accuracy of the data concerning *H. pylori* clarithromycin resistance, resulting in faster and better selection of effective therapy [60, 63].

Metronidazole. Another antimicrobial agent, recommended in the therapy of *H. pylori* infection is metronidazole. Metronidazole has a higher resistance rate than clarithromycin, but it is of secondary importance and can be partly overcome. Treatment with this antimicrobial agent is effective, however, with the exception of the regions where metronidazole resistance reaches 40%. The resistance of *H. pylori* strains to metronidazole amounted to 34.9%, in Europe [5, 61]. In Poland, the resistance rate to metronidazole is higher (46%), according to PSG-E data (2008) [22], whereas in southern Poland, according to our recent study, it is 44% [62].

Common use of metronidazole in parasitic as well as gynecological diseases results in high resistance rates of *H. pylori* strains isolated from both tropical residents and female patients and contributes to overall resistance of the bacterium population [60].

Mechanism of metronidazole resistance in *H. pylori* is not completely understood and, according to some authors, it is related to mutations in *rdx*A (which encodes an oxygen-insensitive NADPH nitroreductase) and *frx*A genes (which encode NADPH flavin oxidoreductase) [60, 64].

Levofloxacin. Levofloxacin is another antimicrobial agent recommended in *H. pylori* treatment, however rapid acquisition of levofloxacin resistance may contribute to the reduction of its future efficiency. In Europe, the resistance rate of *H. pylori* to levofloxacin amounted to 14.4% between 2001 and 2008. Increasing rates of quinolone resistance are attributed to frequent use of these agents in the therapy of the respiratory and urinary tract infections. While in countries with lower quinolone consumption (e.g. Norway) the resistance rate of *H. pylori* strains remains lower, in countries with high use of quinolones (e.g. Italy) the resistance rate is higher [61]. According to data published by PSG-E, the population of *H. pylori* strains in Poland is susceptible to ciprofloxacin [22]. Nevertheless, we reported that levofloxacin resistance rate in southern Poland amounted to 16% in 2011 and in comparison with previous years, the figure had grown [23].

The resistance to fluoroquinolones in *H. pylori* strains is due to the point mutations occurring in *gyr*A gene at the 87 and 91 positions. Furthermore, some studies revealed a correlation between the resistance to levofloxacin and norfloxacin and the point mutation in the position 463 of *gyr*B gene [60, 65].

Amoxicillin and Tetracycline. According to current surveys, the resistance to amoxicillin as well as tetracycline is either very low or even absent, indicating their present clinical irrelevance. While amoxicillin resistance is most likely associated with mutational changes in the penicillin-binding encoding gene (*pbp*D), the tetracycline resistance is based on changes in three nucleotides in the 16S rRNA (AGA 926-928→TTC) [22, 60, 62].

Rifabutin. Rifabutin is one of the antimicrobial agents recommended as an alternative in the third line treatment, after two treatment failures. Prevalence of *H. pylori* resistance to this antibiotic is not well known but it is presumed to be very low, because its use is limited to mycobacterial infection [1]. Moreover, rifabutin is very expensive and causes adverse events like leukopenia, thrombocytopenia or clinically important impairment of liver functions [66, 67]. However, increase in rifabutin consumption may contribute to rapid emergence of resistance. The mechanism of resistance to this antibiotic is mediated by mutations in the *rpo*B gene [1, 60].

1.5. Resistance rate in Poland

Summing up the current and previous data concerning the prevalence of *H. pylori* resistance in Poland, we revealed some differences. The results presented in Polish multi-center study performed between 2000 and 2003 revealed that 28% of the analysed *H. pylori* strains were resistant to clarithromycin, 46% to metronidazole, while all strains were susceptible to amoxicillin and tetracycline [22].

Our studies conducted in the years 2006-2009 and 2010-2012 showed that the resistance rates of *H. pylori* to clarithromycin in southern Poland were 34% and 22%, respectively [23, 62]. Moreover, we reported that the percentage of *H. pylori* strains resistant to metronidazole and levofloxacin accounted for 44% and 6%, respectively. Furthermore, we confirmed the coexistence of resistance to more than one antimicrobial agent: a) resistance to metronidazole and clarithromycin in 23% of the strains, b) resistance to metronidazole, clarithromycin, and levofloxacin in 4% of the strains [62]. Additionally, in our recent studies we demonstrated that in southern Poland the number of *H. pylori* strains resistant to levofloxacin increased significantly; from 5% in the years 2006-2008 to 16% in 2009-2011 [23].

As it was previously emphasized, the Maastricht IV/Florence Consensus Report recommends that treatment regimen should be selected according to areas of low (<20%) and high (>20%) clarithromycin resistance [1]. Referring to available data concerning clarithromycin resistance rates in Poland, this country should be classified as a high clarithromycin resistance region [22, 23, 62].

Although the current Polish guidelines (PSG–E, 2008) on diagnostic and therapeutic approaches to the *H. pylori* infection recommend clarithromycin in the first line treatment, the rationale is to either abandon clarithromycin in an empirical treatment or apply clarithromycin in therapy, but only with prior susceptibility testing.

2. Problem statement

Dynamic growth of *H. pylori* resistance to antimicrobial agents used in empirical treatment becomes an increasingly important problem. While *H. pylori* resistance is often associated with the antibiotic consumption and may vary according to region, it is recommended to constantly monitor the resistance rates of this bacterium. Furthermore, in the areas of high clarithromycin resistance rates as well as increasing resistance to other antibiotics/chemotherapeutics (used in *H. pylori* treatment), it is worth consideration to replace empirical therapy with targeted therapy based on prior susceptibility testing. Moreover, early effective treatment of *H. pylori* infection in patients with peptic ulcer disease can prevent gastric cancer.

3. Aplication area

Data concerning *H. pylori* resistance rates enable to introduce the most effective schemes of infection treatment [5].

4. Research course

1. Monitoring of *H. pylori* resistance to antimicrobial agents used in empirical therapy (according to the Maastricht IV/ Florence Consensus Report) in southern Poland.
2. Selection of the appropriate treatment regimen in *H. pylori* infections in southern Poland, according to the current recommendations and local clarithromycin resistance rates (Maastricht IV/ Florence Consensus Report).
3. Introduction of treatment guided by antimicrobial susceptibility testing in *H. pylori* infections in southern Poland, taking into account: a) high level of clarithromycin resistance, b) increasing resistance rates to levofloxacin, c) persisting high metronidazole resistance rate.
4. Application of molecular method in detection of clarithromycin resistance.

5. Materials and methods

Clinical specimens. The study covered a group of 316 adult dyspeptic patients with therapeutic indications for gastroscopy, who applied to the Falck Medycyna Outpatient Clinic of Gastroenterology (Krakow, Poland) and the Chair of Gastroenterology, Hepatology and Infectious Diseases, Jagiellonian University Medical College (Krakow, Poland).

All patients enrolled to the study underwent gastroscopy in the years 2010-2013. Two biopsy specimens (one from antrum and the second from the body of the stomach) were taken from each patient during gastroscopy. The biopsy specimens were transferred into transport medium (Portagerm Pylori, bioMérieux, France) and transported to the laboratory (Department of Pharmaceutical Microbiology, Jagiellonian University Medical College, Krakow, Poland) for further investigations.

Analysis of endoscopy and histopathological examination enabled to qualify patients into two groups:

1. Subjects with peptic ulcer diseases (PUD) including individuals with peptic and/or duodenal ulcers.

2. Subjects with non-ulcerous dyspepsia (NUD) comprising patients without any pathological changes found in endoscopy and patients with erosive and non-erosive diseases including esophagitis, gastritis or duodenitis.

***H. pylori* microbiological culture and identification.** Gastric biopsy specimens were homogenized in glass sterile mortars and inoculated onto both non selective (Schaedler agar with 5% sheep blood, bioMérieux, France) and selective (Schaedler agar with 5% sheep blood and selective supplement Dent, Oxoid, UK) media. Simultaneously, direct Gram-stained slides and urease tests were performed from the biopsy specimens to confirm the presence of *H. pylori*.

The culture was carried out for 3 to 10 days under microaerophilic conditions at 37°C. The cultured strains were identified according to:

1. Macroscopic appearance of the colonies;
2. Gram–stained slides prepared from bacterial colonies;
3. Biochemical tests (urease, catalase, and oxidase).

The study was approved by the Bioethical Commission of the Jagiellonian University (Krakow, Poland). Before entering our study, each patient signed the informed consent document.

Susceptibility testing. Susceptibility of *H. pylori* strains to the recommended antimicrobial agents (clarithromycin, metronidazole, levofloxacin, tetracycline, and amoxicillin) was quantitatively assessed by the use of strips impregnated with antimicrobial agents gradient (E-test, bioMérieux, France), which enabled to determine the minimal inhibitory concentration (MIC). The colonies from pure *H. pylori* culture were suspended in 0.85% aqueous NaCl solution in order to obtain an equivalent of 3.0 McFarland units. The bacterial suspension was spread onto Schaedler agar medium with 5% sheep blood (bioMérieux, France) with sterile cotton swabs. Single E-test stripes were applied onto the separate, inoculated agar plates and incubated according to the manufacturer recommendations (E-test technical manual, bioMérieux, France).

Results of the susceptibility testing were interpreted according to EUCAST guidelines (breakpoint values were presented in Table 2) [68].

Quality control of the susceptibility testing was performed with *H. pylori* ATCC 43504 strain.

DNA extraction.*H. pylori* culture (incubated for 72 hours on solid medium) was suspended in 1 ml of 0.85% aqueous NaCl solution and centrifuged (12000 rpm/3 min.). Genomic DNA was extracted using the Sherlock AX isolation kit (A&A Biotechnology, Poland) according to the manufacturer's recommendations. DNA quantification was performed by spectrophotometry at 260 nm. The purity of DNA was evaluated by the ratio of the absorbance at 260 and 280 nm (A260/A280). The obtained DNA was stored at -20°C.

PCR identification of *H. pylori*. To confirm *H. pylori* microbiological identification, all analysed strains were subjected to 16S rRNA PCR assay using primers HP-1 and HP-2 described by Kargar et al. [69]. PCR reaction was performed in a final volume of 25 μl containing: 2 μl of genomic DNA, 2 μl of each primer, 5 μl of GoTaq® Flexi Buffer, 1.5 μl of

Antibiotic agent	MIC breakpoints (mg/L)	
	S ≤	R >
Amoxicillin	0.12	0.12
Clarithromycin	0.25	0.5
Levofloxacin	1	1
Metronidazole	8	8
Rifampicin	1	1
Tetracycline	1	1

Table 2. EUCAST clinical breakpoint for *H. pylori* [68].

$MgCl_2$ (25 mM), 0.5 μl of PCR Nucleotide Mix (10 mM each), 0.125 μl of GoTaq® DNA Polymerase (5u/μl) and Nuclease-Free Water (Promega, USA). The following amplification conditions were used: the initial denaturation at 95°C for 2 min., 35 cycles of 95°C for 60 s, 58°C for 60 s, 72°C for 60 s and the final elongation at 72°C for 5 min. The expected 109-base-pair PCR product was visualized after electrophoresis on an 2% agarose gel stained with ethidium bromide.

***cag*A and *vac*A genes detection.** The DNA from analysed *H. pylori* strains was subjected to PCR assay detecting the *cag*A gene with the use of primers D008 and R008 described previously by Chen et al. [70]. The PCR reaction was carried out as described above for the 16s rRNA PCR assay. PCR cycling conditions consisted of initial denaturation at 94°C for 5 min., 33 cycles: 94°C for 60 s, 60°C for 60 s, 62.5°C for 60 s, 72°C for 60 s and the final elongation at 72°C for 5 min. The expected product of 298-base-pairs was visualized after agarose gel electrophoresis. Furthermore, we performed the PCR assay to detect the *vac*A gene. A 229-base-pair fragment of *vac*A was amplified with the primer pair VAC3624F and VAC3853R described previously by Chisholm et al. [71]. The PCR reaction was carried out in the total volume of 25 μl as described above. The following amplification conditions were used: the initial denaturation at 95°C for 2 min., 35 cycles of 95°C for 30 s, 53°C for 30 s, 72°C for 30 s and the final elongation at 72°C for 5 min. The expected product was visualized after agarose gel electrophoresis.

Detection of clarithromycin resistance by RFLP-PCR analysis. The most prevalent point mutations responsible for clarithromycin resistance (A2143G and A2142G) were detected by PCR followed by RFLP analysis. A 425-base-pair fragment of the 23S rRNA was amplified with the primers K1 and K2 described by Agudo et al. [63]. PCR amplification of DNA was performed in a final volume of 25 μl as described above for the 16S rRNA PCR assay. The cycling program was: 1 cycle at 95°C for 2 min.; 35 cycles of 95°C for 30 s, 60°C for 30 s, 72°C for 30 s and a final elongation step at 72°C for 5 min. The amplicon was digested with Eco31I (BsaI) enzyme (Thermo Scientific, USA) for 30 min. at 37°C and 5 min. at 65°C to detect A2143G mutation [63] or with BbsI enzyme (New England Biolabs, USA) for 24 h at 37°C to detect A2142G mutation [72]. The restriction products were analysed by electrophoresis on an 2% agarose gel. Enzyme Eco31I digested the A2143G-positive *H. pylori* PCR amplicon into 304- and 101-base-pair fragments, while BbsI enzyme cut the A2142G-positive *H. pylori* PCR product into 332- and 93-base-pair fragments.

6. Results

Prevalence of *H. pylori* infection. Among 316 patients with dyspeptic symptoms admitted to the study between November 2010 and June 2013, the presence of *H. pylori* infection was confirmed in 73 cases (according to rapid urease test and bacterial culture). Therefore, the prevalence of *H. pylori* infection in patients with dyspeptic symptoms from southern Poland amounted to 23.1% (73/316). Taking into account the analysis of endoscopy and histopathological examination among 73 *H. pylori*-positive patients, 26% (19/73) were qualified into the I group (patients with PUD), whereas 74% (54/73) patients were qualified into the II group (patients with NUD).

Susceptibility testing. The susceptibility testing of 73 *H. pylori* strains to the recommended antimicrobial agents showed that 51.7% of isolates were resistant to one or more drugs, while 49.3% of strains were susceptible to all tested antibiotics/chemotherapeutics. The resistance rates of *H. pylori* strains to the assayed antimicrobial agents were presented in Table 3 (data include strains resistant to one, two or four antibiotics/chemotherapeutics).

The rate of resistance of *H. pylori* strains to clarithromycin amounted to 23.3% (17/73). According to the Maastricht/Florence IV Consensus Report, southern Poland should be qualified as an area of high clarithromycin resistance. Consequently, the use of clarithromycin in *H. pylori* infections in this region should be either abandoned (as an empirical treatment) or applied but only with prior susceptibility testing. Due to this fact, it seems reasonable to change the current Polish recommendation (PSG-E, 2008) concerning clarithromycin use in the treatment of *H. pylori* infections.

Furthermore, the resistance rates to metronidazole and levofloxacin were 39.7% (29/73) and 12.3% (9/73), respectively.

Antimicrobial agents	N (%) of resistant strains (n = 73)
Clarithromycin	17 (23.3)
Metronidazole	29 (39.7)
Levofloxacin	9 (12.3)
Amoxicillin	1 (1.4)
Tetracycline	0 (0)

Table 3. Resistance rates of *H. pylori* to clarithromycin, metronidazole, levofloxacin, amoxicillin, and tetracycline in southern Poland (the data include strains resistant to one, two or four antibiotics/chemotherapeutics).

We also reported the presence of one strain (1,4%; 1/73) resistant to amoxicillin. Resistance to amoxicillin is an uncommon phenomenon and it is the first report of an amoxicillin-resistant strain in southern Poland. All examined *H. pylori* strains were susceptible to tetracycline.

Moreover, we analysed the co-occurrence of resistance to more than one antimicrobial agent among *H. pylori* isolates (Table 4).

Our studies showed the presence of 35.6% (26/73) of single-resistant, 8% (13/73) of double-resistant and 1.4% (1) of quadruple-resistant strains (susceptibility testing for each tested isolate included: clarithromycin, metronidazole, levofloxacin, and amoxicillin).

Antimicrobial agents		N (%) of resistant strainsn n=73
	Clarithromycin	6 (8.2)
single-resistant strains	Metronidazole	16 (21.9)
	Levofloxacin	4 (5.4)
	Clarithromycin + Metronidazole	9 (12.3)
double-resistant strains	Metronidazole + Levofloxacin	3 (4.1)
	Clarithromycin + Levofloxacin	1 (1.4)
quadruple-resistant strains	Clarithromycin + Metronidazole + Levofloxacin + Amoxicillin	1 (1.4)

Table 4. Co-occurrence of resistance to various antibiotics/chemotherapeutics among H. pylori strains isolated in southern Poland.

The MICs obtained in our study ranged from 0.016 mg/L to 256 mg/L for clarithromycin [Figure 3], from 0.016 mg/L to 256 mg/L for metronidazole [Figure 4], from 0.002 mg/L to 12 mg/L for levofloxacin [Figure 5], and from 0.016 mg/L to 0.125 mg/L for both amoxicillin [Figure 6] and tetracycline [Figure 7].

The mean MIC values were as follows: 19.2 mg/L for clarithromycin, 75.2 mg/L for metronidazole, 0.61 mg/L for levofloxacin, 0.018 mg/L for amoxicillin, and 0.024 mg/L for tetracycline.

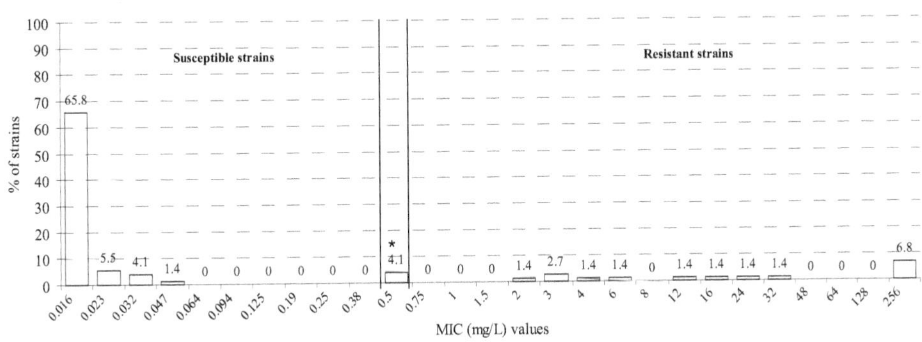

Figure 3. The distribution of clarithromycin MICs among *H. pylori* strains (Clinical breakpoints according to EUCAST: resistant MIC>0.5 mg/L; susceptible MIC≤0.25 mg/L); * strains with MIC value of 0.5 mg/L were considered as resistant to clarithromycin according to the results of PCR–RFLP analysis.

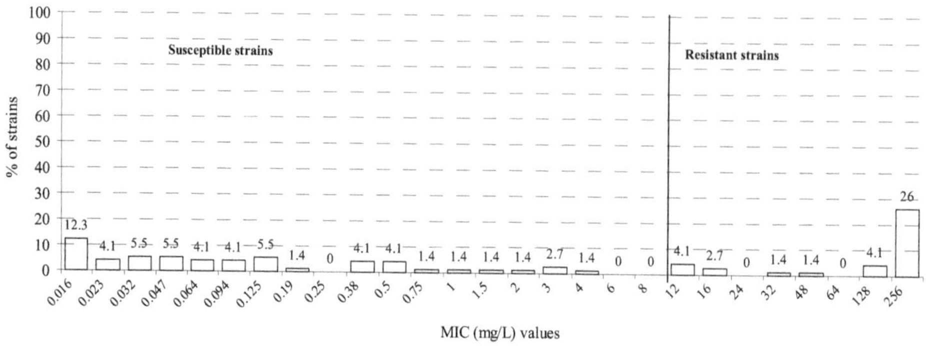

Figure 4. The distribution of MICs among *H. pylori* strains (Clinical breakpoints according to EUCAST: resistant MIC>8 mg/L; susceptible MIC≤8 mg/L).

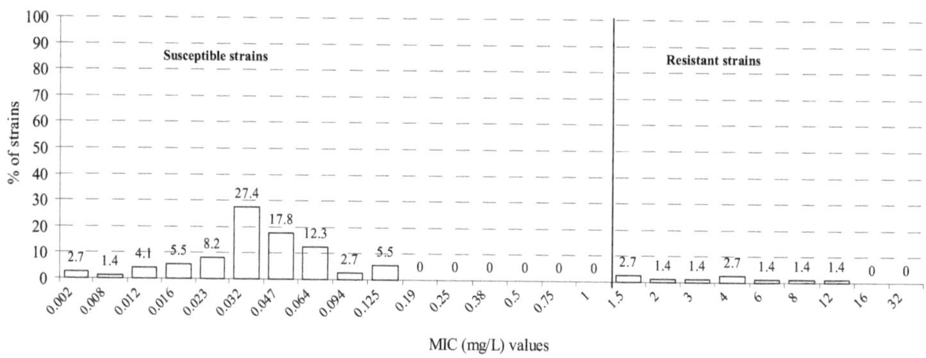

Figure 5. The distribution of levofloxacin MICs among *H. pylori* strains (Clinical breakpoints according to EUCAST: resistant MIC>1 mg/L; susceptible MIC≤1 mg/L).

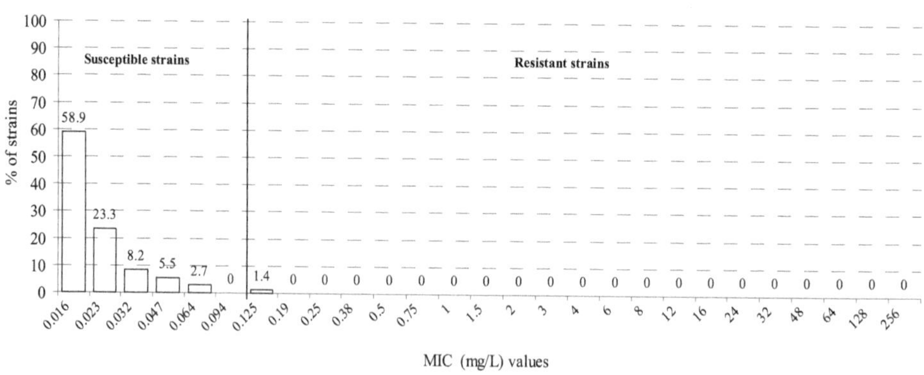

Figure 6. The distribution of amoxicillin MICs among *H. pylori* strains (Clinical breakpoints according to EUCAST: resistant MIC>0.12 mg/L; susceptible MIC≤0.12 mg/L).

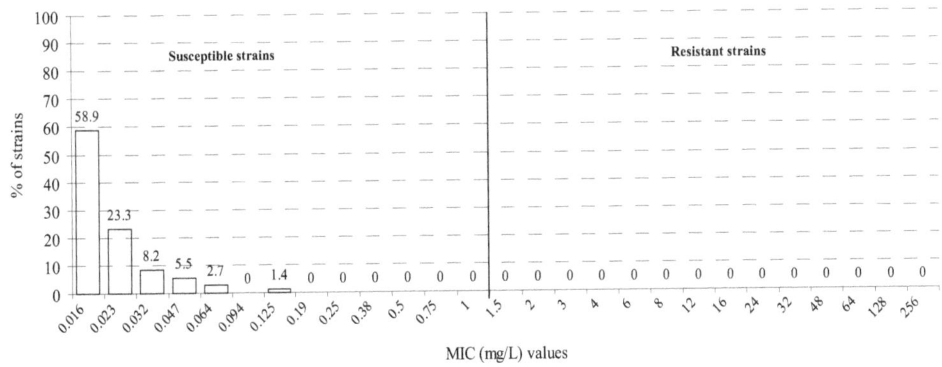

Figure 7. The distribution of tetracycline MICs among *H. pylori* strains (Clinical breakpoints according to EUCAST: resistant MIC>1 mg/L; susceptible MIC≤1 mg/L).

The quantitative E-test method allowed us to observe the dynamically increasing resistance of *H. pylori* to antimicrobials during the monitoring.

In Poland, *H. pylori* resistance rate to clarithromycin exceeded 20% [22, 23, 62]. Our recent study revealed that this rate remained at the same high level or even increased to 23.3%. Therefore the current Polish guidelines (PSG–E, 2008) should be changed according to EHSG (2012). EHSG recommended abandoning clarithromycin in empirical treatment or susceptibility testing prior to the administration of this drug in regions with high prevalence of resistant *H. pylori* strains (>20%).

Moreover, it is worth emphasizing that our study showed that 6.8% of analysed strains demonstrated high clarithromycin MIC values: 256 mg/L.

Furthermore, we revealed persistent, high-level resistance to metronidazole (39.7% of isolates). Twenty-six percent of *H. pylori* strains displayed the metronidazole MIC values as high as 256 mg/L. Additionally, the resistance rate to levofloxacin increased in comparison to our previous studies (5% in the years 2006-2008 [62] *vs.* 12.3% currently).

Although the amoxicillin MIC values are still low, emergence of a resistant *H. pylori* isolate was a new phenomenon. It was the first amoxicillin-resistant *H. pylori* strain isolated in southern Poland.

The reason as to why *H. pylori* resistance to antibiotics/chemotherapeutics has to be monitored, are the results of our study. Moreover, in order to obtain effective regimen for the cure of *H. pylori* infection, it seems reasonable to perform susceptibility testing prior to the treatment.

PCR identification of *H. pylori*. Microbiological identification of all 73 *H. pylori* isolates was confirmed by PCR targeting the 16S rRNA gene (representative samples are presented in Figure 8).

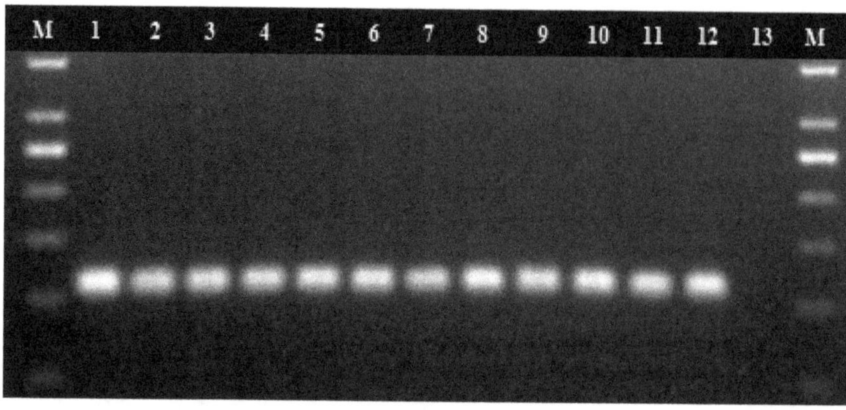

Figure 8. Representative samples of 16S rRNA PCR assay. Lines: 1-11 - selected *H. pylori* strains isolated from patients enrolled to the study, 12 - positive control (109 bp), 13 - negative control; M - molecular weight marker (O'GeneRuler 50 bp DNA Ladder, Thermo Scientific, USA).

***cag*A *and vac*A genes distribution.** *cag*A and *vac*A genes have been identified as being virulence-associated and may have important clinical and epidemiological implications [73]. While *cag*A is carried by 56-90% of *H. pylori* strains [8, 24, 29-32], *vac*A is present in all identified *H. pylori* isolates [74]. The occurrence of *cag*A and *vac*A genes was tested in all 73 strains.

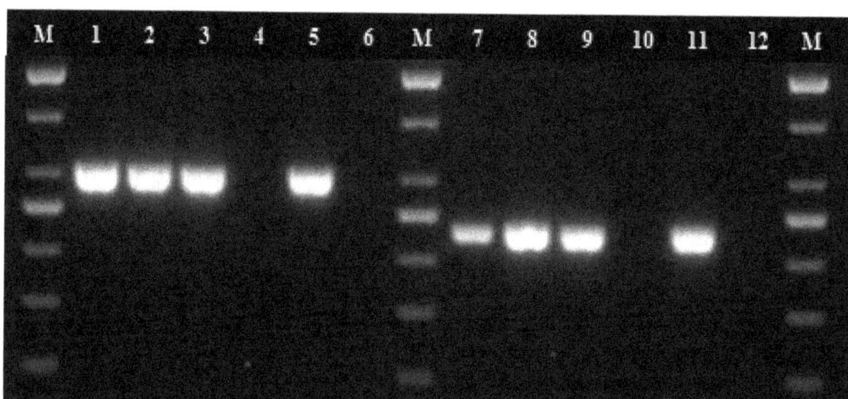

Figure 9. Representative samples of *cag*A and *vac*A genes detection. A) *cag*A detection: lines: 1-4 - selected *H. pylori* strains isolated from patients enrolled to the study, 5 - positive control (298 bp), 6 - negative control; B) *vac*A detection: lines: 7-10 - selected *H. pylori* strains isolated from patients enrolled to the study, 11 - positive control (229 bp), 12 - negative control; M - molecular weight marker (O'GeneRuler 50 bp DNA Ladder, Thermo Scientific, USA).

The cytotoxin associated gene - *cag*A - was detected in 80.8% of *H. pylori* strains (59/73), whereas *cag*A-negative strains accounted for 19.2% (14/73) (representative samples are shown in Figure 9). The occurrence of *vac*A gene was confirmed in 89% (65/73) of strains, while 11% (8/73) of strains were *vac*A-negative. The absence of *vac*A gene in 11% of assayed *H. pylori* strains was associated with limited sensitivity of the method used in this study [71].

Table 5 shows the relationship between the distribution of *cag*A and *vac*A genes and the clinical diagnosis.

Among 19 patients with peptic ulcer disease (PUD), 78.9% (15/19) were infected with *H. pylori cag*A-positive strains, while 21.1% (4/19) with strains *cag*A-negative. Moreover, 84.2% (16/19) of patients with PUD were infected with *H. pylori vac*A-positive strains and 15.8% (3/19) with strains *vac*A-negative. Double positive *H. pylori* strains (*cagA*-positive and *vacA*-positive) occurred in 63.2% (12/19) of patients with peptic ulcer disease.

Among the group of patients with NUD, 81.5% (49/54) of isolated *H. pylori* strains carried *cag*A gene, but only 18.5% (10/54) were *cag*A-negative. Although none of these patients developed ulceration during the study, it is probable that these infections, if untreated, may lead to serious consequences such as peptic ulcer disease or even gastric cancer, due to the fact that the *cag*A-positive *H. pylori* strains increase the likelihood of developing these diseases.

The *cag*A-positive, *vac*A-positive *H. pylori* genotype was the most common one in both: groups of patients: with PUD as well as with NUD, whereas the duble-negative genotype was not found.

Genotype	N (%) of strains	
	PUD n=19	NUD n=54
*cag*A +	15 (78.9)	44 (81.5)
*cag*A -	4 (21.1)	10 (18.5)
*vac*A +	16 (84.2)	49 (90.7)
*vac*A -	3 (15.8)	5 (9.3)
*cag*A + *vac*A +	12 (63.2)	39 (72.5)
*cag*A + *vac*A -	3 (15.8)	5 (9.3)
*cag*A - *vac*A +	4 (21.1)	10 (18.5)
*cag*A - *vac*A -	0 (0)	0 (0)

PUD – peptic ulcer disease

NUD – non-ulcer dyspepsia

Table 5. Relationship between distribution of *cag*A and *vac*A genes and the clinical diagnosis.

PCR-RFLP analysis of *H. pylori* resistance to clarithromycin. Molecular analysis of clarithromycin resistance mechanism was conducted on 73 *H. pylori* strains. The results of PCR-RFLP analysis are shown in Figure 10 and Table 6.

Among the 17 clarithromycin-resistant isolates, Eco31I (BsaI) digested PCR amplicons of 12 (70.6%) strains to 304-base-pair and 101-base-pair, indicating that the strains contained A2143G mutation in the 23S rRNA gene. Furthermore, BbsI enzyme cut products of 3 (17.6%) strains to 332-base-pair and 93-base-pair suggesting that the isolates had A2142G mutation.

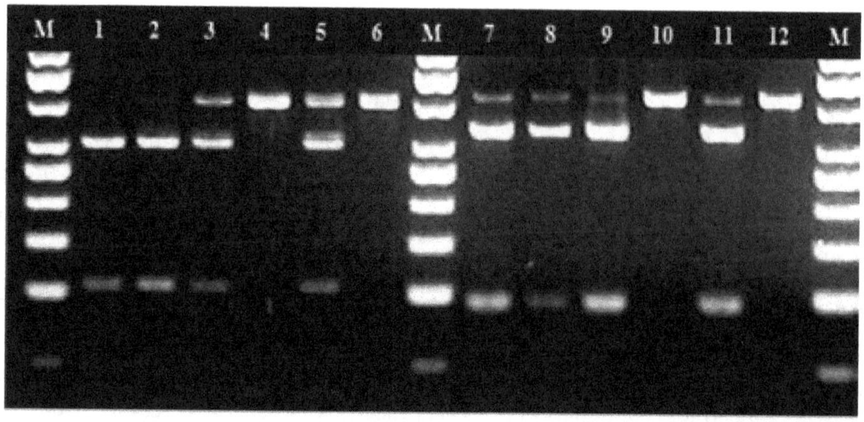

Figure 10. Restriction endonuclease analysis of 23S rRNA amplicons (425 bp) digested with Eco31I (BsaI) and BbsI enzymes. A) detection of A2143G mutation: lines: 1-4 - selected *H. pylori* strains isolated from patients enrolled to the study, 5 - positive control (digestion products of 304 and 101 bp), 6 - negative control; B) detection of A2142G mutation: lines: 7-10 - selected *H. pylori* strains isolated from patients enrolled to the study, 11 - positive control (digestion products of 332 and 93 bp), 12 - negative control; M – Molecular Weight Marker (50 bp O'Gene Ruler, Thermo Scientific, USA).

RFLP analysis of 11.8% (2/17) clarithromycin-resistant isolates gave negative results for both assayed mutations. Resistance to clarithromycin in these isolates (negative for both A2413G and A2142G) might be associated with other mutations in the 23S rRNA such as A2142C, T2245C, T2717C, A2115G, G2141A, T2182G, or T2182C as well as efflux pump [63].

Digestion of PCR products of 100% (56/56) strains not resistant to clarithromycin revealed the absence of the tested mutations. Moreover, our studies suggest that the presence of A2142G mutation is more related to the high clarithromycin MIC level than the A2143G mutation.

Type of mutation	N (%) of strains	
	Clarithromycin–resistant n=17	Clarithromycin–susceptible n=56
A2143G	12 (70.6)	0 (0)
A2142G	3 (17.6)	0 (0)
not detected	2 (11.8)	56 (100)

Table 6. Prevalence of A2143G and A2142G mutations in the group of 73 tested *H. pylori* strains.

7. Conclusions

Results of our studies concerning the resistance rates of *H. pylori* strains isolated from subjects in southern Poland suggest the need for constant monitoring of the resistance to a set of antimicrobial agents routinely used for empirical therapy. We observed high level of clarithromycin resistance rate (>20%), which resulted in the necessity of either to abandon clarithromycin in an empirical treatment or to perform susceptibility testing prior to application of clarithromycin-containing treatment.

We also noted the increase in *H. pylori* resistance to levofloxacin and persistent high level resistance to metronidazole, which resulted in the necessity of treatment guided by antimicrobial susceptibility testing.

To conclude, antimicrobial susceptibility testing can improve treatment outcomes and reduce the outpatient antibiotic consumption, while the introduction of molecular methods for clarithromycin resistance testing allows better and more efficient management of *H. pylori* infections.

8. Further research

Our further investigations will be concerned with the application of the PCR-RFLP method in detection of less frequent 23S rRNA gene mutations associated with clarithromycin resistance. Furthermore, we will focus on direct detection of *H. pylori* in biopsy specimens as well as characterization of the resistance determinants.

Acknowledgements

This work was supported by a research grant funded by the Polish Government in the years 2011-2013 (NN404547640)

Author details

Elżbieta Karczewska[1], Karolina Klesiewicz[1], Paweł Nowak[1], Edward Sito[2], Iwona Skiba[1], Małgorzata Zwolińska–Wcisło[3], Tomasz Mach[3] and Alicja Budak[1]

1 Department of Pharmaceutical Microbiology, Jagiellonian University Medical College, Krakow, Poland

2 Falck Medycyna Outpatient Clinic of Gastroenterology, Krakow, Poland

3 Chair of Gastroenterology, Hepatology and Infectious Diseases, Jagiellonian University Medical College, Krakow, Poland

References

[1] Malfertheiner P, Megraud F, O'Morain CA, Atherton J, Axon AT, Bazzoli F, et al. European Helicobacter Study Group. Management of Helicobacter pylori infection--the Maastricht IV/ Florence Consensus Report. Gut. 2012;61(5):646-664. doi: 10.1136/gutjnl-2012-302084. http://gut.bmj.com/content/61/5/646.long (accessed 10 July 2013).

[2] International Agency For Research on Cancer. IARC. Monograph on the Evaluation of Carcinogenic Risks to Humans, Schistosomes, Liver Flukes and Helicobacter pylori. Lyon, France: IARC, 1994;61:177-242.

[3] Ando T, Goto Y, Maeda O, Watanabe O, Ishiguro K, Goto H. Causal role of Helicobacter pylori infection in gastric cancer. World J Gastroenterol. 2006;12(2):181-186. http://www.wjgnet.com/1007-9327/full/v12/i2/181.htm (accessed 10 July 2013).

[4] Perez-Perez GI, Rothenbacher D, Brenner H. Epidemiology of Helicobacter pylori infection. Helicobacter. 2004;9(Suppl 1):1-6.

[5] Malfertheiner P, Megraud F, O'Morain C, Bazzoli F, El-Omar E, Graham D, et al. Current concepts in the management of Helicobacter pylori infection: the Maastricht III Consensus Report. Gut. 2007;56(6):772-81. doi:10.1136/gut.2006.101634 http://gut.bmj.com/content/56/6/772.long (accessed 10 July 2013).

[6] Goh KL, Chan WK, Shiota S, Yamaoka Y. Epidemiology of Helicobacter pylori infection and public health implications. Helicobacter. 2011;16(Suppl 1):1-9. doi: 10.1111/j.1523-5378.2011.00874.x. http://onlinelibrary.wiley.com/doi/10.1111/j.1523-5378.2011.00874.x/full (accessed 12 July 2013).

[7] Wroblewski LE, Peek Jr. RM, Wilson KT. Helicobacter pylori and Gastric Cancer: Factors That Modulate Disease Risk. Clin. Microbiol. Rev. 2010;23(4)713-739. doi: 10.1128/CMR.00011-10. http://cmr.asm.org/content/23/4/713.full (accessed 11 July 2013).

[8] Konturek PC, Konturek SJ, Brzozowski T. Helicobacter pylori infection in gastric cancerogenesis. J Physiol Pharmacol. 2009;60(3):3-21.

[9] Venerito M, Selgrad M, Malfertheiner P. Helicobacter pylori: Gastric Cancer and Extragastric Malignancies - Clinical aspects. Helicobacter. 2013;18(Suppl 1):39-43.

[10] Wotherspoon AC, Ortiz-Hidalgo C, Falzon MR, Isaacson PG. Helicobacter pylori-associated gastritis and primary B-cell gastric lymphoma. Lancet 1991;338:1175-1176.

[11] Gisbert JP, Calvet X. Review article: common misconceptions in the management of Helicobacter pylori-associated gastric MALT-lymphoma. Aliment Pharmacol Ther. 2011;34(9):1047-1062. doi: 10.1111/j.1365-2036.2011.04839.x. http://onlinelibrary.wiley.com/doi/10.1111/j.1365-2036.2011.04839.x/full (accessed 10 July 2013).

[12] Pellicano R, Franceschi F, Saracco G, Fagoonee S, Roccarina D, Gasbarrini A. Helicobacters and extragastric diseases. Helicobacter. 2009;14(Suppl 1):58-68.

[13] Qu XH, Huang XL, Xiong P, Zhu CY, Huang YL, Lu LG, et al. Does Helicobacter pylori infection play a role in iron deficiency anemia? A meta-analysis. World J Gastroenterol. 2010;16(7):886-896.

[14] Figura N, Franceschi F, Santucci A, Bernardini G, Gasbarrini G, Gasbarrini A. Extragastric manifestations of Helicobacter pylori infection. Helicobacter. 2010;15(Suppl 1):60-68.

[15] Banić M, Franceschi F, Babić Z, Gasbarrini A. Extragastric manifestations of Helicobacter pylori infection. Helicobacter. 2012;17(Suppl 1):49-55.

[16] Pellicano R, Franceschi F, Saracco G, Fagoonee S, Roccarina D, Gasbarrini A. Helicobacters and extragastric diseases. Helicobacter. 2009;14(Suppl 1):58-68.

[17] Kowalski M, Konturek PC, Pieniazek P, Karczewska E, Kluczka A, Grove R, et al. Prevalence of Helicobacter pylori infection in coronary artery disease and effect of its eradication on coronary lumen reduction after percutaneous coronary angioplasty. Dig Liver Dis. 2001;33(3):222-229.

[18] Pieniazek P, Karczewska E, Duda A, Tracz W, Pasowicz M, Konturek SJ. Association of Helicobacter pylori infection with coronary heart disease. J Physiol Pharmacol. 1999;50(5):743-751.

[19] Miendje Deyi VY, Vanderpas J, Bontems P, Van den Borre C, De Koster E, Cadranel S, et al. Marching cohort of Helicobacter pylori infection over two decades (1988-2007): combined effects of secular trend and population migration. Epidemiol Infect. 2011;139(4):572-580.

[20] Tonkic A, Tonkic M, Lehours P, Mégraud F. Epidemiology and diagnosis of Helicobacter pylori infection. Helicobacter. 2012;17(Suppl 1):1-8.

[21] Bureš J, Kopáčová M, Koupil I, Seifert B, Skodová Fendrichová M, Spirková J, et al. Significant decrease in prevalence of Helicobacter pylori in the Czech Republic. World J Gastroenterol. 2012;18(32):4412-4418. doi: 10.3748/wjg.v18.i32.4412. http://www.wjgnet.com/1007-9327/full/v18/i32/4412.htm (accessed 11 July 2013).

[22] Dzieniszewski J, Jarosz M, Grupa Robocza PTG-E do spraw zakażenia Helicobacter pylori. Ustalenia Grupy Roboczej PTG-E dotyczące postępowania w zakażeniu Helicobacter pylori - consensus 2008. Gastroenterologia Polska 2008;15(5):323-331; Article In Polish.

[23] Karczewska E, Klesiewicz K, Skiba I, Wojtas-Bonior I, Sito E, Czajecki K, et al. Variability in Prevalence of Helicobacter pylori Strains Resistant to Clarithromycin and Levofloxacin in Southern Poland. Gastroenterol Res Pract. 2012;2012:418010. doi: 10.1155/2012/418010. http://www.hindawi.com/journals/grp/2012/418010/ (accessed 10 July 2013).

[24] Jaguszyn-Krynicka EK, Gajkowska A, Godlewska R. Virulence factors of Helicobacter pylori. Mikrobiol Med 1999;3(20):3-13 Article In Polish.

[25] Jagusztyn-Krynicka EK, Godlewska R, Laniewski P. Helicobacter pylori - patogen roku 2005. Kosmos 2005;54:307-319. Article In Polish.

[26] Malfertheiner P, Sipponen P, Naumann M, Moayyedi P, Mégraud F, Xiao SD, et al. H. pylori-Gastric Cancer Task Force. Helicobacter pylori eradication has the potential to prevent gastric cancer: a state-of-the-art critique. Am J Gastroenterol. 2005;100(9): 2100-2115.

[27] Peek RM Jr, Crabtree JE. Helicobacter infection and gastric neoplasia. J Pathol. 2006;208(2):233-248.

[28] Konturek PC, Konturek SJ, Brzozowski T. Gastric cancer and Helicobacter pylori infection. J Physiol Pharmacol. 2006;57(Suppl 3):51-65.

[29] Karczewska E, Wojtas I, Sito E, Trojanowska D, Budak A, Zwolinska-Wcislo M, et al. Assessment of co-existence of Helicobacter pylori and Candida fungi in diseases of the upper gastrointestinal tract. J Physiol Pharmacol. 2009;60(Suppl 6):33-39.

[30] Palli D, Masala G, Del Giudice G, Plebani M, Basso D, Berti D, et al. CagA+ Helicobacter pylori infection and gastric cancer risk in the EPIC-EURGAST study. Int J Cancer. 2007;120(4):859-867.

[31] Portal-Celhay C, Perez-Perez GI. Immune responses to Helicobacter pylori colonization: mechanisms and clinical outcomes. Clin Sci (Lond). 2006;110(3):305-314.

[32] Essawi T, Hammoudeh W, Sabri I, Sweidan W, Farraj MA. Determination of Helicobacter pylori Virulence Genes in Gastric Biopsies by PCR. ISRN Gastroenterol. 2013;2013:606258. doi: 10.1155/2013/606258. http://www.hindawi.com/isrn/gastroenterology/2013/606258/ (accessed 15 July 2013).

[33] Crabtree JE, Covacci A, Farmery SM, Xiang Z, Tompkins DS, Perry S, et al. Helicobacter pylori induced interleukin-8 expression in gastric epithelial cells is associated with CagA positive phenotype. J Clin Pathol. 1995;48(1):41-5.

[34] Gocki J, Bartuzi Z, Dziedziczko A. Cytotoxity genes of Helicobacter pylori. Annales Academiae Medicae Bydgostiensis. 2003, 17(2):65-70. Article In Polish.

[35] Huklińska U, Łasica AM, Jagusztyn-Krynicka EK. Białko CagA Helicobacter pylori-pierwsza zidentyfikowana bakteryjna onkoproteina. Post. Mikrobiol 2011;50(2): 97-106. Article In Polish.

[36] Figueiredo C, Machado JC, Yamaoka Y. Pathogenesis of Helicobacter pylori Infection. Helicobacter. 2005;10(Suppl 1):14-20.

[37] Wen S, Moss SF. Helicobacter pylori virulence factors in gastric carcinogenesis. Cancer Lett. 2009;282(1):1-8.

[38] Delahay RM, Rugge M. Pathogenesis of Helicobacter pylori infection. Helicobacter. 2012;17(Suppl 1):9-15. doi: 10.1111/j.1523-5378.2012.00976.x.

[39] Atherton JC, Cao P, Peek RM Jr, Tummuru MK, Blaser MJ, Cover TL. Mosaicism in vacuolating cytotoxin alleles of Helicobacter pylori. Association of specific vacA types with cytotoxin production and peptic ulceration. J Biol Chem. 1995;270(30): 17771-17777.

[40] Atherton JC, Peek RM Jr, Tham KT, Cover TL, Blaser MJ. Clinical and pathological importance of heterogeneity in vacA, the vacuolating cytotoxin gene of Helicobacter pylori. Gastroenterology. 1997;112(1):92-99.

[41] Wen S, Moss SF. Helicobacter pylori virulence factors in gastric carcinogenesis. Cancer Lett. 2009;282(1):1-8. doi: 10.1016/j.canlet.2008.11.016.

[42] Garner JA, Cover TL. Analysis of genetic diversity in cytotoxin-producing and non-cytotoxin-producing Helicobacter pylori strains. J Infect Dis. 1995;172(1):290-293.

[43] Skouloubris S, Labigne A, De Reuse H. Identification and characterization of an aliphatic amidase in Helicobacter pylori. Mol Microbiol. 1997;25(5):989-998.

[44] Langton SR, Cesareo SD. Helicobacter pylori associated phospholipase A2 activity: a factor in peptic ulcer production? J Clin Pathol 1992;45:221-224.

[45] Slomiany BL, Murty VL, Piotrowski J, Liau YH, Sundaram P, Slomiany A. Glycosulfatase activity of Helicobacter pylori toward gastric mucin. Biochem Biophys Res Comm 1992;183:506-513.

[46] Dzierżanowska-Fangrat K, Dzierżanowska D. Helicobacter pylori: Microbiology and Interactions with Gastrointestinal Microflora. J Physiol Pharmacol. 2006;57(Suppl 3): 5-14.

[47] Spigelhalder CB, Gerstenecker A, Kersten, Schiltz E, Kist M. Purification of Helicobacter pylori superoxide dismutase and cloning and sequencing of the gene. Infect Immun 1993;61:5315-5325.

[48] Hazell SL, Evans DJ Jr, Graham DY. Helicobacter pylori catalase. J Gen Microbiol 1991;137:57-61.

[49] Sidebotham RL, Batten JJ, Karim QN, Spencer J, Baron JH. Breakdown of gastric mucus in presence of Helicobacter pylori. J Clin Pathol. 1991;44(1):52-57.

[50] Evans DJ Jr, Evans DG. Helicobacter pylori adhesins: review and perspectives. Helicobacter. 2000;5(4):183-195.

[51] Testerman TL, McGee DJ, Mobley HLT. Adherence and Colonization. In: Mobley HLT, Mendz GL, Hazell SL, editors. Helicobacter pylori: Physiology and Genetics. Washington (DC): ASM Press; 2001. Chapter 34. Available from: http://www.ncbi.nlm.nih.gov/books/NBK2437/ (accessed 20 July 2013).

[52] Cid TP, Fernández MC, Benito Martínez S, Jones NL. Pathogenesis of Helicobacter pylori Infection. Helicobacter. 2013;18(Suppl 1):12-17. doi: 10.1111/hel.12076.

[53] D Scott, D Weeks, K Melchers, G Sachs. The life and death of Helicobacter pylori. Gut. 1998;43(Suppl 1):56-60.

[54] Matsuura M. Structural Modifications of Bacterial Lipopolysaccharide that Facilitate Gram-Negative Bacteria Evasion of Host Innate Immunity. Front Immunol. 2013;4:109. doi: 10.3389/fimmu.2013.00109. http://www.frontiersin.org/Journal/10.3389/fimmu.2013.00109/full (accessed 25 July 2013).

[55] Moran AP. Relevance of fucosylation and Lewis antigen expression in the bacterial gastroduodenal pathogen Helicobacter pylori. Carbohydr Res. 2008;343(12): 1952-1965. doi: 10.1016/j.carres.2007.12.012.

[56] Dzieniszewski J, Jarosz M, Grupa Robocza PTG-E. Postępowanie w zakażeniu Helicobacter pylori (Rok 2004). Wytyczne opracowane przez Grupę Roboczą Polskiego Towarzystwa Gastroenterologii Gastroenterol Pol. 2004;11:41-48. Article In Polish.

[57] Grupa Robocza PTG-E do spraw zakażenia Helicobacter pylori: http://www.ptg-e.org.pl/helico.php

[58] European Helicobacter Study Group Current European concepts in the management of Helicobacter pylori infection. The Maastricht Consensus Report. Gut 1997;41:8-13.

[59] Malfertheiner P, Mégraud F, O'Morain C, Hungin AP, Jones R, Axon A, et al. European Helicobacter Pylori Study Group (EHPSG). Current concepts in the management of Helicobacter pylori infection-the Maastricht 2-2000 Consensus Report. Aliment Pharmacol Ther. 2002;16(2):167-180.

[60] Mégraud F. H pylori antibiotic resistance: prevalence, importance, and advances in testing. Gut. 2004;53(9):1374-1384.

[61] Megraud F, Coenen S, Versporten A, Kist M, Lopez-Brea M, Hirschl AM, Andersen LP, Goossens H, Glupczynski Y; Study Group participants. Helicobacter pylori resistance to antibiotics in Europe and its relationship to antibiotic consumption. Gut. 2013;62(1):34-42. doi: 10.1136/gutjnl-2012-302254. http://gut.bmj.com/content/62/1/34.long (accessed 13 July 2013).

[62] Karczewska E, Wojtas-Bonior I, Sito E, Zwolińska-Wcisło M, Budak A. Primary and secondary clarithromycin, metronidazole, amoxicillin and levofloxacin resistance to Helicobacter pylori in southern Poland. Pharmacol Rep. 2011;63(3):799-807.

[63] Agudo S, Pérez-Pérez G, Alarcón T, López-Brea M. Rapid detection of clarithromycin resistant Helicobacter pylori strains in Spanish patients by polymerase chain reaction-restriction fragment length polymorphism. Rev Esp Quimioter. 2011;24(1):32-36.

[64] Yang YJ, Wu JJ, Sheu BS, Kao AW, Huang AH. The rdxA gene plays a more major role than frxA gene mutation in high-level metronidazole resistance of Helicobacter pylori in Taiwan. Helicobacter. 2004;9(5):400-407.

[65] Rimbara E, Noguchi N, Kawai T, Sasatsu M. Fluoroquinolone resistance in Helicobacter pylori: role of mutations at position 87 and 91 of GyrA on the level of resistance and identification of a resistance conferring mutation in GyrB. Helicobacter. 2012;17(1):36-42.

[66] Gisbert JP, Calvet X. Review article: rifabutin in the treatment of refractory Helicobacter pylori infection. Aliment Pharmacol Ther. 2012;35(2):209-221.

[67] Gisbert JP. Rescue Therapy for Helicobacter pylori Infection 2012. Gastroenterol Res Pract. 2012;2012:974594. doi: 10.1155/2012/974594. http://www.hindawi.com/journals/grp/2012/974594/ (accessed 10 July 2013).

[68] European Committee on Antimicrobial Susceptibility Testing. Breakpoint tables for interpretation of MICs and zone diameters. Version 3.1. Available from: http://www.eucast.org/fileadmin/src/media/PDFs/EUCAST_files/Breakpoint_tables/Breakp (accessed 10 July 2013).

[69] Kargar M, Ghorbani-Dalini S, Doosti A, Souod N. Real-time PCR for Helicobacter pylori quantification and detection of clarithromycin resistance in gastric tissue from patients with gastrointestinal disorders. Res Microbiol. 2012;163(2):109-113.

[70] Chen XJ, Yan J, Shen YF. Dominant cagA/vacA genotypes and coinfection frequency of H. pylori in peptic ulcer or chronic gastritis patients in Zhejiang Province and correlations among different genotypes, coinfection and severity of the diseases. Chin Med J (Engl). 2005;118(6):460-467. http://www.cmj.org/ch/reader/view_abstract.aspx?volume=118&issue=6&start_page=460 (accessed 15 July 2013).

[71] Chisholm SA, Owen RJ, Teare EL, Saverymuttu S. PCR-Based Diagnosis of Helicobacter pylori Infection and Real-Time Determination of Clarithromycin Resistance Directly from Human Gastric Biopsy Samples. J Clin Microbiol. 2001;39(4):1217-1220.

[72] Occhialini A, Urdaci M, Doucet-Populaire F, Bébéar CM, Lamouliatte H, Mégraud F. Macrolide resistance in Helicobacter pylori: rapid detection of point mutations and assays of macrolide binding to ribosomes. Antimicrob Agents Chemother. 1997;41(12):2724-2728.

[73] van Doorn LJ. Detection of Helicobacter pylori virulence-associated genes. Expert Rev Mol Diagn. 2001;1(3):290-298.

[74] Palframan SL, Kwok T, Gabriel K. Vacuolating cytotoxin A (VacA), a key toxin for Helicobacter pylori pathogenesis. Front Cell Infect Microbiol. 2012;2:92. doi: 10.3389/fcimb.2012.00092.

7

The Mechanisms of Action and Resistance to Fluoroquinolone in *Helicobacter pylori* Infection

Carolina Negrei and Daniel Boda

1. Introduction

The discovery of the *Helicobacter pylori* (*H. pylori*) infection and its role in various diseases (from chronic gastritis to gastric cancer) has been a radical change in the therapeutic conduct of patients suffering from this condition [1, 2].

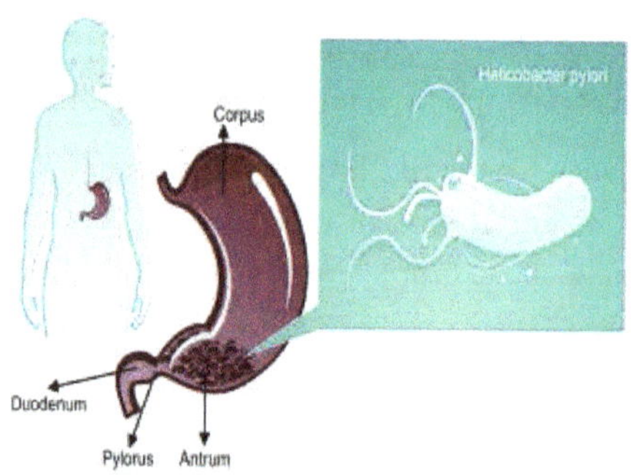

Figure 1. *Helicobacter pylori* infection

Unfortunately though, the purpose of inducing a cure of all first intention treated patients, as is the case in most ordinary infectious diseases, has not occurred in the *H. pylori* infection (Figure 1).

Current guidelines recommend triple therapy of a double dose proton pump inhibitor and two antibiotics chosen from among amoxicillin, clarithromycin and metronidazole for four to seven days, which is conducive to an eradication rate between 70-80%. Resistance to antibiotics, to clarithromycin and metronidazole in particular, is a major factor contributing to failure of the therapy [3, 4]; resistance to clarithromycin may lead to a decrease in efficiency to 70%, whereas the infection may persist up to about 20% of patients under treatment [5]. Such limitations have resulted in development of alternative therapies - "rescue" therapies – using medicines which have not been used as a first or second intention, such as fluoroquinolones (moxifloxacin, levofloxacin) and rifabutin (a derivative of rifamycin), which are commonly used in treatment of mycobacterial infections and are also highly efficient against *H. pylori* [5, 6].

Quinolones have been the focus of considerable scientific and clinical interest, since their very development in the early 1960s. This happened because such drugs possess many of the attributes of an ideal antibiotic, combining high potency, a broad spectrum of activity, good bioavailability, oral and intravenous formulations, high serum levels, a large volume of distribution, indicating concentration on a tissue level and potential low incidence of adverse reactions.

Nalidixic acid was the first quinolone to be developed. Subsequent medicines have been derived by manipulation at the level of their side chain and nucleus [7]. Development of the fluoroquinolone class may be described in terms of generations, each generation sharing similar characteristics or antimicrobial spectrum. The activity of first-generation medicines is more effective against gram-negative aerobic bacteria and less effective against gram-positive aerobic bacteria or anaerobic bacteria. Original fluoroquinolones are second-generation agents and they owe their name to the addition of a fluorine atom in the C6 position; they provide improved coverage against gram-negative bacteria and moderately improved coverage against gram-positive ones. Third-generation agents have greater efficacy against gram-positive bacteria, particularly against pneumococci, which is combined with good activity against anaerobic bacteria. Fourth generation fluoroquinolones provide superior coverage against pneumococci and anaerobic bacteria [8].

2. Clinical indications of fluoroquinolones

Fluoroquinolones such as levofloxacin are indicated in: acute bacterial sinusitis (diagnosed according to national guidelines on treatment of infections of the respiratory tract and where use of antibacterial agents commonly recommended for initial treatment of this infection is considered inappropriate or in case of their failure to cure the infection), acute bacterial exacerbations of chronic bronchitis (diagnosed according to national guidelines on treatment of respiratory tract infections and where use of antibacterial agents commonly recommended for initial treatment of this infection is considered inappropriate or in case of their failure to cure the infection), community acquired pneumonia (where use of antibacterial agents commonly recommended for initial treatment of this infection is considered inappropriate), uncomplicated urinary tract infections (including pyelonephritis), chronic bacterial prostatitis and skin and soft tissue infections.

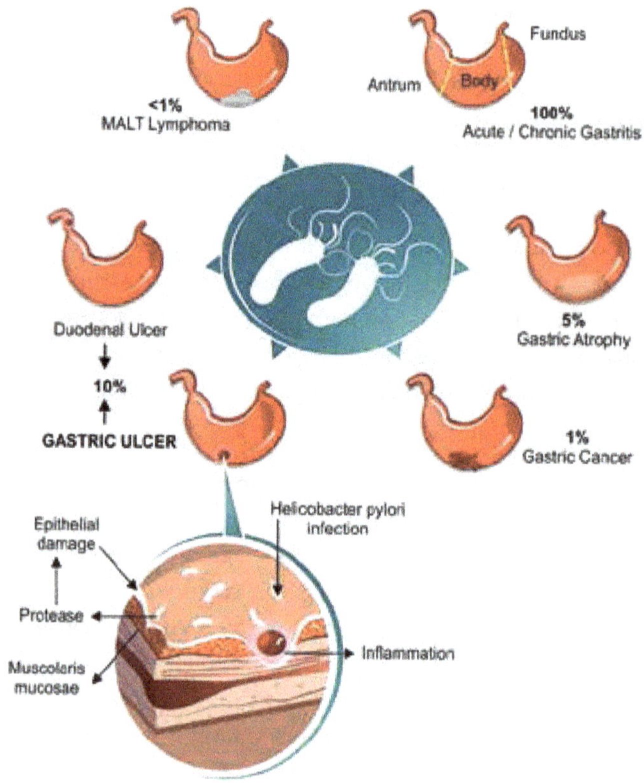

Figure 2. Diseases involving *Helicobacter pylori*

At the same time, as mentioned before, fluoroquinolones are implicated in *H. pylori* eradication. Indications for a *H. pylori* eradication therapy are defined in consensus guidelines. These indications include peptic ulcer disease, low-grade gastric mucosa-associated lymphoid tissue lymphoma, atrophic gastritis and after resection of early gastric cancer (Figure 2).

The following are included in the *H. pylori* elimination:

First-line treatment: should be considered as the first-line therapy in areas with high prevalence of *H. pylori* resistance to clarithromycin, in the frame of the new sequential ten-day scheme. Sequential therapy includes a dual therapy (proton pump inhibitor and amoxicillin for five days), followed by triple therapy with a proton pump inhibitor, clarithromycin and metronidazole for five days. The eradication rate achieved by sequential therapy has shown higher values, than those obtained with standard therapy [9, 10]. However, sequential therapy has been shown ineffective in eradicating *H. pylori* in patients with dual resistance to clarithromycin and metronidazole [11, 12]. A new aspect of the scheme as concomitant therapy is a fourth medicine – a non-bismuth-containing regimen (proton pump inhibitor, clarithromycin, amoxicillin and metronidazole), which seems more appropriate for patients in highly endemic areas and with dual resistance. Clinically speaking, this is much easier than sequential therapy and can improve compliance, because medicines are administered concurrently, instead of changed in mid therapy An intention-to-treat analysis demonstrated that sequential or concomitant therapy with a PPI, amoxicillin, clarithromycin and an imidazole agent has similar rates for eradication of *H. pylori* infection [10]. As far as dual resistance is concerned, several attempts have been made such as extension of sequential therapy and continuation with amoxicillin therapy for all 14 days, in order to improve effectiveness of standard triple therapy and proton pump inhibitors. A hybrid sequential-concomitant therapy has been recently designed by Hsu et al. [13]. Data have shown promising success rate: 99% by per-protocol analysis and 97% by intention-to-treat analysis. However, it should be noted this may not be effective in all geographic areas and results will have to be confirmed in areas where different patterns of resistance are present.

Second-line therapy: bismuth is a component of quadruple therapy and/or rescue therapy recommended by the Maastricht IV/Florence Consensus Report [7]. Several multicentre studies regarding quadruple therapy using a single triple medicine (bismuth, metronidazole and tetracycline), in a capsule pharmaceutical formulation together with a proton pump inhibitor have shown good efficacy in *H. pylori* eradication [14-16]. With regard to adverse reactions, bismuth induced toxic effects are still one of the unnecessary safety concerns in relation to quadruple therapy [17]; therefore, a reasonable bismuth dose regimen needs to be established to ensure maximum eradication. In patients where first-line treatment has failed, e.g., clarithromycin-based triple therapy, levofloxacine-based triple therapy (levofloxacin, amoxicillin and a proton pump inhibitor), a meta-analysis has shown this therapy to be superior to quadruple therapy and be accompanied by fewer adverse reactions than rescue therapy [18]. In addition, the study has shown that antibiotics (e.g., levofloxacin) in this triple therapy should not be changed randomly and then switched to first-line treatment. As far as antibiotic resistance is concerned, growth rates of levofloxacin resistance, particularly in developing countries, are to be taken into account, since resistance to quinolones is related to the status of patients having used fluoroquinolones for other indications [19].

Third-line treatment: the third-line treatment standard for refractory *H. pylori* infection has not been established. The Maastricht IV/Florence Consensus Report recommends conducting anti-*H. pylori* therapy according to results of susceptibility testing after failure of second-line therapy, whenever possible [7]. Unfortunately, antimicrobial sensitivity data for patients in whom eradication therapy has failed are not yet widely available in clinical practice.

Practitioners need a few simple strategies for empirical management. A prospective study has assessed the efficacy and safety of levofloxacin, amoxicillin, bismuth and rabeprazole, as a quadruple therapy, with regard to third-line treatment in patients where eradication of *H. pylori* infection has failed. In this study, the ten-day quadruple rescue therapy, based on levofloxacin and amoxicillin, ensured better eradication with a significant additional clinical benefit involving improvement of tolerability due to fewer adverse reactions [18]. Other alternative agents that are candidates for third-line treatment are rifabutin and quinolones, which also have promising results [20-22], although the optimal dose and the combination require further study (Table 1).

Treatment			Regimens									Duration of treatment
			A	C	M	T	L	R	F	B	PPI	
First line therapy	Standard triple therapy		1g b.i.d.	0. 5g b.i.d.							SD b.i.d.	7-14 days
	Concomitant therapy		1g b.i.d.	0. 5g b.i.d.	0. 5g b.i.d.						SD b.i.d.	7-10 days
	Bismuth-containing quadruple therapy				0. 25g q.i.d.	0. 5g q.i.d.				0. 48g q.i.d.	SD b.i.d.	10-14 days
	Sequential therapy	First phase	1g b.i.d.								SD b.i.d.	5 days
		Second phase		0. 5g b.i.d.	0. 5g b.i.d.						SD b.i.d.	5 days
	Hybrid therapy	First phase	1g b.i.d								SD b.i.d.	7 days
		Second phase	1g b.i.d.	0. 5g b.i.d.	0. 5g b.i.d.						SD b.i.d.	7 days
Second line therapy	Bismuth-containing quadruple therapy				0. 5g t.i.d.	0. 5g q.i.d.				0. 48g q.i.d.	SD b.i.d.	10-14 days
	Levofloxacin-based triple therapy		0. 5g b.i.d.				0. 5g q.i.d.				SD b.i.d.	10 days
Third line therapy	Culture guided therapy		Sensitivity tests – two antibiotics selected							0. 48 q.i.d.	SD b.i.d.	NA
	Levofloxacin-based quadruple therapy		0. 5g q.i.d.				0. 5g q.i.d.			0. 48 q.i.d.	SD b.i.d.	10 days
	Rifabutin-based triple therapy		1g b.i.d.					0. 15g b.i.d.			SD b.i.d.	14 days
	Furazolidone-based quadruple therapy					1g b.i.d.			0. 2g b.i.d.	0. 24g b.i.d.	SD b.i.d.	NA

A = amoxicillin, C = clarithromycin, M = metronidazole, T = tetracycline, L = levofloxacin, R = rifabutin, F = furazolidone, SD = standard dose, B = bismuth, PPI = proton pump inhibitor

Table 1. Recommended regimens for the treatment of *H. pylori* infections in adults

3. Safety of fluoroquinolones

3.1. Overview

As a class of medicines, fluoroquinolones are generally well tolerated; most adverse reactions are mild, self-limiting and rarely require treatment discontinuation [23]. The most frequently occurring adverse reactions class consists of gastrointestinal trouble (nausea, vomiting, diarrhoea, constipation and abdominal pain, about 7% of all adverse reactions). Less common are adverse reactions include those involving the central nervous system (less than 5%), kidney disorders (approximately 4. 5%), skin hypersensitivity reactions and photosensitivity reactions (approximately 2%). In rare cases, convulsions, psychosis and tendonitis have been reported [24]. Some of these events may not be directly attributed to fluoroquinolone therapy, but to other underlying conditions in the patient, including additional therapies not related to the microbial infection but still contributing to adverse reactions. Phototoxicity could be observed over a longer period in relation to administration of lomefloxacin, sparfloxacin and clinafloxacine, which has been determined to be a dose-dependent phenomenon requiring direct or indirect exposure to UVA rays and also closely correlated with the presence of a habide in the C8 position.

Serious adverse reactions have been developed following introduction to the use of the following three agents: temafloxacin, grepafloxacin and trovafloxacine.

Temafloxacin syndrome has been characterized by haemolytic anaemia, renal failure, hepatotoxicity, disseminated intravascular coagulation and hypoglycaemia [28]. Approximately two thirds of patients with "temafloxacin syndrome" develop acute renal failure. In addition, slight hepatobiliary changes have been observed in half of patients, whereas coagulopathy has been observed in a third of patients. Development of such adverse reactions resulted in withdrawal of temafloxacin from the market in 1992 [26]. Adverse reactions to temafloxacin not shown in the clinical trials conducted were observed at a rate of 1/3500 patients after placement on the market. In contrast, rare adverse reactions similar to those seen in temafloxacin have been reported with ciprofloxacin. This is significant, considering that ciprofloxacin has the largest database regarding fluoroquinolone safety information. Further analysis of such specific temafloxacin events have demonstrated that data involving norfloxacin and ofloxacin have been similar to those of ciprofloxacin. Specifically, such effects have been observed in 1/17000 patients treated with ciprofloxacin, in 1/25000 patients treated with norfloxacin and in 1/30000 patients treated with ofloxacin [25].

Grepafloxacin was placed on the market in 1997 and subsequently withdrawn in 1999 because of serious cardiovascular reports of adverse reactions in patients who had been administered this medicine [27]. The association between grepafloxacin and serious cardiovascular adverse reactions became evident after extended clinical use. Starting with grepafloxacin placement on the market to its withdrawal in 1999, torsades de pointes were observed in 7/3.7 million patients [27]. Trovafloxacin was authorized based on clinical efficacy trials conducted on batches including more than 6000 patients treated with this medicine. In these studies, 5% of patients discontinued trovafloxacin treatment because of adverse events, the most common of which included those on the central nervous system and gastrointestinal tract levels. As with temafloxacin, adverse reactions had not been clearly associated with use of the medicinal product before extended clinical use. Serious adverse reactions associated with trovafloxacin included liver eosinophilia and hypoglycaemia [29], observed post-marketing.

All the adverse reactions described above have resulted in limiting the use of these medicines to hospital use only, in cases of severe life-threatening infections [29]. Whereas withdrawal of temafloxacin and grepafloxacin from the market has raised concerns about the safety of fluoroquinolones, in considering the evaluation of their safety and efficacy, several aspects have required balancing. Despite rigorous preclinical studies, once a medicine is placed on the market for widespread clinical use, the likelihood of observing rare but serious adverse reactions is significantly increased [29]. It is important to recognize the low incidence of adverse reactions and serious adverse reactions in other agents of the same class, which generally demonstrates the relative safety of this class of medicines [23].

3.2. Categorization of adverse effects

Adverse reactions of levofloxacin consist of: disorders such as tachycardia, ventricular arrhythmia and torsades de pointes (reported predominantly in patients with risk factors for QT prolongation), ECG QT prolonged, leukopoenia, eosinophilia, thrombocytopenia, neutropoenia, dizziness, headaches, drowsiness, convulsion, tremors, paraesthesia, vertigo, impaired hearing, bronchospasm, dyspnoea, diarrhoea, nausea, vomiting, abdominal pain, dyspepsia, flatulence, constipation, increased blood creatinine, rashes, pruritis, urticaria, tendon disorders including tendinitis (e.g., in the Achilles tendon), arthralgia, myalgia, anorexia, fungal infections (and proliferation of other resistant microorganisms), hypotension, asthenia, increased hepatic enzymes (aspartate aminotransferase/alanine aminotransferas, alkaline phosphatise and gamma-glutamyl transpeptidase) and increased blood bilirubin [30].

Many of the fluoroquinolone adverse reactions are associated with quinolone pharmacore in positions one, seven and eight. In the following sections, the discussion focuses on class specific reactions regarding structural modifications in positions one, seven and eight [25].

Adverse reactions on the central nervous system level: although much information about the pathophysiology of fluoroquinolone induced central nervous system adverse reactions remain less well defined, one hypothesis suggests that drug interactions with the gamma-aminobutyric acid (GABA) receptor, an inhibitory neurotransmitter, may explain the stimulant effects at this level.

Affinity for the GABA receptor seems to be triggered by the R7 side chain substituent, unsubstituted piperazinyl and pyrrolidinyl moieties in particular. In this respect, agents with an unsubstituted piperazinyl ring (ciprofloxacin, enoxacine and norfloxacin) display high-affinity binding to GABA as well as interference with GABA binding to its receptor. It has been demonstrated that biphenyl acetic acid, which is an active metabolite of fenbufen, a nonsteroidal anti-inflammatory medicine, enhances binding of fluoroquinolones to GABA receptors.

Concurrent administration of fenbufen and fluoroquinolones has been shown to be capable of inducing seizures in mice; certain researchers however have observed that alterations in GABA receptor binding mediated by quinolone are weak and may not fully explain reactions at the central nervous system level [31]. It was noted that seven Japanese patients developed seizures following concurrent administration of enoxacine and fenbufen. Studies have also shown that penetration of quinolones at the CNS level does not seem to be correlated with the incidence of adverse reactions at this level [25]. A possible understanding of such discrepancies is that fluoroquinolones may also induce excitatory effects by means of direct activation of N-methyl-D-aspartate (NMDA) and adenosine-receptor mechanisms. It is therefore possible that the events mentioned may occur at this level only under special circumstances, when sufficient penetration is possible in the CNS, coupled with threshold antagonism of inhibitory pathways (GABA) and stimulation of excitatory pathways (NMDA, adenosine).

Ofloxacin and levofloxacin, its levorotatory isomer, have been observed to induce a number of adverse reactions at the central nervous system level, including headaches (9% ofloxacin, 6% levofloxacin), dizziness (5% ofloxacin, 3% levofloxacin) and less common events such as confusion, impaired thinking, insomnia and psychosis, in rare cases. Such reactions were induced even in the absence of concomitant medications such as NSAIDs [25] and they tend to occur more frequently with ofloxacin than levofloxacin.

Genetic Toxicology: quinolones have been shown to inhibit mammalian cell topoisomerase II, a mechanism correlating with the occurrence of in vitro cytotoxicity, on the level of these cells [30]. Substitutions and positions one, seven and eight have the greatest potential cytotoxicity and the effect is additive. However, chromosomal disruption or clastogenicity usually occurs only at very high concentrations of the medicine (300 to 10000 times the therapeutic dose) and in post-marketing studies was not shown to have carcinogenic potential.

Cardiovascular adverse reactions: cardiovascular adverse reactions, particularly prolongation of the heart rate corrected QT interval (the QTc interval) have been reported with quinolone therapy [30]. Sparfloxacin increases the QTc interval in up to 3% of patients [32]. Such significant results involving serious cardiac events have led to the withdrawal of grepafloxacin. Sparfloxacin is not recommended for administration in patients with a history of QT prolongation or patients receiving concomitant therapy likely to increase the interval, induce bradycardia or cause torsades de pointes (e.g., class Ia and III antiarrhythmics, bepridil, cisapride, erythromycin, terfenadine or tricyclic antidepressants). It seems possible that this effect may be more predictable with medicines administered concurrently with quinolones inhibiting cytochrome P450-mediated metabolizing, because of drug accumulation. So far, no specific structural change has been associated with adverse cardiovascular outcomes, including those possibly affecting cytochrome P450-involving metabolism. Currently, the only possible specific structural changes that may be associated with increased incidence of serious cardiovascular events in relation to grepafloxacin or sparfloxacin therapy consist of a methyl or amino moiety in position C5 (of grepafloxacin, sparfloxacin, respectively) [32]. In light of experience acquired with sparfloxacin and grepafloxacin concerning adverse cardiovascular outcomes, more recent members of this class of medicines have been studied with particular focus on these reactions [30].

4. Basic antimicrobial activity

4.1. Pharmacokinetics

Fluoroquinolones have favourable pharmacokinetic properties, which have encouraged their extensive use. They are well absorbed and show good tissue penetration, which favours their use in many clinical syndromes. Whereas ciprofloxacin requires frequent administration, the long half-life of new generation fluoroquinolones allows use in daily single doses.

Most fluoroquinolones are eliminated renally. Moxifloxacin elimination involves the liver and this is one of the fluoroquinolones lacking effectiveness in treatment of genitourinary infections. In general, because they are not as highly bound to plasma proteins and because of CYP1A2 enzyme-limited inhibition of CYP450, drug interactions are somewhat minimized [33-35]. Fluoroquinolones have been shown to interact with xanthines, theophylline and caffeine, which is matter of concern with older generation agents [36]. Concurrent use of fluoroquinolone and warfarin may result in excessive anticoagulation [37]. Probably the most common interactions involve cationic di- and trivalents. Administration with antacids may result in subtherapeutic fluoroquinolone levels, thus raising potential therapeutic failure. This may be particularly relevant in an "inpatient setting", because of the frequent fluoroquinolone and antacids association; co-administration of agents mentioned previously has raised the issue of emergence of resistance to fluoroquinolones [38, 39].

In terms of levofloxacin involved in *H. pylori* eradication therapy, oral administration is rapidly and almost completely followed by levofloxacin absorption, with a peak concentration achieved within one hour. Absolute bioavailability is approximately 100% and food has a low impact on levofloxacin absorption.

Approximately 30-40% of levofloxacin is bound to plasmatic proteins and a therapy involving a 500mg dose once daily for several days has shown non-significant accumulation. However, there is modest but predictable accumulation after therapy involving 500mg twice daily, with a balance reached within three days. Levofloxacin metabolism is very scarce and its metabolites are "desmethyl-levofloxacine" and "levofloxacin N-oxide". These metabolites contribute to less than 5% of the urine-excreted dose. Levofloxacin is stereochemically stable and undergoes no chiral inversion. Following oral or intravenous administration, levofloxacin is relatively slowly eliminated from plasma (t1/2 = 6-8 hours). The chief route of excretion is mainly renal (>85% of the dose administered). There are no major differences in levofloxacin pharmacokinetics in terms of oral versus intravenous administration, which leads to the conclusion that oral and intravenous administration are interchangeable.

4.2. Pharmacodynamics

Pharmacokinetics (PK) regards the time course of antimicrobial concentrations in the body; on the other hand, pharmacodyamics (PD) provides insight into the relationship between such concentrations and the effect on antimicrobial level.

Traditionally, doses of antibiotic therapeutic schemes only determined the pharmacokinetics; however, pharmacodynamics plays an equally, if not more important, role.

In this period of increased antimicrobial resistance, pharmacodynamics is becoming perhaps the most important because it can be used in the design of a dosage regimen to prevent resistance [40, 41].

The primary parameter of antibiotic activity is the minimum inhibitory concentration (MIC). MIC is the lowest concentration of an antibiotic able to completely inhibit in vitro microorganism growth. Whereas MIC is a reliable indicator of antibiotic potency, it has no relevance in terms of the time course of antimicrobial activity.

Pharmacokinetic parameters quantify the time course of an antibiotic level. The three pharmacokinetic parameters most important in evaluating effectiveness of the antibiotic are the peak serum level (Cmax), the minimum level (Cmin) and the area under the serum concentration time curve (AUC). Whereas these parameters quantify the serum level over a certain period of time, they describe the destruction activity of an antibiotic.

Integration of pharmacokinetic parameters and MIC provides three pharmacokinetic/ pharmacodynamic (PK/PD) parameters quantifying the activity of an antibiotic: the peak/MIC ratio, the T>MIC and the ratio 24h-AUC/MIC

- the peak / MIC ratio is Cmax divided by MIC
- the T>MIC (time above MIC) is the percentage of a dosing interval when the serum level reaches MIC
- the 24h-AUC/MIC ratio is determined by dividing the 24-hour-AUC by MIC [40, 41].

The three pharmacodynamic properties of antibiotics best describing the destruction activity are time-dependent, concentration-dependent and the presence of persistent effects. The destruction rate is determined by either the time needed for destruction (time-dependent) or the effect of increased concentration (concentration-dependent). Persistent effects include post-antibiotic effect, which is the persistence of suppression of bacterial growth after exposure to antibiotics.

For fluoroquinolones, the best dosing regimen would maximize the concentration, as higher concentrations cause a superior and faster degree of destruction, therefore the "24h-AUC/MIC ratio" and the "peak/MIC ratio" are important predictors for antibiotic efficacy.

In this case, as far as fluoroquinolones are concerned, the "24h-AUC/MIC ratio" for Gram-negative bacteria (*H. pylori* included) is about 125 and 40, respectively, for Gram-positive bacteria. For Gram-negative bacteria, however, the "24h-AUC/MIC ratio" for the group of medicines described above, the reports vary widely in the literature [40, 41].

4.3. Mechanisms of action

The process of fluoroquinolone interference in cell replication, transcription and DNA repair consists in disabling DNA gyrase (previously topoisomerase II) and topoisomerase IV, two processes essential to bacterial enzymes (Figure 3).

Essentially a tetramer of two A and two B subunits, DNA gyrase is subject to encoding performed by gyrA and gyrB [42]. It brings in negative DNA supercoils, also removing both positive and negative supercoils and acts on chromosomal material by catenating and decatenating it [43].

The other bacterial enzyme mentioned above is topoisomerase IV, which is a homologue of DNA gyrase. This consists of two E and two E subunits, both subject to parC- and parE-encoding [42]. Similarly to its homologue, topoisomerase IV this is also able to remove both negative and positive supercoils; however, its main involvement remains contribution to separating of the daughter chromosome [33, 43] (Figure 4).

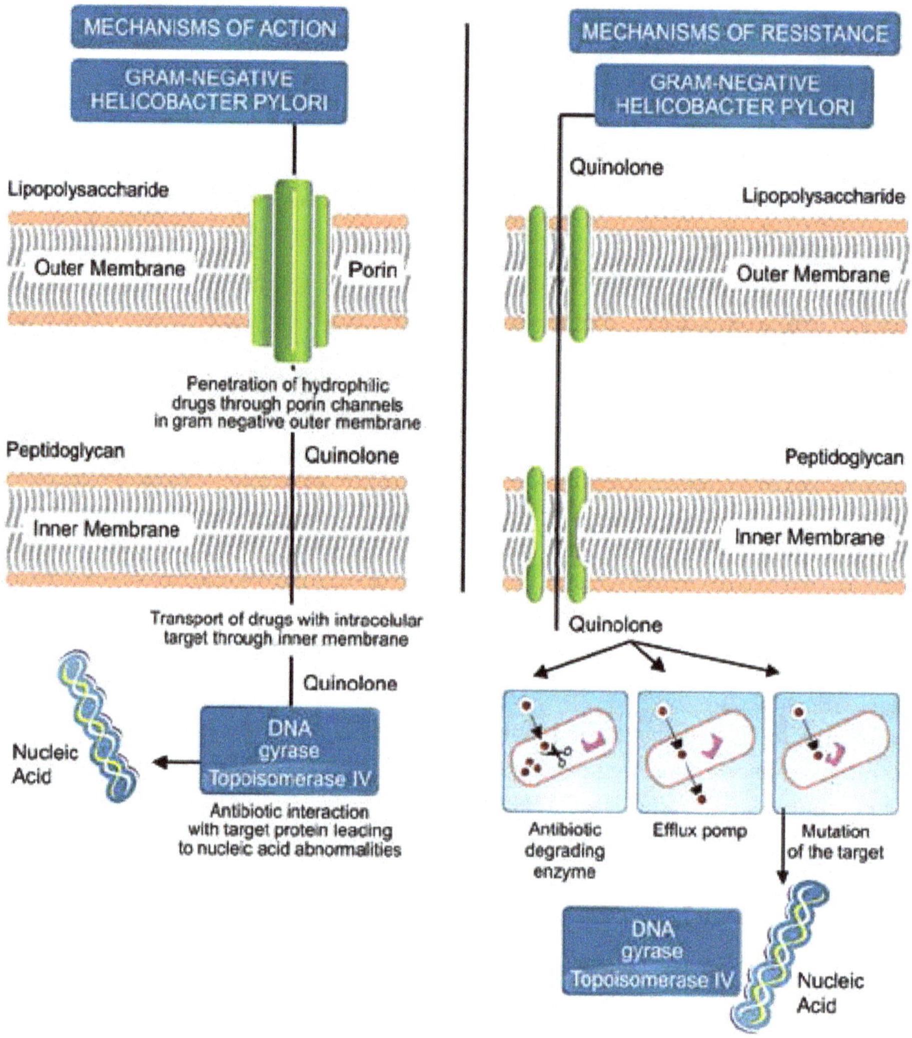

Figure 3. Mechanisms of action/Mechanisms of resistance

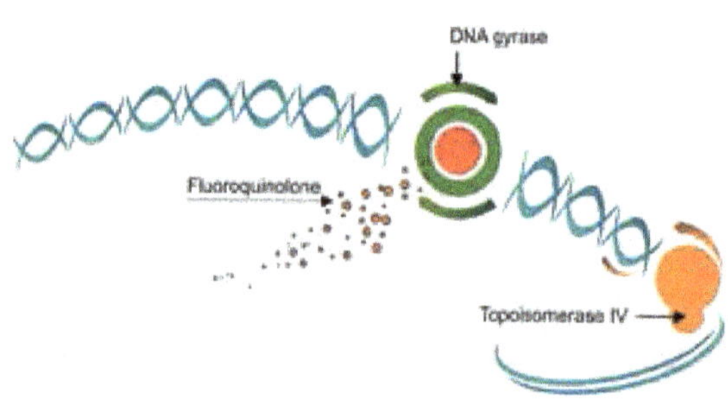

Figure 4. Fluoroquinolones bind the two nuclear enzymes, inhibiting DNA replication

The binding of fluoroquinolones to the complex made up of enzyme–DNA determines the change in enzyme conformation. This results in enzyme cleaving of the DNA, while ligation of broken DNA strands is prevented by the continued presence of the fluoroquinolone. Continuation of DNA replication is inhibited by the process in which the enzyme on the DNA is "trapped" by fluoroquinolone as a complex of fluoroquinolone–enzyme–DNA. DNA cleavage is generally held responsible for the destructive action of fluoroquinolones on bacteria [42, 43].

5. General mechanisms of fluoroquinolone resistance

Regarding quinolone resistance reported during treatment, it has been observed that, in the context of its rather extended use during the twenty years after its placement on the market, it was not commonly observed except for cases involving Staphylococcus aureus and notably P. aeruginosa and S. aureus, which were resistant to methicillin.

These two species have been observed to rapidly develop resistance to fluoroquinolones, which has been attributed to clonal spread occurring in immunocompromised patients and nursing home settings [44].

Starting around 1995 however, increased quinolone resistance has been noted in most Gram-negative (*H. pylori*) and Gram-positive species. At the same time, it has become evident that species were broadly varied (from ≤0.015 up to ≥128 mg/l [45-47]) by minimal concentrations (MICs) that inhibited 90% of the strains under study; this showed the common character of resistant subpopulations over the same period of time after placement on the market, which had however not been noticed.

In light of more recent studies involving surveillance of the issue, resistance rates have been shown to further increase and therefore have an impact on the management of patients.

5.1. Interaction with bacterial DNA gyrase and topoisomerase IV

From among antimicrobial agents in common clinical use, fluoroquinolones are the only class that directly inhibit synthesis of bacterial DNA. There are two bacterial enzymes with distinct and essential roles in DNA replication, called DNA gyrase and topoisomerase IV, which are inhibited by fluoroquinolones. The respective process involves binding quinolones to the complex with DNA of each such enzyme, which results in a ternary complex of topoisomerase-quinolone-DNA. Subsequently, this complex induces the generation of double-stranded breaks in DNA, further blocking progress of the DNA replication enzyme complex.

The final result of this action is damaged bacterial DNA and ultimately death of bacterial cells [48-51].

The responsibility for quinolones resistance lies with mutation in chromosomal genes. This occurs by means of two mechanisms: the altered target mechanism, on one hand, involving encoding DNA-gyrase and topoisomerase IV subunits and the altered permeation mechanism, on the other hand, regulating expression of proteins or cytoplasmic membrane efflux pumps, both of which make up the channels for outer membrane diffusion.

A further mechanism for the generation of low-level quinolone resistance has been considered, reduced target expression [52].

5.2. Response of the SOS gene network

Inhibition of bacterial type II topoisomerases activates repair mechanisms in response. This is because each piece of DNA damage activates an SOS gene network, which initiates the generation of repair proteins of various kinds [53-57]. There are over 40 genes making up this so-called SOS system, which is under the control of regulatory RecA and LexA proteins. The former is in charge of generating a signal triggering the SOS response, whereas the latter has a repressor function. The process consists of gene repressor LexA binding, which results in the unmasking of its autoproteolytic activity and subsequent ending of repression of the 40 SOS genes. The respective LexA binding takes place in the sequence up from qnrB (but not qnrS or qnrA). Therefore, in response to DNA damage, the SOS-system regulates qnrB as well [58]. Furthermore, the SOS response has recently been shown to promote qnrB expression [59].

Bacterial DNA-topoisomerases are protected from quinolone inhibition by the QnrB peptide, which also renders low-level resistance to quinolone. On the contrary, high-level resistance emerges with facilitation of the Qnr-determinants. It should also be noted that, in the case of *E. coli*, this particular effect directly depends on the increased ability for mutation due to action of nonessential polymerases Pol II, Pol IV and Pol V over the de-repression of the genes polB, dinB and umuDC, respectively, mediated by the LexA-cleavage.

In this way, the same signal of the SOS response triggers both increased mutation ability and qnrB-mediated quinolone resistance.

Because of the RecA/LexA-dependent manner in which ciprofloxacin upregulates the qnrB quinolone resistance gene, the development of quinolone resistance is integral to their action mode in bacteria harbouring qnrB.

LexA positive wild-type strains are much more liable to elicit ciprofloxacin resistant mutants than their mutant counterparts [60, 61]. The reverse is also true – prevention of LexA cleavage results in bacterial inability to develop fluoroquinolone resistance [60, 61].

The ability of the SOS response to induce persistent fluoroquinolone should also be mentioned [62].

From the above outcomes inference may occur in the role of fluoroquinolones as more than simply selectors of resistant variants, as well as on the active role of bacteria themselves in their own genomes' mutation.

Resistance to quinolone is acquired by means of both mutations in the target site and by the SOS system induced de-repression of genes, whose products increase rates of mutation.

The emergence of resistance may generally be reduced by interference with the response of bacterial stress [63].

In *E. coli*, ciprofloxacin has recently been shown to stimulate recombination of divergent DNA sequences that is independent from the SOS system.

Genetic variation may also be increased by fluoroquinolones by means of a second mechanism, which is SOS independent [64] and may also favour acquisition, evolution and the spread of resistance determinants.

Besides quinolones as DNA damaging agents, the SOS gene network response is triggered by other factors as well, such as beta-lactams interfering with penicillin binding protein 3 [65, 66], zidovudine or trimethoprim [67] and rifampicin [60].

As shown by these data, persistence and evolution of resistance in general is facilitated by induction of the SOS response by means of any of these medicines classes.

Given the above, speculation becomes possible concerning the ability of these agents to also affect quinolone activity and/or development of resistance via the expression of qnrB as promoted by the SOS system.

In turn, the SOS system further promotes horizontal dissemination of antibiotic-resistance genes [68] or mutations, thus contributing to the spread of antibiotic resistance.

5.3. Plasmid mediated resistance

Usually, genetic information for the efflux resistance mechanisms or the targeted site is chromosomally encoded.

In this context however, there have been reports of resistance to fluoroquinolones mediated by plasmids, which renders such resistance transferable (Figure 5).

This involves a number of mechanisms, such as:

1. Qnr
2. Aminoglycoside acetyltransferase AAC(6_)-Ib-cr
3. OqxAB, QepA [69-72]

Plasmid-mediated resistance to quinolone was first found in 1998, emerging in strains of Klebsiella pneumoniae in one US region [73]. The emergence was determined to be induced by one of the members of the pentapeptide repeat (PPR) family of proteins, Qnr (subsequently referred to as QnrA).

Later on, several related plasmid-mediated Qnr determinants were communicated in Enterobacteriaceae (QnrB, QnrC, Qnr D, QnrS) that were distantly related [74, 75].

These have been further found in the entire world and almost invariably in association with expanded spectrum β-lactamases production [76-78].

Gram-positive bacteria M. smegmatis Mycobacterium tuberculosis, M. avium [79], E. faecalis [80], C. perfringens, Listeria monocytogenes, C. difficile and E. faecium [81] have been found to display Qnr-like peptides (that share a 16 to 22% amino-acid identity with QnrA).

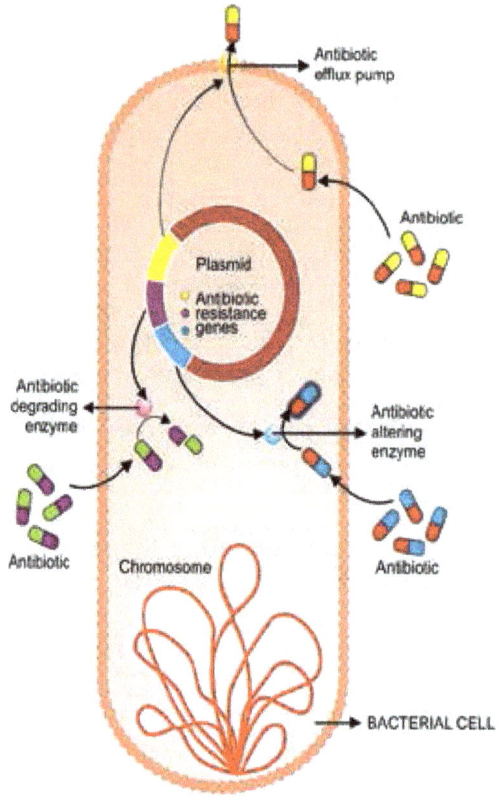

Figure 5. Plasmid mediated resistance

Stenotrophomonas maltophilia has recently shown the emergence of a new quinolone resistance gene of the PPR family that was chromosomally encoded, which has accordingly been called Smqnr [82]. Serratia marcescens has never been found to display the smaqnr gene[83].

Quinolone inhibition is prevented by the interaction of topoisomerase IV and DNA-gyrase with Qnr [69, 84].

The Qnr protein induces resistance to nalidixic acid and diminished susceptibility to fluoroquinolone resistance or low-levels of fluoroquinolone resistance [84].

Identification of Qnr-genes in isolates susceptible to ciprofloxacin and isolates displaying resistance to quinolones has made it possible to infer from laboratory results that because of chromosomal mutation, presence of Qnr-genes promotes higher-level resistance.

That is why there exists the possibility that development of quinolone resistance in clinically relevant species of both Gram-negative and Gram-positive bacteria can be fostered by presence of qnr genes.

In addition, the qnrA and qnrB genes usually make up integrons containing genes such as aminoglycoside inactivating enzymes or β-lactamases, which are responsible for resistance to other antibiotics.

Integrons do not contain qnrS genes, but these genes however associate with TEM-1 type β-lactamases-containing transposons [85].

As a result, the association of genes that encode resistance to both quinolone and other medicine classes like aminoglycosides and β-lactams are favourable to selection and subsequent dissemination by chemically unrelated medicines classes of strains that are resistant to fluoroquinolones.

The reverse is also found concerning fluoroquinolones selecting and disseminating aminoglycoside or β-lactam resistant strains (please see the sections related to resistance to fluoroquinolones for issues regarding the tight correlation between and quinolone resistance and production of extended spectrum β-lactamases (ESBL)).

The chromosome of Shewanella algae, a bacterium found in environmental water has also been found to display Qnr genes.

The discovery of other qnr homologs in the genome sequences characterizing several Photobacterium profundum and Vibrio spp. suggests the possibility of water-borne Vibrionaceae as a source of qnr genes and also a reservoir [86-88].

Recent in vitro tests have shown the possibility for transfer of the plasmid borne Shewanella algae qnr gene to Enterobacteriaceae [86].

A further discovery envisages a plasmid-encoded determinant of resistance to quinolones, a variant of the aac(6_)Ib gene that encodes an aminoglycoside acetyltransferase.

The process of acetylation of both medicine classes is catalysed by AAC(6_)-Ib-cr, the bifunctional fluoroquinolone and aminoglycoside active variant [89].

This variant enzyme has become able to acetylate norfloxacin and ciprofloxacin as well as to determine a fourfold reduction of ciprofloxacin activity [90, 91].

Because of the absence in position C-7 of a piperazinyl substituent, levofloxacin and moxifloxacin do not undergo acetylation.

Interestingly, S. marcescens, the first clinical isolate determined as ciprofloxacin resistant, was found prior to the introduction of quinolone treatment in a patient treated with an aminoglycoside and a β-lactam. In that context, ciprofloxacin MIC during pre-therapy was 0.06, whereas the respective post-therapy MIC was 4mg/L.

The strain in question underwent changes in the composition of its outer-membrane and produced an aminoglycoside acetyltransferase [92].

It is possible that Qnr- determinants are less widespread than AAC(6_)-Ib-cr.

ESBL production is associated with the production of both AAC(6_)-Ib-cr- and Qnr-, which may therefore be considered a second mechanism for co-selection of drug-resistance induced by exposure to agents that are chemically unrelated.

A third type of plasmid-mediated resistance to quinolones has been recently identified, consisting of the quinolone efflux pumps Qep and OqxAB, [70-72, 93, 94].

The QepA and OqxAB proteins are responsible for the induction of resistance to hydrophilic fluoroquinolones such as ciprofloxacin, norfloxacin and enrofloxacin, leading to a 32- to 64-fold MIC increase [93-96].

As far as QepA is concerned, in addition to quinolones, this extrudes a restricted range of agents such as ethidium bromide, erythromycin and acrifliavine.

In turn, OqxAB is responsible for the export of a wider range of agents among which are tetracyclines, chloramphenicol, ethidium bromide, olaquindox, trimethoprim and disinfectants such as triclosan [85, 96, 97].

However, the issue here is the presence of a transposable element also consisting of an aminoglycoside ribosome methyltransferase and the qepA gene [94]. This allows for the possibility for both aminoglycosides to select QepA determinants and for quinolones to select aminoglycoside resistance, which is also true in what concerns aac(6_)Ib gene mediated resistances.

A third mechanism for cross-resistance consists of extrusion by efflux-pumps of chemically unrelated agents.

To conclude, it appears that, even in the absence of exposure to this medicine, class resistance to fluoroquinolones can emerge. This can be explained by the action of several co-selection mechanisms, which all support emergence of quinolone resistance.

Identification in 50–70% of *E. coli* clinical isolates displaying high-level quinolone resistance (MICs up to 1500-fold higher than expected) of the multidrug efflux pump AcrAB, as well as of known plasmid- and chromosomally- mediated resistance mechanisms, makes it reasonable to infer the existence of additional mechanisms inducing quinolone resistance that have yet to be discovered

5.4. Other resistance mechanisms

In order to reach its target, all antibacterial agents that interact with an intracellular target have to cross the bacterial cell wall and then the cytoplasmic membrane. The process continues with active efflux of most antibacterial agents taken up.

This explains why permeation barriers and efflux pumps affect fluoroquinolones as well, whether accompanied by target modifications or just by themselves.

As indicated earlier, there are many, many Gram- positive and Gram-negative mutant strains resistant to fluoroquinolone, which did not display mutation in the region determining quinolone resistance (QRDR).

For instance, absence of classical QRDR mutations was observed in 70% of *E. coli* mutant variants recovered from besifloxacin selection plates [99]. At the same time, 39% of wild type *E. coli* accumulated higher levels of ciprofloxacin than high-level ciprofloxacine-resistant isolates. To this, one must add the gyrA mutations detected in all [100].

In addition, fluoroquinolone susceptibilities of *E. coli* were also affected by chemically unrelated substances such as salicylate, tetracycline and cyclohexane.

In this respect, it was determined that 21 of 57 clinical isolates of *E. coli* showing high level fluoroquinolone-resistance displayed tolerance to cyclohexane, which suggests a presence of elevated broad spectrum efflux activity [101]. Efflux of a wide range of chemically unrelated compounds, among which are different medicine classes of antibacterials, is determined by the so-called mar (multiple antibiotic resistance) genes [102], which suffer the influence of an assortment of chemically unrelated substances.

The role of the mar genes is the regulation of accumulation of quinolones and thus their intracellular concentrations, which is achieved by changing the expression of efflux pumps and porins [100, 102].

To this, one must add the extrusion of quinolones out of the bacteria by AcrAB, a different efflux pump.

The mar gene exerts partial control over the pump, which seems the most important mechanism of resistance for mar mutant variants [103].

Salicylate stimulates fluoroquinolone resistance selection because the production of MarA, a positive regulator of acrAB transcription, is induced by salicylate and tetracycline.

Resistance is visible in either mar expression alone or if combined with type II topoisomerase mutations [102]. The combination of topoisomerase mutations with AcrAB over-expression results in high-level resistance to fluoroquinolone. In this respect, increased production of AcrA has been noted in over 60% of high-level ciprofloxacine-resistant isolates [104-106].

Patterns of quinolone resistance may be altered by further nontopoisomerase resistance mechanisms, over which the mar exerts no control. The quinolone entry into the cell is decreased because of the nfxB gene action to code for a modified outer cell membrane protein F [107].

Fluoroquinolone activity is further affected by the action of soxRS gene products involved in bacterial adaptation to superoxide stress [101].

Fluoroquinolone-resistant *E. coli*, other Enterobacteriaceae and nonfermenters display a relatively wide range of diminished antibiotic accumulation, efflux and target enzyme modification [100, 108].

Because of their limited substrate specificity, increased expression of efflux pumps is associated with cross-resistance between fluoroquinolones and antibacterials of chemically unrelated medicine classes. This is the case of, for instance, MexAB, which induces resistance to nonfluorinated and fluoroquinolones, chloramphenicol and tetracycline in MexCD, rendering resistance to fluoroquinolones, trimethoprim, triclosan and erythromycin in MexEF and providing resistance to triclosan, imipenem, chloramphenicol and triclosan in MexXY, which gives resistance to fluoroquinolones, aminoglycosides and erythromycin.

There are a number of reviews available, which provide a comprehensive view on the impact of fluoroquinolone resistance and extrusion [108-111].

A fourth type of cross-resistance can be represented by the selection of a fluoroquinolone resistant or even multidrug-resistant phenotype by exposure to a broad range of chemically unrelated drug classes. All the above are illustrations which underline the complex character of mechanisms inducing resistance to fluoroquinolone, selection by fluoroquinolones and co-selection of resistance by chemically unrelated classes of antibacterials and antiseptics.

All general mechanisms of fluoroquinolone resistance have been presented for an overview of the issue. Regarding fluoroquinolone resistance in the case of *H. pylori* infection, this is due mainly (99%) to mutations in the QRDR of gyrA (Figure 3).

Antibiotic bacterial resistance is a result of the inhibition of binding between the enzyme and the antibiotic, determined by point mutations in QRDR of gyrA. In various studies, the following *H. pylori* loci have been found to be involved: (1) position 88 (Ala88Val), (2) position 91 (Asp91Gly, Asn, Ala, or Tyr) and (3) position 87 (Asn87Lys). In 100% of levofloxacin resistant isolates there have been observed mutations in both position 91 and 87. In addition, a new mutation has been identified, which consists of Tyr substituting Asn in position 87. Position 86 (Asp86Asn) is involved in infrequent mutations; the same position usually associates with mutations at positions 87 and 91, which diminishes its role in MIC values. In a similar manner, it is most likely that gyrB constantly associating with gyrA 87-91 mutations reduce to a minimum the role gyrB mutations hold in emergence of quinolone resistance. Actually, the involvement of gyrA and gyrB gene mutations has been observed in levofloxacin resistance as 83.8% and 4.4%, respectively.

There are also other factors that are involved in levofloxacin resistance, such as occurrence in codon 87 of gyrA of an amino acidic polymorphism, which consists of the presence of various asparagine-threonine residues. Specifically, presence of threonine in the J99 strain and asparagine residues in the 26695 strain associated with a higher antibiotic susceptibility has been identified due to the complete sequencing genome of two strains, namely the J99 and the 26695. Other Helicobacter types interestingly preserve the presence of threonine residue in codon 87, which therefore indicates the likelihood of the occurrence of a "philogenic" type evolution of the Helicobacter species.

6. Clinical and social implications of fluoroquinolone resistance

The increased incidence of fluoroquinolone resistance is a major reason for concern in medicine. Identification of and subsequent familiarisation with plasmid-mediated quinolone resistance (PMQR) has revealed a new and more dangerous mechanism of resistance allowing bacteria to adapt to and survive therapeutic concentrations of fluoroquinolones. As mentioned above, PMQR only provides low-level resistance, not enough to enable classification as clear resistance (MIC ≥4g/ml), according to the Clinical and Laboratory Standards Institute (CLSI) breakpoint criteria for quinolone resistance. With these low MICs, such isolates, although transporting mutations conferring low sensitivity to quinolones, are to be classified as sensitive (MIC ≥1g/ml), meaning that physicians can further prescribe this class of medicines.

This in itself is a dilemma, because PMQR allows such "sensitive" organisms to survive even under therapeutic concentrations, easily circulating their genes afterwards. Continued exposure to these antibiotics determines high selection for plasmid-carrying pathogens, then rapidly conducing to general development of high-level clinically significant degrees of resistance. It has been shown that PMRQ-conferred low resistance levels can still remain undetected by current CLSI criteria and therefore are still conducive to failure of therapy. This is reason for concern with regard to the safety of prescribing fluoroquinolones for treatment of PMRQ gene-bearing organisms, even if they do not qualify as "resistant".

In such cases, the problem arises whether clinical breakpoints should be reviewed with regard to plasmid-carrying pathogens.

There is a strong association between fluoroquinolone resistance and resistance to other antibiotics, particularly wide spectrum β-lactamases and aminoglycosides. This indicates that gene-carrying plasmid organisms conferring quinolone resistance increase the likelihood of developing multi-drug resistant bacteria and prescription of a quinolone may be selective of not only quinolone resistance but also resistance to other classes of medicines.

The discovery of plasmid-mediated resistance genes in some non-Typhi serotypes of Salmonella enterica in animals has raised a major public health concern. The presence of such resistance genes from plasmid-mediated resistance genes in some non-Typhi serotypes of Salmonella enterica suggests an unsettling potential for horizontal transmission of resistance genes among animals and of infection-causing human pathogens, by means of food. Fluoroquinolone resistance prolongs hospitalisation and may further determine complications because of the selected therapy. The following can be mentioned among strategies implemented in some geographic areas: prohibited use as animal food and restricted use of fluoroquinolones in agriculture and their use for therapeutic purposes only, development of programmes for antibiotics management in hospitals (by drug rotation, cycling and restriction) as well as carrying out educational campaigns addressing physicians and patients, whose aim should be to increase awareness of inappropriate antibiotics.

The current breakpoints allow continuation of the quinolone treatment, whereas the organisms carrying these plasmid-mediated resistance genes remain undetected, which results in further dissemination of these plasmids, because of the selection pressure. The aim is a review of CLSI quinolone and fluoroquinolone breakpoints, against the background of the new mechanism (PMQR). Lower clinical breakpoints will help physicians to detect the low-level-resistance phenotype as rendered by such genes as well as avoidance of resumed prescription of quinolones as a treatment.

Identification of the PMQR mechanism is indicative of an increased risk of spreading resistance not only to fluoroquinolones but also, because of co-transmission, to other significant antimicrobial classes. Tackling this issue by judicious use of antibacterials and re-evaluation of clinical breakpoints will constitute an important step in preserving the efficiency of this important class of medicines.

Concerning the *H. pylori* infection, an encouraging strategy to approach cases of multiple failures in prior *H. pylori* eradication is quinolone-based treatment as a rescue therapy. According to European guidelines, before selecting a third-line treatment, which is based on microbial sensitivity to antibiotics, culture is recommended. Quinolones for third-line therapy should be selected based on results of drug susceptibility tests or analysis of gyrA.

If available, further alternatives have also been suggested for rescue therapy, consisting of furazolidone-based therapy, triple rifabutin-based therapy or high-dose amoxicillin/PPI therapy.

Author details

Carolina Negrei[1*] and Daniel Boda[2]

*Address all correspondence to: carol_n2002@hotmail.com

1 Department of Toxicology, "Carol Davila" University of Medicine and Pharmacy, Bucharest, Romania

2 Dermato-oncology Excellence Research Center "Carol Davila" University of Medicine and Pharmacy, Bucharest, Romania

References

[1] Go M. F. Natural history and epidemiology of *Helicobacter pylori* infection. Alimentary Pharmacology and Therapeutics 2002; 16 (Suppl. 1): 3–15.

[2] Suerbaum S., Michetti P. *Helicobacter pylori* infection. New England Journal of Medicine 2002; 347: 1175–1186.

[3] Dore M. P., Leandro G., Realdi G., Sepulveda A. R., Graham D. Y. Effect of pretreatment antibiotic resistance to metronidazole and clarithromycin on outcome of *Helicobacter pylori* therapy: a meta-analytical approach. Digestive Diseases and Sciences 2000; 45: 68–76.

[4] Jenks P. J. Causes of failure of eradication of *Helicobacter pylori*. British Medical Journal 2002; 325: 3–4.

[5] Gisbert J. P., Pajares J. M. *Helicobacter pylori* "rescue" therapy after failure of two eradication treatments. Helicobacter 2005; 10: 363–372.

[6] Toracchio S., Capodicasa S., Soraja D.B., Cellini L., Marzio L. Rifabutin based triple therapy for eradication of *H. pylori* primary and secondary resistant to tinidazole and clarithromycin. Digestive and Liver Disease 2005; 37: 33–38.

[7] Malfertheiner P., Megraud F., O'Morain C. A., Atherton J., Axon A. T., Bazzoli F., Gensini G. F., Gisbert J. P., Graham D. Y., Rokkas T., El-Omar E. M., Kuipers E. J. Management of *Helicobacter pylori* infection–the Maastricht IV/ Florence Consensus Report. Gut 2012; 61: 646–664.

[8] Hsu P. I., Wu D., Chen A. et al. Quadruple rescue therapy for *Helicobacter pylori* infection after two treatment failures, European Journal of Clinical Investigation 2008; 38(6):404-409.

[9] Gisbert J. P, Calvet X., O'Connor A., Megraud F., O'Morain C.A. Sequential therapy for *Helicobacter pylori* eradication: a critical review, Journal of Clinical Gastroenterology 2010; 44(5): 313-325.

[10] Vaira D., Zullo A., Vakil N. et al. Sequential therapy versus standard triple-drug therapy for *Helicobacter pylori* eradication: a randomized trial, Annals of Internal Medicine 2007; 146(8): 556-563.

[11] Megraud F. *H. pylori* antibiotic resistance: prevalence, importance and advances in testing," Gut 2004; 53(9): 1374-1384.

[12] Wu D. C., Hsu P. I., Wu J. Y. et al. Sequential and concomitant therapy with four drugs is equally effective for eradication of H pylori infection, Clinical Gastroenterology and Hepatology 2010; 8(1): 36-41.

[13] Hsu P. I., Wu D. C., Wu J. Y., Graham D. Y. Modified Sequential *Helicobacter pylori* therapy: proton pump inhibitor and amoxicillin for 14 days with clarithromycin and metronidazole added as a quadruple (hybrid) therapy for the final 7 days, Helicobacter 2011; 16(2): 139-145.

[14] O'Morain C., Borody T., Farley A. et al. Efficacy and safety of single-triple capsules of bismuth biskalcitrate, metronidazole and tetracycline, given with omeprazole, for the eradication of *Helicobacter pylori*: an international multicentre study, Alimentary Pharmacology and Therapeutics 2003; 17(3): 415-420.

[15] Laine L., Hunt, R., El-Zimaity H., Nguyen B., Osato M., Spenard J. Bismuth-based quadruple therapy using a single capsule of bismuth biskalcitrate, metronidazole, and tetracycline given with omeprazole versus omeprazole, amoxicillin, and clarithromycin for eradication of *Helicobacter pylori* in duodenal ulcer patients: a prospective, randomized, multicenter, North American trial, American Journal of Gastroenterology 2003; 98(3): 562-567.

[16] Malfertheiner P., Bazzoli F., Delchier J. C. et al. *Helicobacter pylori* eradication with a capsule containing bismuth subcitrate potassium, metronidazole, and tetracycline

given with omeprazole versus clarithromycin-based triple therapy: a randomised, open-label, non-inferiority, phase 3 trial, The Lancet 2011; 377(9769): 905-913.

[17] Phillips R. H., Whitehead M. W., Doig L. A. et al. Is eradication of *Helicobacter pylori* with colloidal Bismuth subcitrate quadruple therapy safe? Helicobacter 2001; 6(2): 151-156.

[18] Liou J. M., Lin J. T., Chang C. Y. et al. Levofloxacin-based and clarithromycin-based triple therapies as first-line and secondline treatments for *Helicobacter pylori* infection: a randomised comparative trial with crossover design, Gut 2010; 59(5): 572-578.

[19] Chey W. D., Wong B. C. Y. American College of Gastroenterology guideline on the management of *Helicobacter pylori* infection. The American Journal of Gastroenterology 2007; 102(8): 1808-1825.

[20] Nishizawa T., Suzuki H., Hibi T. Quinolone-based thirdline therapy for *Helicobacter pylori* eradication. Journal of Clinical Biochemistry and Nutrition 2009; 44(2): 119-124.

[21] Van Der Poorten D., Katelaris P. H. The effectiveness of rifabutin triple therapy for patients with difficult-to-eradicate *Helicobacter pylori* in clinical practice. Alimentary Pharmacology and Therapeutics 2007; 26(11-12): 1537-1542.

[22] Toracchio S., Capodicasa S., Soraja D. B., Cellini L., Marzio L. Rifabutin based triple therapy for eradication of *H. pylori* primary and secondary resistant to tinidazole and clarithromycin. Digestive and Liver Disease 2005; 37(1): 33-38.

[23] Ball P., Mandell L., Niki Y., Tillotson G. Comparative tolerability of the newer fluoroquinolone antibacterials. Drug Safety 1999; 21: 407-21.

[24] Childs S. Safety of the fluoroquinolone antibiotics; focus on the molecular structure. Infections in Urology 2000; 13: 3-10.

[25] Mandell L., Tillotson G. Safety of fluoroquinolones: An update. Canadian Journal of Infectious Diseases 2002; 13(1): 54-61.

[26] Finch R. G. The withdrawal of temafloxacin; Are there implications for other quinolones? Drug Safety 1993; 8: 9-11.

[27] GlaxoWellcome voluntarily withdraws Raxar (grepafloxacin). Press Release, October 26, 1999, http://www. fda. gov/medwatch/safety/1999/raxar. html.

[28] Trovafloxacin (Trovan) package insert. New York: Pfizer, 1998

[29] Chen J. L., MacLean J. A. Trovafloxacin associated eosinophilic hepatitis. New England Journal of Medicine 2000; 342: 359-60.

[30] The electronic Medicines Compendium (eMC), Levofloxacin, http://www. medicines. org. uk/emc/ (accessed 1 June 2013).

[31] Hori S., Shimada J., Saito A. Comparison of the inhibitory effects of new quinolones on gamma-aminobutyric-acid receptor binding in the presence of anti-inflammatory drugs. Reviews of infectious diseases 1989; 5: 1397-1398.

[32] Fish D. N. Fluoroquinolone Adverse Effects and Drug Interactions. Pharmacotherapy. 2001; 21: 10.

[33] O'Donnell J. A., Gelone S. P. The newer fluoroquinolones. Infectious Disease Clinics of North America 2004; 18(3): 691–716.

[34] Ball P. The quinolones: history and overview. In: Andriole VT. (ed) The quinolones. 3rd edition. San Diego (CA): Academic Press; 2000; 1–33.

[35] Stahlman R., Lode H. Safety overview: toxicity, adverse effects, and drug interactions. In: Andriole, V. T. (ed) The quinolones. 3rd edition. San Diego (CA): Academic Press; 2000; 397–453.

[36] Niki Y., Hashiguchi K., Okimoto N. et al. Quinolone antimicrobial agents and theophylline [letter]. Chest 1992; 101(3): 881.

[37] Carroll D. N., Carroll D. G. Interactions between warfarin and three commonly prescribed fluoroquinolones. Annals of Pharmacotherapy 2008; 42(5): 680–5.

[38] Barton T. D., Fishman N. O., Weiner M. G. et al. High rate of coadministration of di- or trivalent cation-containing compounds with oral fluoroquinolones: risk factors and potential implications. Infection Control and Hospital Epidemiology 2005; 26(1): 93–9.

[39] Cohen K. A., Lautenbach E, Weiner M. G. et al. Coadministration of oral levofloxacin with agents that impair absorption: impact on antibiotic resistance. Infection Control and Hospital Epidemiology 2008; 29(10): 975–7.

[40] Bolon M. K. The Newer Fluoroquinolones. Medical Clinics of North America 2011; 95: 793–817.

[41] Andriole V. T. The Quinolones: Past, Present, and Future Clinical Infectious Diseases 2005; 41: S113–9.

[42] Hawkey P. M. Mechanisms of quinolone action and microbial response Journal of Antimicrobial Chemotherapy 2003; 51(Suppl 1): 29–35.

[43] Jacoby G. A. Mechanisms of resistance to quinolones. Clinical Infectious Diseases 2005; 41(Suppl 2): S120–6.

[44] Dalhoff A. Quinolone resistance in Pseudomonas aeruginosa and Staphylococcus aureus. Development during therapy and clinical significance. Infection 1994; 22(2): S111–S121.

[45] Thauvin-Eliopoulos C., Eliopoulos G. M. Activity in vitro of the quinolones, in: Hooper D.C., Rubinstein E., Quinolone Antimicrobial Agents, 3rd edition, (ed.) ASM Press, Washington, DC, USA. 2003; 91-111.

[46] Dalhoff A. In vitro activities of quinolones. Expert Opinion on Investigational Drugs 1999; 8(2): 123-137.

[47] Dalhoff A, Schmitz F. J. In vitro antibacterial activity and pharmacodynamics of new quinolones. European Journal of Clinical Microbiology and Infectious Diseases 2003; 22(4): 203-221.

[48] Drlica K., Malik M., Kerns R. J., Zhao X. Quinolonemediated bacterial death. Antimicrobial Agents and Chemotherapy 2008; 52(2): 385-392.

[49] Drlica K., Zhao X, DNA gyrase, topoisomerase IV, and the 4-quinolones. Microbiology and Molecular Biology Reviews 1997; 61(3): 377-392.

[50] Zhao X., Xu C., Domagala J., Drlica K. DNA topoisomerase targets of the fluoroquinolones: a strategy for avoiding bacterial resistance. Proceedings of the National Academy of Sciences of the United States of America 1997; 94(25): 13991–13996.

[51] Hooper D.C. Mechanisms of fluoroquinolone resistance. Drug Resistance Updates 1999; 2(1): 38–55.

[52] Ince D., Hooper D. C. Quinolone resistance due to reduced target enzyme expression. Journal of Bacteriology 2003; 185(23): 6883–6892.

[53] Walker G. C. Mutagenesis and inducible responses to deoxyribonucleic acid damage in Escherichia coli. Microbiological Reviews 1984; 48(1): 60–93.

[54] Fernandez De Henestrosa A. R, Ogi T, Aoyagi S. et al. Identification of additional genes belonging to the LexA regulon in Escherichia coli. Molecular Microbiology 2000; 35(6): 1560–1572.

[55] Courcelle J., Kodursky A., Pete, B., Brown P., Hanawalt P. Comparative gene expression profiles following UV exposure in wild-type and SOS-deficient Escherichia coli. Genetics 2001; 158(1): 41–64.

[56] Ysern P., Clerch B., Castano M., Gibert I., Barbe J., Llagostera M. Induction of SOS genes in Escherichia coli and mutagenesis in Salmonella typhimurium by fluoroquinolones. Mutagenesis 1990; 5(1): 63–66.

[57] Malik M., Zhao X., Drlica K. Lethal fragmentation of bacterial chromosomes mediated by DNA gyrase and quinolones. Molecular Microbiology 2006; 61(3): 810–825.

[58] Wang M., Jacoby G. A., Mills D. M., Hooper. D. C. SOS regulation of qnrB expression. Antimicrobial Agents and Chemotherapy 2009; 53(2): 821–823.

[59] Da Re S., Garnier F., Guerin E., Campoy S., Denis F., Ploy M. C. The SOS response promotes qnrB quinoloneresistance determinant expression. EMBO Reports 2009; 10(8): 929–933.

[60] Cirz R. T., Chin J. K., Andes D. R., de Crecy-Lagard V., Craig. W. R. Inhibition of mutation and combating the evolution of antibiotic resistance. PLoS Biology 2005; 3(6): 175.

[61] Cirz R. T., Jones M. B., Gingles N. A. et al. Complete and SOS-mediated response of Staphylococcus aureus to the antibiotic ciprofloxacin. Journal of Bacteriology 2007; 189(2): 531–539.

[62] Dorr T., Lewis. K., Vulic M. SOS response induces persistence to fluoroquinolones in Escherichia coli. PLoS Genetics 2009; 5(12):1-9 e1000760. http://www. northeastern. edu/adc/publications/sostobidorr. pdf (accessed 9 June 2013).

[63] Avison M. B. New approaches to combating antimicrobial drug resistance. Genome Biology 2005; 6(13): 243.

[64] Lopez E., Elez M., Matic I., Bl′azquez J. Antibioticmediated recombination: ciprofloxacin stimulates SOS independent recombination of divergent sequences in Escherichia coli. Molecular Microbiology 2007; 64(1): 83–93.

[65] Miller C., Thomsen L. E., Gaggero C., Mosseri R., Ingmer H., Cohen S.N. SOS response induction by β-lactams and bacterial defence against antibiotic lethality. Science 2004; 305(5690): 1629–1631.

[66] Maiques E., U′ beda C., Campoy S. et al. β-lactam antibiotics induce the SOS response and horizontal transfer of virulence factors in Staphylococcus aureus. Journal of Bacteriology 2006; 188(7): 2726–2729.

[67] Lewin C. S., Amyes S. G. B. The role of the SOS response in bacteria exposed to zidovudine or trimethoprim. Journal of Medical Microbiology 1991; 34(6): 329–332.

[68] Beaber J. W., Hochhut B., Waldor M. K. SOS response promotes horizontal dissemination of antibiotic resistance genes. Nature 2004; 427(6969): 72–74.

[69] Tran J. H., Jacoby G. A. Mechanism of plasmid-mediated quinolone resistance. Proceedings of the National Academy of Sciences of the United States of America 2002; 99(8):5638–5642.

[70] Strahilevitz J., Jacoby G. A, Hooper D. C., Robicsek A. Plasmid-mediated quinolone resistance: a multifaceted threat. Clinical Microbiology Reviews 2009; 22(4): 664–689.

[71] Poirel L., Cattoir V., Nordmann P., Plasmid-mediated quinolone-resistance; interactions between human, animal, and environmental ecologies. Frontiers in Microbiology 2012; 3: 1-7.

[72] Rodriguez-Martinez J. M., Cano M. E., Velasco C., Martinez-Martinez L., Pascual A. Plasmid-mediated quinolone resistance: an update. Journal of Infection and Chemotherapy 2011; 17(2): 149-182.

[73] Martinez-Martinez L., Pascual A., Jacoby G.A. Quinolone resistance from a transferable plasmid. The Lancet 1998; 351(9105): 797-799.

[74] Jacoby G., Cattoir V., Hooper D. et al. qnr gene nomenclature. Antimicrobial Agents and Chemotherapy 2008; 52(7): 2297-2299.

[75] Baquirin M. H. C., Barlow M. Evolution and recombination of the plasmidic qnr alleles. Journal of Molecular Evolution 2008; 67(1): 103-110.

[76] Robicsek A., Jacoby G. A., Hooper D.C. The worldwide emergence of plasmid-mediated quinolone resistance. The Lancet Infectious Diseases 2006; 6(10): 629-640.

[77] Poirel L., Rodriguez-Martinez J. M., Mammeri H., Liard A., Nordmann P. Origin of plasmid-mediated quinolone resistance determinant QnrA. Antimicrobial Agents and Chemotherapy 2005; 49(8): 3523-3525.

[78] Poirel L., Van De Loo M., Mammeri H., Nordmann P. Association of plasmid-mediated quinolone resistance with extended-spectrum β-lactamase VEB-1. Antimicrobial Agents and Chemotherapy 2005; 49(7): 3091-3094.

[79] Montero C., Mateu G., Rodriguez R., Takiff H. Intrinsic resistance of Mycobacterium smegmatis to fluoroquinolones may be influenced by new pentapeptide protein MfpA. Antimicrobial Agents and Chemotherapy 2001; 45(12): 3387-3392.

[80] Arsene S., Leclercq R. Role of a qnr-like gene in the intrinsic resistance of Enterococcus faecalis to fluoroquinolones. Antimicrobial Agents and Chemotherapy 2007; 51(9): 3254-3258.

[81] Rodriguez-Martinez J. M., Velasco C., Briales A., Garcia I., Conejo M. C., Pascual A. Qnr-like pentapeptide repeat proteins in Gram-positive bacteria. Journal of Antimicrobial Chemotherapy 2008; 61(6): 1240-1243.

[82] Shimizu K., Kikuchi K., Sasaki T. et al. Smqnr, a new chromosome-carried quinolone resistance gene in Stenotrophomonasmaltophilia. Antimicrobial Agents and Chemotherapy 2008; 52(10): 3823-3825.

[83] Velasco C., Rodriguez-Martinez J. M., Briales A., Diaz de Alba P., Calvo J., Pascual A. Smaqnr, a new chromosome-encoded quinolone resistance determinant in Serratia marcescens. The Journal of antimicrobial chemotherapy 2010; 65(2): 239-242.

[84] Nordmann P., Poirel L. Emergence of plasmid-mediated resistance to quinolones in Enterobacteriaceae. Journal of Antimicrobial Chemotherapy 2005; 56(3): 463-469.

[85] Hernandez A., Sanchez M. B., Martinez J. L. Quinolone-resistance: much more than predicted. Frontiers in Microbiology 2011; 2: 1-6.

[86] Lascols, C., Podglajen I., Verdet C. et al. A plasmid-borne Shewanella algae gene, qnrA3, and its possible transfer in vivo between Kluyvera ascorbata and Klebsiella pneumoniae. Journal of Bacteriology 2008; 190(15):5217-5223.

[87] Cattoir V., Poirel L., Aubert C., Soussy C.J., Nordmann P. Unexpected occurrence of plasmid-mediated quinolone resistance determinants in environmental Aeromonas spp.. Emerging Infectious Diseases 2008; 14(2): 231-237.

[88] Poirel L., Liard A., Rodriguez-Martinez J.M., Nordmann P. Vibrionaceae as a possible source of Qnr-like quinolone resistance determinants. Journal of Antimicrobial Chemotherapy 2005; 56(6): 1118–1121.

[89] Vetting M. W., Chi H. P., Hegde S. S., Jacoby G. A., Hooper D. C., Blanchard J. S. Mechanistic and structural analysis of aminoglycoside N-acetyltransferase AAC(6_)-Ib and its bifunctional, fluoroquinolone-active AAC(6_)-Ib-cr variant. Biochemistry 2008; 47(37): 9825–9835.

[90] Ruiz E., Ocampo-Sosa A. A., Alcoba-Florez J. et al. Changes in ciprofloxacin resistance levels in Enterobacter aerogenes isolates associated with variable expression of the aac(6_)-Ibcr gene. Antimicrobial Agents and Chemotherapy 2012; 56(2): 1097–1100.

[91] Frasson I., Cavallaro A., Bergo C., Richter S. N., Palu G. Prevalence of aac(6_)-Ib-cr plasmid-mediated and chromosome-encoded fluoroquinolone resistance in Enterobacteriaceae in Italy. Gut Pathogens 2011; 3(1):12 doi:10. 1186/1757-4749-3-12. http:// www. gutpathogens. com/content/3/1/12 (accessed 9 June 2013).

[92] Sanders C. C., Watanakunakorn C. Emergence of resistance to β-lactams, aminoglycosides, and quinolones during combination therapy for infection due to Serratia marcescens. Journal of Infectious Diseases 1986; 153(3): 617–619.

[93] Perichon B., Courvalin P., Galimand M. Transferable resistance to aminoglycosides by methylation of G1405 in 16S rRNA and to hydrophilic fluoroquinolones by QepA-mediated efflux in Escherichia coli. Antimicrobial Agents and Chemotherapy 2007; 51(7):2464–2469.

[94] Yamane K., Wachino J. I., Suzuki S. et al. New plasmid-mediated fluoroquinolone efflux pump, QepA, found in an Escherichia coli clinical isolate. Antimicrobial Agents and Chemotherapy 2007; 51(9): 3354–3360.

[95] Kim H. B., Wang M., Park C. H., Jacoby G. A., Hooper D. C. oqxAB encoding a multidrug efflux pump in human clinical isolates of Enterobacteriaceae. Antimicrobial Agents and Chemotherapy 2009; 53(8): 3582–3584.

[96] Hansen L. H., Jensen L. B., Sørensen H. I., Sørensen S. J. Substrate specificity of the OqxAB multidrug resistance pump in Escherichia coli and selected enteric bacteria. Journal of Antimicrobial Chemotherapy 2007; 60(1): 145–147.

[97] Hansen L. H., Johannesen E., Burmølle M., Sørensen A. H., Sørensen S. J. Plasmid-encoded multidrug efflux pump conferring resistance to olaquindox in Escherichia coli. Antimicrobial Agents and Chemotherapy 2004; 48(9): 3332–3337.

[98] Morgan-Linnell S. K., Boyd L. B., Steffen D., Zechiedrich L. Mechanisms accounting for fluoroquinolone resistance in Escherichia coli clinical isolates. Antimicrobial Agents and Chemotherapy 2009; 53(1): 235–241.

[99] Cambau E., Matrat S., Pan X. S. et al. Target specificity of the new fluoroquinolone besifloxacin in Streptococcus pneumoniae, Staphylococcus aureus and Escherichia coli. Journal of Antimicrobial Chemotherapy 2009; 63(3): 443–450.

[100] Everett M. J., Jin Y. F., Ricci V., Piddock L. J. V. Contributions of individual mechanisms to fluoroquinolone resistance in 36 Escherichia coli strains isolated from humans and animals. Antimicrobial Agents and Chemotherapy 1996; 40(10): 2380–2386.

[101] Oethinger M., Podglajen I., Kern W. V., Levy S. B. Overexpression of the marA or soxS regulatory gene in clinical topoisomerasemutants of Escherichia coli. Antimicrobial Agents and Chemotherapy 1998; 42(8): 2089–2094.

[102] Goldman J. D., White D. G., Levy S. B. Multiple antibiotic resistance (mar) locus protects Escherichia coli from rapid cell killing by fluoroquinolones. Antimicrobial Agents and Chemotherapy 1996; 40(5): 1266–1269.

[103] Okusu H., Ma D., Nikaido H. AcrAB efflux pump plays a major role in the antibiotic resistance phenotype of Escherichia coli multiple-antibiotic-resistance (Mar) mutants. Journal of Bacteriology 1996; 178(1): 306–308.

[104] Mazzariol A., Tokue Y., Kanegawa T. M., Cornaglia G., Nikaido H. High-level fluoroquinolone-resistant clinical isolates of Escherichia coli overproduce multidrug efflux protein AcrA. Antimicrobial Agents and Chemotherapy 2000; 44(12): 3441–3443.

[105] Oethinger M., Kern W. V., Jellen-Ritter A.S., McMurry L. M., Levy S. B. Ineffectiveness of topoisomerase mutations in mediating clinically significant fluoroquinolone resistance in Escherichia coli in the absence of the AcrAB efflux pump. Antimicrobial Agents and Chemotherapy 2000; 44(1): 10–13.

[106] Wang H., Dzink-Fox J. L., Chen M., Levy S. B. Genetic characterization of highly fluoroquinolone-resistant clinical Escherichia coli strains from China: role of acrR mutations. Antimicrobial Agents and Chemotherapy 2001; 45(5): 1515–1521.

[107] Truong Q. C., Van Nguyen J. C., Shlaes D., Gutmann L., Moreau N. J. A novel, double mutation in DNA gyrase A of Escherichia coli conferring resistance to quinolone antibiotics. Antimicrobial Agents and Chemotherapy 1997; 41(1): 85–90.

[108] Hooper D. C. Mechanism of quinolones resistance, in Hooper, D. C., Rubinstein E. Quinolone Antimicrobial Agents, 3rd edition. (ed.) ASM Press, Washington, DC, USA; 2003; 41–67.

[109] Hooper D. C. Efflux pumps and nosocomial antibiotic resistance: a primer for hospital epidemiologists. Clinical Infectious Diseases 2005; 40(12): 1811–1817.

[110] Van Bambeke F., Pages, J. M., Lee, V. J. Inhibitors of bacterial efflux pumps as adjuvants in antibacterial therapy and diagnostic tools for detection of resistance by efflux. Frontiers in Anti-Infective Drug Discovery 2010; 1: 138–175.

[111] Piddock L. J. V. Multidrug-resistance efflux pumps—not just for resistance. Nature Reviews Microbiology 2006; 4(8): 629–636.

8

Molecular Epidemiology of *Helicobacter pylori* in Brazilian Patients with Early Gastric Cancer and a Review to Understand the Prognosis of the Disease

Bruna Maria Roesler and
José Murilo Robilotta Zeitune

1. Introduction

Helicobacter pylori (*H. pylori*) is an universally distributed bacterium that affects more than half of the world population and is considered an important public health problem. Although colonization with *H. pylori* is not actually a disease, it is a condition that affects the relative risk of developing various clinical disorders of the upper gastrointestinal tract, as chronic gastritis, peptic ulcer disease, mucosa-associated lymphoid tissue (MALT lymphoma) and gastric adenocarcinoma, and, possibly, extradigestive diseases.

Colonization with *H. pylori* virtually leads to infiltration of the gastric mucosa in both antrum and corpus with neutrophilic and mononuclear cells. Gastritis can be classified as an acute or chronic gastritis and it can involve all parts of the stomach or just the fundus, corpus or antrum. The chronic active gastritis is the primary condition related to *H. pylori* colonization, and other *H. pylori*-associated disorders, in particular, resulting from this chronic inflammatory process, as atrophic gastritis, causing an elevated risk of gastric cancer. Considering this association, in 1994 the bacterium was classified as a group I carcinogen by the International Agency for Research on Cancer, World Health Organization.

Molecular techniques have revealed that *H. pylori* possesses a remarkable degree of genetic diversity, which could be responsible for its adaptation in the host stomach and for its pathological characteristics, in addition to the clinical outcome of the infection, although this aspect remains unclear.

In Brazil, it is estimated that only about 10 to 15% of the gastric cancer cases are diagnosed at an early stage, aspect that directly impact the prognosis of the disease, which presents low survival rates. Unlike patients with advanced gastric cancer, that ones diagnosed at the early stage of the disease present an excellent prognostic, in which a five-year survival rate is more than 90%.

Many early gastric cancers are believed to go through a life cycle consisting of ulcerations, followed by healing, then reulceration, and some tumors remain at this early stage for years even without treatment. Nevertheless, some of these tumors rapidly advanced, perhaps one of the principal questions concerning the gastric carcinogenesis.

Consequently, some questions can be considered about it. Is the *H. pylori* presence important for the evolution of the early lesions in advanced ones? To what extent *H. pylori* eradication could prevent the progression of lesions from one to another stage? Are the genetic characteristics of *H. pylori* strain that is colonizing the patient with early gastric cancer important for the progression of the disease in a faster or in a slower way?

The principal aim of our book chapter is to identify the genetic characteristics of *H. pylori* strains in Brazilian patients diagnosed with early distal type intestinal gastric adenocarcinoma, trying to determine the genotypic pattern of bacterium in our population through molecular techniques. Besides, other aim of our study is to discuss the principal aspects of the *H. pylori* infection and then correlate them with the development of the precancerous lesions and the development of the early gastric cancer properly, trying to understand to what extent the microorganism eradication treatment could be important to preventing the disease progression.

2. *Helicobacter pylori*

2.1. General characteristics

Helicobacter pylori (H. pylori) is a spiral-shaped Gram-negative flagellate bacterium that colonizes the human stomach and can establish a long-term infection of the gastric mucosa [1]. In gastric biopsy specimens, *H. pylori* organisms are 2.5 to 5.0 μm long and 0.5 to 1.0 μm wide, with four to six unipolar sheated flagella, which are essential for bacterial motility. When cultured on solid medium, the bacteria assume a rod-like shape and spiral shapes are infrequent or absent [2]; after prolonged culture on solid or liquid medium, coccoid forms, that are metabolically active, tipically predominate [3].

Gastric colonization with *H. pylori* affects at least half the world´s population, and, while the infection is on a fast decline in most of the western countries, mainly due to the success of therapeutic regimens and improved personal and community hygiene that prevents reinfection, the situation is exactly opposite in many of the developing countries due to failure of treatment and emergence of drug resistance [4,5]. Most studies suggest that males and females are infected at approximately the same rates [6] and, probably, the infection occurs in the childhood. In developed countries, persons of higher socioeconomic status have lower infection rates, although among certain ethnic minorities, high rates persist despite economic advancement [7].

The routes of transmission of *H. pylori* still remain unclear. Person-to-person transmission and intrafamilial spread seem to be the main route, based on the intrafamilial clustering observed in some studies [8,9]. Children are often infected by a strain which a genetic fingerprint identical to that of their parents, and they maintain this genotype even after moving to a different environment [10]. Animals harbor organisms that resemble *H. pylori,* but with the exception of nonhuman primates [11] and, under particular circumstances, perhaps cats [12] and houseflies (*Musca domestica*) [13], none harbor *H. pylori.* In the same way, food-borne transmission has not been substantiated [14]. Nevertheless, the waterborne infection remains possible [15,16].

H. pylori remains one of the most common worldwide human infections and its isolation by Marshall and Warren (1984) [17] has markedly improved our understanding about the nature of chronic gastritis and other important upper gastrointestinal disorders, such as peptic ulcer disease, mucosa-associated lymphoid tissue (MALT) lymphoma and gastric adenocarcinoma [18]. In 1994, the bacterium was classified as a group I carcinogen by the International Agency for Research on Cancer and is regarded as a primary factor for gastric cancer development [19]. For their revolutionary discovery, Marshall and Warren received the Nobel Prize in Physiology or Medicine in 2005.

In addition, in the last years, *H. pylori* infection has also been associated with some extradigestive diseases, such as iron-deficiency anemia [20], idiopathic thrombocytopenic purpura [21,22], cardiovascular diseases [23,24], hepatobiliary diseases [25,26], and diabetes mellitus [27], among others.

2.2. Virulence factors of *H. Pylori*

H. pylori populations are highly diverse and constantly change their genome, which can be an important factor in its adaptation to the host stomach and also for the clinical outcome of the infection. The changes in its genome occur mainly due to point mutations, substitutions, insertions, and/or deletions of their genome. Moreover, mixed infections are frequent and lead to exchange of DNA fragments between different *H. pylori* strains in a single host [28,29]. Experience with other bacterial pathogens suggests that *H. pylori*-specific factors may exist that influence the microorganism pathogenicity, and, these factors, together with the host genetic characteristics and the external environment, can contribute to the clinical outcome of the infection. Among the most studied virulence factors of *H. pylori* are the urease gene, the vacuolating cytotoxin gene (vacA), the cytotoxin associated gene-Pathogenicity Island (cagPAI) and the duodenal ulcer promoting gene (dupA).

Urease is an important enzyme which is produced by *H. pylori* to counteract the acidic environment of the stomach. Urease causes damage to the epithelium through the production of ammonia, that, in conjunction with neutrophil metabolites, forms carcinogenic agents that might participate in the development of gastric malignances [30,31]. Ammonia is capable to cause different cell alterations, including swelling of intracellular acidic compartments, alterations of vesicular membrane transport, repression of protein synthesis and ATP production, and cell-cycle arrest [32]. Urease might also help to the recruitment of neutrophils and monocytes in the mucosa and to the production of proinflammatory cytokines

[33]. It has been demonstrated that this enzyme plays and important hole in the *H. pylori* colonization, being observed that urease-defective bacteria mutants are not able to colonize the gastric environment [32].

VacA is a cytotoxin secreted from *H. pylori* as a large 140kd polypeptide and latter trimmed at both ends to finally deliver it in an active form to host cells, where it exerts its activity [34]. The gene encoding VacA is present in all *H. pylori* strains and displays allelic diversity in three main regions: s (signal), i (intermediate) and m (middle); consequently, the activity of the toxin varies between strains [35]. Different combinations of two major alleles of each region (s1, s2, i1, i2, m1, m2) may exist, which results in VacA toxins with distinct capability of inducing vacuolating in epithelial cells [36]. VacA induces multiple cellular activities, including the alteration in the endosomal maturation which consequently leads to vacuolating of epithelial cells, the induction of membrane-channel formation, the cytochrome c releasing from mitochondria and the binding to cell-membrane receptors activating a proinflammatory response [35].

The cagPAI is a 40kb region of chromosomal DNA encoding approximately 31 genes that forms a type IV secretion system that forms a pilus that delivers CagA, an oncoprotein, into the cytosol of gastric epithelial cells through a rigid needle structure covered by CagY, a VirB10-homologous protein and CagT, a VirB7-homologous protein, at the base [37,38]. cagA is a polymorphic gene that presents different numbers of repeat sequences located in its 3′region and each repeat region of the CagA protein contains Glu-Pro-IIe-Tyr-Ala (EPIYA) motifs, including a tyrosine phosphorylation site [39]. Upon delivery into host cells, CagA undergoes Src-dependent tyrosine phosphorylation and activates an eukaryotic phosphatase (SHP-2), leading to dephosphorylation of host cell proteins and cellular morphologic changes [40]. CagA has also been shown to dysregulate β-catenin signaling [41] and apical-junctional complexes [42], events that have been linked to increased cell motility and oncogenic transformation in a variety of models [43]. In addition, some studies have been reported that the cagPAI appears to be involved in the induction of gastric interleukin-8 (IL-8) production, a potent neutrophil-activating chemokine [44]. Consequently, the presence of the cagA gene has been associated with higher grades of inflammation, which may lead to the development of the most severe gastrointestinal diseases, such as peptic ulcer disease and gastric cancer [45-48].

H. pylori duodenal ulcer promoting gene (dupA), located in the plasticity region of bacterium genome, has been initially described as a risk marker for duodenal ulcer development and a protective factor against gastric cancer [49]. It was the first putative specific marker whose association was described using strains obtained from in both Asian (Japan and Korea) and Western (Colombia) regions and it is though to be a *vir*B4 homologue [49, 50]. dupA gene encompasses two continuous sequences, jhp0917 and jhp0918, as described in strain J99. The jhp0917 gene encodes a protein of 475 amino acids, but lacks a region homologous to the C-terminus of *vir*B4, while jhp0918 gene encodes a product of 140 amino acids that is homologous to the missing *vir*B4 region [51]. Since its discovery, dupA gene has been studied by various authors, and the results of their researches suggest that, in some places, dupA gene is not associated with an specific disease [52], or it is suggested that it can be associated with gastric cancer development [53-55], or it is directly associated with the development of duodenal ulcer disease [50,56]. Considering all these results, it is suggested that there must be diversity in gene content that can contribute to bacterial adaptation to genetically different ethnic groups that make up de human population [57].

3. Gastric cancer

3.1. Epidemiology

Cancer is a worldwide full-scale problem as it will affect one in three men and one in four women during their lifetime [58]. Nowadays, this disease represents one in eight deaths around the world. The global cancer rate has doubled in the last 30 years of the 20th century, and will almost triple by 2030, a year in which it is foreseen that 20.3 million people will be diagnosed cancer and 13.2 million will die as a result of this disease [59].

World Health Organization estimates that 43% of cancer deaths are due tobacco, diet and infection. One-fifth of cancers worldwide are due to chronic infections, mainly from hepatitis viruses (liver), papillomaviruses (cervix), *H. pylori* (stomach), schistosomes (bladder), the liver fluke (bile duct), and human immunodeficiency virus (Kaposi sarcoma and lymphoma) [60].

Gastric cancer continues to be a major global health problem [61] and, despite the decreasing incidence and mortality rates observed worldwide over the last 50 years, it still ranks as a leading cause of cancer-related deaths in many parts of the world [62]. As symptoms are often absent or nonspecific in patients with the early stages of the disease, gastric cancer is usually diagnosed in an advanced stage, when curative options are limited. With exceptions in countries that have developed screening programs for early diagnoses, as example Japan, most patients reach treatment with cancers already in advanced stages [63]. Consequently, gastric cancer carries a poor prognosis, with an overall five-year survival rate of less than 20% [64].

Besides, one study assessed the survival of gastric cancer in population-based registries obtained in cities from four continents and concluded that the large differences observed among these areas were exclusively due to the different types of stomach cancer, highlighting the importance of the stage of the disease as an indicator of the effect of delayed diagnosis on the prognosis of these patients [65].

In Brazil, in 2005, the highest incidence rates, adjusted by age, were found in São Paulo (male, 38,8/100.000; female, 15,0/100.000) and the Federal District (male, 32,7/100.000; female 14,7/100.000) [66]. The National Institute of Cancer in Brazil estimates that, in 2014, there will occur 580.000 new cases of cancer. The most frequent cancers in Brazilian population will be non-melanoma skin (182.000), prostate (69.000), breast (57.000), colon and rectum (33.000), lung (27.000) and stomach (20.000). Considering Brazilian regions and gender, gastric cancer will be the fourth most common cancer in Brazil. In male gender, it is the second most common tumour in the North (11/100.000 cases) and Northeast (10/100.000 cases) regions; it is the fourth most common tumour in the Midwest (11/100.000 cases) and in the South (16/100.000) regions and the fifth most common in the Southeast region (15/100.000 cases). Concerning the female gender, gastric cancer is the fifth most common cancer in Brazil, the third most frequent in the

North region (6/100.000 cases), and the fifth most frequent in the Northeast (6/100.000 cases) and Southeast (8/100.000 cases) regions [67].

The chances of surviving the onset of some common cancers depend largely on how early they are detected and how well they are treated. Early detection is based on the observation that treatment is more effective when cancer is detected early. It includes awareness of early signs and symptoms of cancer and screening, which is the mass testing of people who appear to be healthy. In many developing countries, where these are not feasible, several other low technology approaches are being studied and look promising. The success of public health programmes in detecting cancer early depends on the allocation of resources, availability of qualified specialists and access to follow-up treatment [60].

3.2. Classification of gastric cancer

The vast majority of gastric cancers are adenocarcinomas. Two histologically distinct variants of gastric adenocarcinoma have been described, each with different pathophysiological features: the diffuse type and the intestinal type [68], which corresponds, respectively, to the undifferentiated or poorly-differentiated type and to the well-differentiated type, in the Japanese classification [69].

Diffuse type gastric adenocarcinoma is often associated with familial distribution and more commonly affects younger people. It consists of individually infiltrating neoplastic cells that do not form glandular structures and arises closer to the advancing border of inflammation but without any identifiable histological precursor lesion [62,70,71].

Gastric adenocarcinoma of the intestinal type is preceded by a prolonged precancerous process. In 1975, Correa and colleagues proposed a model of gastric carcinogenesis, postulating that the intestinal type of gastric cancer was the end result of progressive changes in the gastric mucosa, starting with chronic gastritis, followed by multifocal atrophic gastritis and intestinal metaplasia [72]. This model was updated in 1988 and 1992 [73,74] and the following steps were recognized: normal gastric mucosa → superficial gastritis (later renamed non-atrophic gastritis) → multifocal atrophic gastritis without intestinal metaplasia → intestinal metaplasia of the complete (small intestine) type → intestinal metaplasia of the incomplete (colonic) type → low-grade dysplasia (low-grade noninvasive dysplasia) → high-grade dysplasia (high-grade noninvasive dysplasia) → invasive adenocarcinoma [75]. These lesions are well-characterized histopathologically and represent a continuum of changes depicting multiple events that increase in intensity and extension with time [76].

Both diffuse and intestinal types are associated with *H. pylori* infection, which plays an initiating role in the pathogenesis of gastric cancer by changing many important factors, including antioxidant agents, reactive oxygen metabolites, and the balance between epithelial cell proliferation and apoptosis [77]. *H. pylori* infection induces cell apoptosis, stimulates cell proliferation in the gastric epithelium, and causes alterations or mutations of apoptosis/proliferation-related genes [78].

3.3. *Helicobacter pylori* and gastric cancer — The precancerous cascade

Exposure of gastric epithelial cells to *H. pylori* results in an inflammatory reaction with the production of reactive oxygen species and nitric oxide that, in turn, deaminates DNA causing mutations [62]. The complex interplay among *H. pylori* strain, inflammation and host characteristics, besides the external environment, may directly promote diffuse type gastric cancer or induce the cascade of morphological events that leads to intestinal type gastric cancer.

Specifically regarding to intestinal type gastric adenocarcinoma, evidence that *H. pylori* increases the risk of gastric cancer development via the sequence of atrophy and metaplasia originates from various studies, in which it was shown that *H. pylori* positive subjects develop these conditions more often than do uninfected controls [79]. Consequently, since *H. pylori* isolation, many investigators have emphasized its role in gastric carcinogenesis [80,81]. Epidemiological studies have determined that the attributable risk for gastric cancer conferred by *H. pylori* is approximately 75% [82]. Besides, in respect to localization in the stomach, premalignant lesions are most frequently localized in the antrum in the transitional zone between the antrum and corpus [83].

As explained before, Correa and colleagues (1975) proposed a model of gastric carcinogenesis, considering that the intestinal type gastric cancer probably is the result of histological continuum changes that occur especially due to *H. pylori* infection: chronic active nonatrophic gastritis, multifocal atrophic gastritis, intestinal metaplasia, dysplasia, and, finally, invasive adenocarcinoma. Consequently, the principal characteristics of each one of these stages are report below.

3.3.1. Chronic active non-atrophic gastritis

Gastritis is characterized by increased infiltration of the lamina propria with mononuclear leukocytes (chronic inflammation) and polymorphonuclear neutrophils (acute inflammation). Additionally, scattered eosinophils and mast cells can be observed. The gastritis is called "active" when polymorphonuclear neutrophils are found, representing acute inflammation. This phase of the precancerous process does not show loss of glands (atrophy) and is called "nonatrophic gastritis" in the updated Sydney classification of gastritis, adopted by most pathologists (Figure 1) [84].

The most frequent cause of gastritis is *H. pylori* infection and the severity of inflammation may vary according to the infected *H. pylori* strain [75].

3.3.2. Multifocal atrophic gastritis

Loss of normal glandular tissue is the first specific recognizable step in the precancerous cascade. Usually it is the result of a prolonged inflammatory process and tends to be multifocal, giving rise to the so-called multifocal atrophic gastritis (Figure 2). The foci of atrophy are present in the mucosa of gastric antrum and body, and their extension progresses with time [75]. More virulent bacterial strains and a permissive host immune response are strongly associated with atrophy and progression to severe disease [84].

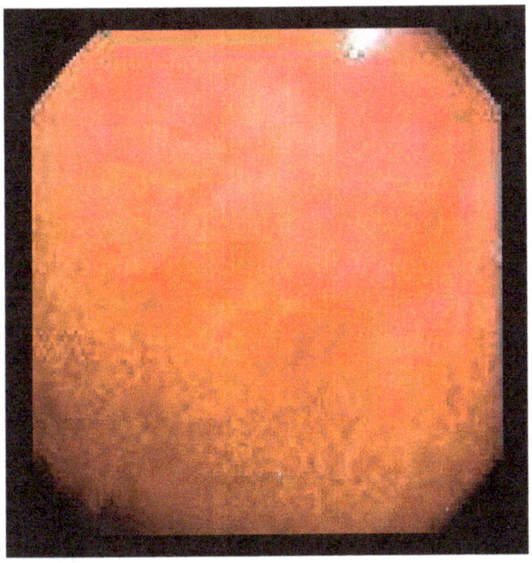

Figure 1. Chronic gastritis

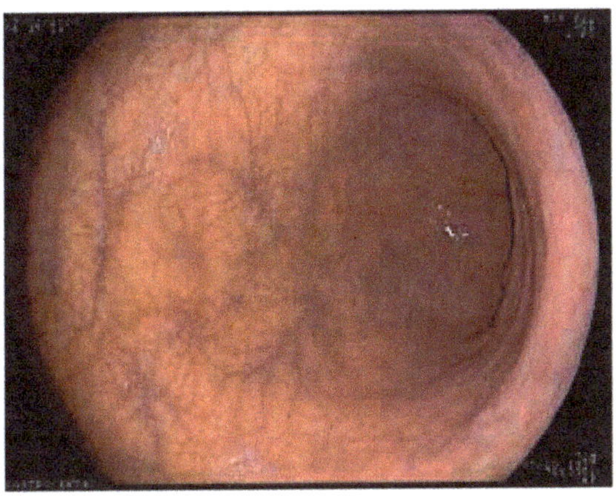

Figure 2. Atrophic gastritis

3.3.3. Intestinal metaplasia

At this stage of the gastric precancerous process, the original glands and the foveolar epithelium are replaced by cells with intestinal phenotype [84]. Intestinal metaplasia (Figure 3) is considered to be an advanced stage of atrophy because the metaplastic glands replace the original glands and chronologically the metaplastic glands appear after the gastric glands are lost. Intestinal metaplasia has been classified on the basis of morphology and enzyme histochemistry in two main types: the small intestine or complete type, and the colonic or incomplete type [75].

Up to this point in the cascade, the epithelium in the atrophic and metaplastic lesions remains well differentiated, with normal nuclear-cytoplasmic ratio, normal nuclear morphology, and normal tissue architecture. The dynamics of the precancerous process to this point shows a gradual phenotypic transformation from normal epithelium to metaplastic cells with small intestinal morphology and then to cells resembling colonic mucosa, additionally expressing gastric and colonic mucins. This process usually takes decades and is progressive, supporting the notion that although environmental alterations (bacterial factors and cytokine environment, loss of cell signaling) may have initially driven differentiation decisions, with time, permanent changes in the stem cell compartment have occurred. In some patients with incomplete metaplasia, a mild degree of nuclear atypia and architectural distortion is observed, leading some investigators to consider incomplete metaplasia as a mild form of dysplasia [84,85].

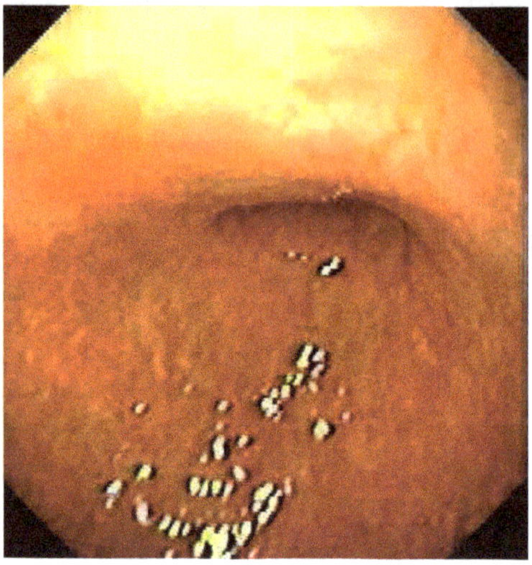

Figure 3. Intestinal metaplasia (antrum)

3.3.4. *Dysplasia*

Also called intraepithelial neoplasia or noninvasive neoplasia, dysplasia is characterized by a neoplastic phenotype, both in terms of cell morphology and architectural organization [75]. The nuclei of the dysplastic epithelium are enlarged, hyperchromatic, irregular in shape, and devoid of polarity [84]. The Padova classification is focused on gastric dysplasia and was developed by an international group of experienced gastrointestinal pathologists and recognizes five categories of lesions, utilizing mostly western nomenclature and grouping them numerically following the prevailing Japanese system: 1. negative for dysplasia; 2. indefinite for dysplasia; 3. noninvasive neoplasia (sub-classified in low grade or high grade); 4. suspicious for invasive carcinoma; and 5. invasive carcinoma [86].

The management of low-grade dysplasia is not well defined and there is a recommendation of annual endoscopic monitoring with rebiopsy [87]. Nevertheless, patients with high-grade dysplasia confirmed at least two gastrointestinal pathologists should undergo surgical or endoscopic resection because of the high probability of coexisting or metachronous invasive carcinoma [88].

3.3.5. Invasive adenocarcinoma

Invasive adenocarcinoma is the next stage in the cascade and requires the penetration of neoplastic cells into the surrounding stroma (Figure 4). Recent evidence suggests that this step demands that neoplastic cells acquire the capability of degrading the stromal matrix surrounding the neoplastic cells [75.

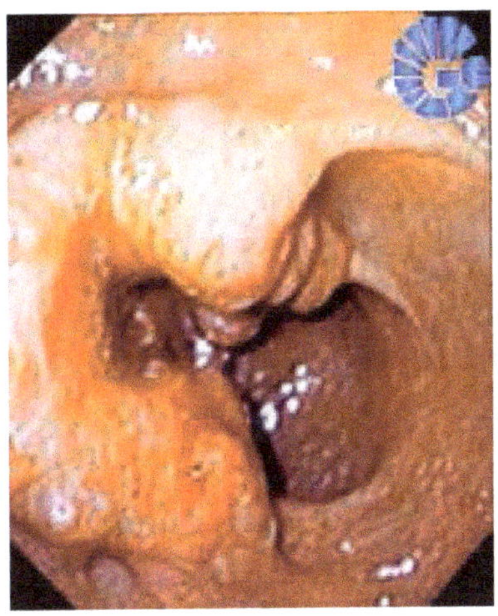

Figure 4. Gastric adenocarcinoma

3.4. Early and advanced lesions

Follow-up of patients with precursor lesions in populations at high gastric cancer risk has thrown light on the dynamics of the process. The progression of the precursor lesions described before follows a pattern of steady state, with episodes of progression to more advanced lesions and episodes of regression to less advanced lesions.

Unlike patients with advanced gastric cancer, patients diagnosed in an early stage of the disease present an excellent prognostic, in which a five-year survival rate is more than 90%. Early gastric cancer lesions are defined as the adenocarcinoma that is confined to the mucosa or submucosa, irrespective of lymphonode invasion (Figure 5). Many early gastric cancers are believed to go through a life cycle consisting of ulcerations, followed by healing, then reulceration, and some lesions remain at this early stage for years even without treatment [89]. Nevertheless, some early tumours rapidly became advanced and it is one of the principal questions concerning the gastric carcinogenesis. Are *H. pylori* virulence factors important to influence these alterations? To what extent *H. pylori* eradication treatment would be important to prevent the continued progression of the disease? To what extent *H. pylori* eradication in the early stage of cancer would be important to prevent the appearance of new lesions?

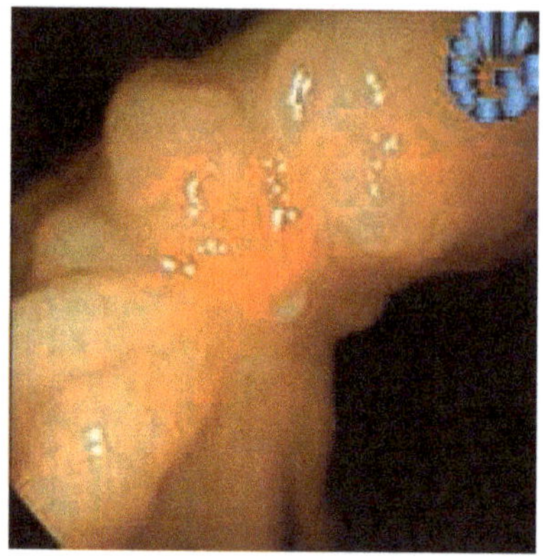

Figure 5. Early gastric adenocarcinoma

Considering these important questions, our chapter is divided into two sections: 1. the identification of the principal genetic characteristics of *H. pylori* strains in Brazilian patients with early distal type intestinal gastric adenocarcinoma, in order to determine the genotypic pattern of bacterium in our population through molecular techniques; 2. the discussion of the principal studies concerning *H. pylori* eradication and its importance to prevent the progression of precancerous lesions and the importance of *H. pylori* eradication in the early gastric cancer to prevent the development of new cancerous lesions.

4. Materials and methods

4.1. Determination of principal genotypes of *H. Pylori* in Brazilian patients with early gastric adenocarcinoma

4.1.1. Clinical samples

Clinical isolates of *H. pylori* analyzed in this study were obtained from the Laboratory of Pathology of the Center of Diagnosis of Digestive Diseases, Faculty of Medical Sciences, State University of Campinas (Campinas, São Paulo, Brazil). Third one paraffin wax-embedded specimens of gastric tissue were analyzed from a total of 31 patients with early distal type intestinal gastric adenocarcinoma. All the gastric tissue samples were obtained from endoscopic biopsy and were positive for *H. pylori* by histological analysis. Samples from gastric tissue obtained from endoscopic biopsy of patients with chronic gastritis and peptic ulcer disease and positive for *H. pylori* were used as positive controls for all the reactions carried out in this study. The study was approved by the Ethics Committee of the Faculty of Medical Sciences, State University of Campinas.

4.1.2. Methods

Paraffin wax-embedded tissue DNA extraction was carried out with xylene and ethanol washes for paraffin removal; successive steps using proteinase K, phenol, chloroform, and isoamyl alcohol were carried out in order to isolate and purify the DNA [90]. Quantification of the obtained product and polymerase chain reaction (PCR) for human betaglobin gene [91] were carried out to guarantee the quality of all the results.

After DNA extraction, PCR for ureaseC [92], vacA (s and m) [93,94,95], cagA [96], cagT [97] and dupA (jhp0917 and jhp0918) [49] genes were performed. Primers pairs for all the genes as well as the length of the fragments are described in Table 1. PCR for ureaseC gene was carried out to confirm the positivity for *H. pylori* in all the samples.

After amplification, each PCR product was analyzed by eletrophoresis on a 2% agarose gel stained with ethidium bromide with a 0.5 X tris-acetate-EDTA buffer. A 100-bp ladder was used as standard.

Gene	Strand	Primer sequence (5´ - 3´)	Length (bp)
betaglobin	+	ACAAACTGTGTTCACTAGC	110
	-	CAACTTCATCCACGTTTCACC	
ureaseC	+	AAGCTTTAGGGGTGTTAGGGGTTT	294
	-	AAGCTTACTTTCTAACACTAACGC	
vacA (s1/s2)	+	ATGGAAATACAACAAACACAC	s1: 259
	-	CTGCTTGAATGCGCCAAAC	s2: 286
vacA m1	+	GGTCAAAATGCGGTCATGG	290
	-	CCATTGGTACCTGTAGAAAC	
vacA m2	+	ATGCTTTAATATCGTTGAGA	198
	-	GAACATGTTTTAGTGAAAGC	
cagA	+	GATAACAGGCAAGCTTTTGAGG	349
	-	CTGCAAAAGATTGTTTGGCAGA	
cagT	+	CCATGTTTATACGCCTGTGT	301
	-	CATCACCACACCCTTTTGAT	
dupA (jhp0917)	+	TGGTTTCTACTGACAGAGCGC	307
	-	AACACGCTGACAGGACAATCTCCC	
dupA (jhp0918)	+	CCTATATCGCTAACGCGCGCTC	276
	-	AAGCTGAAGCGTTTGTAACG	

Table 1. Sequence of synthetic oligonucleotide primers used to characterization of *H. pylori* strains

Then, for each specific reaction, products obtained were classified in vacA s1m1, s2m1, s1m2 or s2m2; cagA positive or negative; cagT positive or negative; and dupA positive or negative. dupA gene was considered positive when its two regions (jhp0917 and jhp0918) were positive simultaneously.

After all amplifications, a table with absolute frequencies (n) and percentages (%) was made in order to determine genotypes combinations.

4.2. Analysis of the principal manuscript references concerning the study of eradication treatment of *H. pylori* in precancerous lesions and early gastric cancer

After determination of the principal genotype presented in Brazilian patients with early gastric cancer, a review concerning the importance of eradication of *H. pylori* in precancerous lesions and in early gastric adenocacinoma was done.

5. Results

5.1. Determination of principal genotypes of *H. Pylori* in Brazilian patients with early gastric adenocarcinoma

PCR for ureaseC gene of *H. pylori* was positive for all 31 samples obtained from patients with early distal type intestinal gastric adenocarcinoma. As regards to vacA gene region s, of 31 samples, 71.0% (22 cases) were s1 and 29.0% (9 cases) were s2. Related to the vacA region m, all the samples were m1. Following this analysis, samples were classified in s1m1 or s2m1. So, 71.0% (22 cases) were s1m1 and 29.0% (9 cases) were s2m1.

Classification	
UreaseC	31 (100.0%)
vacA s1	22 (71.0%)
vacA s2	9 (29.0%)
vacA m1	31 (100.0%)
vacA m2	0 (0.0%)
vacA s1m1	22 (71.0%)
vacA s2m1	9 (29.0%)
cagA positive	19 (61.3%)
cagA negative	12 (38.7%)
cagT positive	17 (54.8%)
cagT negative	14 (45.2%)
dupA (jhp0917/jhp0918) positive	11 (35.5%)
dupA (jhp0917/jhp0918) negative	20 (64.5%)
Total	31 (100.0%)

Table 2. Frequencies and percentages of the principal genes of *H. pylori* studied in samples of early gastric cancer

As regards to gene cagA, 61.3% (19 cases) were cagA positive and, for cagT gene, 54.8% (17 cases) were positive. For dupA (jhp0917/jhp0918) gene, there were 35.5% (11 cases) of positivity. All these results can be seen in Table 2.

Genotypes combinations where then analyzed and the most prevalent genotype for gastric samples obtained from Brazilian patients with early distal type intestinal gastric adenocarcinoma was vacA s1m1, cagA positive, cagT positive and dupA negative (Table 3).

Genotype combinations: vacA s/m cagA cagT dupA (jhp0917/jhp0918)	Early gastric cancer
s1m1 neg neg neg	4 (12.90)
s1m1 neg neg pos	1 (3.23)
s2m1 neg neg neg	1 (3.23)
s2m1 neg neg pos	0 (0.00)
s1m1 neg pos neg	2 (6.45)
s1m1 neg pos pos	1 (3.23)
s2m1 neg pos neg	2 (6.45)
s2m1 neg pos pos	1 (3.23)
s1m1 pos neg neg	3 (9.68)
s1m1 pos neg pos	2 (6.45)
s2m1 pos neg neg	2 (6.45)
s2m1 pos neg pos	1 (3.23)
s1m1 pos pos neg	5 (16.13)
s1m1 pos pos pos	4 (12.90)
s2m1 pos pos neg	2 (6.45)
s2m1 pos pos pos	0 (0.00)
Total	**31**

Table 3. Genotype combinations for early gastric adenocarcinoma samples

5.2. Analysis of the principal manuscript references concerning the study of eradication treatment of *H. pylori* in precancerous lesions and early gastric cancer

Epidemiological studies have established a strong causal relationship between *H. pylori* infection and gastric cancer. *H. pylori* eradication is therefore likely to be one of the most promising approaches to gastric cancer prevention. Animal studies have shown that eradication of *H. pylori* infection, especially at the early stage, is effective in preventing *H. pylori*-related gastric carcinogenesis. However, the available data from human studies show that *H. pylori* eradication does not completely prevent gastric cancer and that it might be useful in patients without atrophic gastritis or intestinal metaplasia at baseline [77].

Considering these important issues, the present chapter book analized and discussed some studies that assessed the possible relationship between the eradication of *H. pylori* infection and the prevention of gastric cancer even if the precancerous cascade has started. Obviously, there should be a point which there is no return in this process and the presence of *H. pylori* could not be more decisive to continue the progression of the precancerous lesions. With the aim to analyze these topics, we discussed some important questions concerning *H. pylori* infection, precancerous cascade and *H. pylori* eradication treatment, both in the precancerous lesions (atrophic gastritis, metaplasia intestinal and dysplasia) and in the early gastric cancer stage.

6. Discussion

Molecular techniques may be applied to the measurement of host or agent factors and of exposures. Molecular techniques help to stratify and to refine data by providing more sensitive and specific measurements, which facilitate epidemiologic activities, including disease surveillance, outbreak investigations, identifying transmission patterns and risk factors among apparently disparate cases, characterizing host-pathogen interactions, detecting uncultivatable organisms, providing clues for possible infectious causes of cancer and other chronic diseases, and providing better understanding of disease pathogenesis at the molecular level [98].

Our study determined the principal genotype of *H. pylori* strains in Brazilian patients with early distal type intestinal gastric adenocarcinoma, which is vacA s1m1, cagA positive, cagT positive and dupA negative. It provides to the scientific community important information concerning the epidemiology of gastric cancer in Brazil, as regards to the infecting strains. This principal *H. pylori* genotype was also the principal found in advanced gastric cancer samples, but, when considering the cagA gene in an isolate evaluation, it was more incident in patients with advanced gastric cancer [48].

Many factors, including a high-salt diet [99], genetic abnormality [100] and autoimmune gastritis [101], among others, have been reported concerning gastric carcinogenesis; however, it is clear that *H. pylori* infection is the most important gastric carcinogen [60, 102].

Currently recommended anti-*H. pylori* infection therapies achieve eradication rates of up to 90% [103]. Several studies have indicated that *H. pylori* screening and eradication is a cost-effective strategy for the prevention of gastric cancer in middle-aged adults, even if the treatment prevents only 20%-30% of *H. pylori*-associated cancers, and that the strategy is particularly beneficial in high-risk populations and in the long term [77,104,105,106], although the feasibility, safety and appropriated timing of this strategy for cancer prevention in the general population remains to be determined [77].

Some studies focused on patients with gastric precancerous lesions such as gastric atrophy, intestinal metaplasia and dysplasia and evaluated the effect of eradicating *H. pylori* on the intermediate lesions in the carcinogenic cascade rather than using gastric cancer as the primary end points [107].

Conflicting results have been reported on whether or not these precancerous lesions were reversible following successful eradication of *H. pylori* infection.

The investigation of Uemura et al. (2001) [108] is considered the first study providing some evidence that *H. pylori* eradication has an impact in gastric cancer. In this study, none of the 253 treated patients developed cancer, whilst there were 36 gastric cancer cases among 993 untreated patients. However, it is of note that the mean duration of follow-up after eradication was significantly shorter than the mean duration for patients who were not treated (4,8 vs. 8,5 years; $p < 0.001$). Therefore, the risk of gastric cancer development could have been understated in the treated group [107].

In a randomized placebo controlled study in China, gastritis (acute and chronic) decreased in both the antrum and the corpus at one year after *H. pylori* eradication and a slight regression of intestinal metaplasia was observed [109]. With similar results, a follow-up study developed by Zhou et al. (2003) [110] demonstrated that *H. pylori* eradication significantly reduced the severity and activity of chronic gastritis. Besides, while the proportion of intestinal metaplasia in the *H. pylori* positive group increased significantly, intestinal metaplasia in the antrum either regressed or had no progression in the *H. pylori* negative group.

In Colombia, a randomized, controlled chemoprevention trial with patients with confirmed multifocal nonmetaplastic atrophy and/or intestinal metaplasia demonstrated that, after *H. pylori* eradication therapy and/or dietary supplementation with ascorbic acid or beta-carotene, or their placebos, it was observed a significant increase in the rate of regression of the precursos lesions [111].

Other follow-up studies also identified that *H. pylori* eradication in patients with intestinal metaplasia could be important in the regression of the lesions [112-118]. In the same way, other randomized studies identified that *H. pylori* eradication in intestinal metaplasia could be important in the regression of this precancerous lesion [76,109-111,119,120]. Oppositely, other trials, both follow-up and randomized control, had not identified regression of intestinal metaplasia when *H. pylori* eradication was administrated [121-129].

Concerning to patients with gastric atrophy, the most part of the studies have identified that this lesion presents a regression when *H. pylori* eradication occurs [76, 109, 111, 119, 120, 128-130]. In Japan, where there is a significant ability in diagnostic, with a detection of 94% of early gastric cancers, one important multicenter randomized controlled trial by the Japan Gast Study Group enrolled patients undergoing previous endoscopic therapy for gastric cancer and demonstrated that eradication therapy significantly reduced the prevalence of secondary gastric cancer in a 3-year follow-up period [131]. However, this study does not demonstrate that eradication therapy can prevent newly developed gastric cancer even in secondary cancer, because the follow-up period was too short.

As well as other authors mentioned before, Ito (2009) [132] considered that theoretically *H. pylori* eradication therapy should be beneficial for cancer prevention. However, attention should be drawn to the fact that the gastric cancer risk is not similar between noninfected and eradicated people. Until now, many human studies have demonstrated that some patients develop gastric cancer even if they have undergone successful eradication therapy [133]. Considering it, we can conclude that eradication therapy may have an effect on cancer prevention if the therapy is administrated before a single cancer cell has transformed or before cancer tissue shows invasive growth. It is likely that eradication therapy has no effect if the cancer has progressed to an advanced stage.

Wong et al. (2004) [134], with the aim to determine whether eradication of *H. pylori* infection reduces the incidence of gastric cancer, carried out a randomized, placebo controlled trial with 1630 *H. pylori* infected patients in a high-risk region of China. Their results indicated that *H. pylori* eradication can reduce the incidence of gastric cancer in patients without precancerous lesions at entry. Besides, the eradication therapy had no statistically significant effect on the incidence of gastric cancer in patients with precancerous lesions on presentation. It appears that there is a point of no return for patients with precancerous lesions and a chemoprevention strategy may work only in a subset of *H. pylori* infected subjects [135].

As regards to animal models, they are useful because they represent tractable systems that permit insights into the effects of host, pathogen and environmental factors on gastric carcinogenesis [136]. Nevertheless, the use of animals does not completely reflect *H. pylori*-induced cancer in humans. Romero-Gallo et al. (2008) [137], using a population of gerbils that received antibiotics for *H. pylori* treatment, demonstrated that the timing of intervention influences the magnitude of suppression of pro-inflammatory cytokine expression, inflammation, pre-malignant, and neoplastic lesions. These findings have demonstrated that treatment of *H. pylori* decreases the incidence and the severity of pro-inflammatory cytokine expression, as well as premalignant and malignant lesions. However, the effectiveness of eradication is dependent upon the timing of intervention [137].

A 5-year study in Japanese monkeys (*Macaca fustata*) demonstrated that *H. pylori* infection can cause gastric atrophy, increased cell proliferation, and mutation of *p53* in gastric epithelial cells [138]. In other study, with Mongolian gerbils, it was demonstrated that the resulting pathological changes in gastric mucosa are similar to those in humans [139]. Some studies demonstrated that when the animals were infected with *H. pylori* together with a carcinogen (N-methyl-N-nitrosourea or N-methyl-N-nitro-N-nitrosoguanidine), they developed gastric cancer (both diffuse and intestinal types) that were at significantly higher frequencies than animals receiving either *H. pylori* or the carcinogen alone [140-142]. Gastric cancer incidence was reduced at 75 weeks to 6.7%, 27.3%, and 38.2% in Mongolian gerbils receiving eradication treatment at early (15 weeks), middle (35 weeks) and late (55 weeks) stages, respectively. These results suggest that eradication at an early stage might be effective in preventing carcinogenesis. Other study demonstrated that application of antimicrobial therapy at 8 weeks postinoculation of bacterium attenuated inflammation, but did not completely prevent the development of premalignant and malignant lesions, indicating that the *H. pylori* eradication therapy is effective when administered at an early stage after infection [143]. Nevertheless, it is important to remember that the carcinogenic potential of *H. pylori* is strain dependent and some results of these studies could be caused by the use of an *H. pylori* strain that lacked carcinogenic potential.

In the mouse model, both *H. pylori* infection and gastric atrophy increase the serum concentration of polypeptide hormone gastrin, a hormone that controls secretion of gastric acid by the stomach´s parietal cells and hypergastrinemia is regarded to play a role in the development.

The results obtained indicated that the timing of antimicrobial eradication therapy is very important as early application can prevent the progression of gastric cancer [144].

Finally, for cancers detected early, endoscopic mucosal resection can conserve the noncancerous gastric mucosa, but it can not eliminate the recurrence of metachronous gastric cancer [145]. Fukase et al. (2008) [131], in a randomized control trial, studied a group of patients submitted to *H. pylori* eradication therapy following endoscopic resection of early gastric cancer. These patients were monitored at different time intervals: at 3 years, metachronous gastric cancer had developed in 9 of 225 patients in the eradication group compared with 24 of 250 patients in the control group, suggesting that prophylactic eradication of *H. pylori* in a high-risk population can substantially reduce gastric cancer rates.

Briefly, the most part of the studies suggests that *H. pylori* eradication is able to induce regression of precancerous lesions in most of the treated subjects, and particularly in those with baseline, early and non-severe lesions. However, it also seems that a proportion of treated subjects will still show progression of preneoplastic lesions. So, we can consider that they really are other factors that contribute to the progression of these lesions. So, *H. pylori* eradication is an effective strategy in reducing the risk of gastric cancer; however, it is not efficient enough to eradicate gastric cancer. Prevention of the infection, *H. pylori* immunization, *H. pylori* eradication in the youth, selection of the high-risk population, and alternative chemopreventive measures may be essential for optimal management of malignancy of the stomach.

7. Conclusions

All the available evidence suggests that *H. pylori* eradication might represent a primary chemopreventive strategy in a subset of subjects. However, *H. pylori* eradication in those patients who have already developed advanced preneoplastic lesions does not prevent gastric cancer development, and endoscopic follow-up should always be performed.

More research is needed to elucidate mechanisms underlying the *H. pylori*-induced gastric carcinogenesis. As the infection usually depends on the characteristics of the infecting strain, studies that determine the genotypes in gastric cancer, as we presented in our study, are necessary. Besides, more trials concerning the interaction among the infecting strain, the host characteristics and the external environment are also needed to explaining the complex gastric carcinogenesis. An understanding of biochemical, genetic and epigenetic changes following eradication therapy would be helpful to develop strategies to identify high-risk individuals, thereby contributing to effective management in gastric cancer prevention.

Finally, it is important to gain more insight into the pathogenesis of H. pylori-induced gastric adenocarcinoma, not only to develop more effective treatments for this cancer, but also because it might serve as a paradigm for the role of chronic inflammation in the genesis of other malignancies.

Author details

Bruna Maria Roesler and José Murilo Robilotta Zeitune

*Address all correspondence to: roeslerbruna@gmail.com

Department of Internal Medicine, Center of Diagnosis of Digestive Diseases, Faculty of Medical Sciences – State University of Campinas – UNICAMP, Campinas, São Paulo, Brazil

References

[1] Kusters JG, van Vliet AHM, Kuipers EJ. Pathogenesis of *Helicobacter pylori* infection. Clinical Microbiology Reviews 2006; 19(3): 449-490.

[2] Goodwin CS, Armstrong JA. Microbiological aspects of *Helicobacter pylori* (*Campylobacter pylori*). European Journal of Clinical Microbiology 1990; 9(1): 1-13.

[3] Bode G, Mauch F, Malfertheiner P. The coccoid forms of *Helicobacter pylori*. Criteria for their viability. Epidemiology and Infection 1993; 111(3): 483-490.

[4] Blaser MJ. An endangered species in the stomach. Scientific American 2005; 292(2): 38-45.

[5] Ahmed N. 23 years of the discovery of *Helicobacter pylori*: Is the debate over? Annals of Clinical Microbiology and Antimicrobials 2005; 4: 17-19.

[6] Replogle ML, Glaser SL, Hiatt RA, Parsonnet J. Biologic sex as a risk factor for *Helicobacter pylori* infection in healthy young adults. American Journal of Epidemiology 1995; 142(8): 856-863.

[7] Graham DY, Malaty HM, Evans DG, Evans DJ, Klein PD, Adam E. Epidemiology of *Helicobacter pylori* in an asymptomatic population in the United States. Gastroenterology 1991; 100(6): 1495-1501.

[8] Urita Y, Watanabe T, Kawagoe N, Takemoto I, Tanaka H, Kijima S, Kido H, Maeda T, Sugasawa Y, Miyazaki T, Honda Y, Nakanishi K, Shimada N, Nakajima H, Sugimoto M, Urita C. Role of infected grandmothers in transmission of *Helicobacter pylori* to children in a Japanese rural town. Journal of Paediatrics and Child Health 2013; 49(5): 394-398.

[9] Bastos J, Carreira H, La Vecchia C, Lunet N. Childcare attendance and *Helicobacter pylori* infection: systematic review and meta-analysis. European Journal of Cancer Prevention 2013; 22(4): 311-319.

[10] Covacci A, Telford JL, Del Giudice G, Parsonnet J, Rapuolli R. *Helicobacter pylori* virulence and genetic geography. Science 1998; 284(5418): 1328-1333.

[11] Dubois A, Fiala N, Heman-Ackah LM, Drazek ES, Tarnawski A, Fishbein WN, Perez-Perez GI, Blaser MJ. Natural gastric infection with *Helicobacter pylori* in monkeys: a model for spiral bacteria infection in humans. Gastroenterology 1994; 106(6): 1405-1417.

[12] Fox JG, Batchelder M, Marini R, Yan L, Handt L, Li X, Shames B, Hayward A, Campbell J, Murphy JC. *Helicobacter pylori*-induced gastritis in the domestic cat. Infection and Immunity 1995; 63(7): 2674-2681.

[13] Grubel P, Hoffman JS, Chong FK, Burstein NA, Mepani C, Cave DR. Vector potential of houseflies (*Musca domestica*) for *Helicobacter pylori*. Journal of Clinical Microbiology 1997; 35(6): 1300-1303.

[14] Dunn BE, Cohen H, Blaser MJ. *Helicobacter pylori*. Clinical Microbiology Reviews 1997; 10(4): 720-741.

[15] Lu Y, Redlinger TE, Avitia R, Galindo A, Goodman K. Isolation and genotyping of *Helicobacter pylori* from untreated municipal wastewater. Applied and Environmental Microbiology 2002; 68(3): 1436-1439.

[16] Bahrami AR, Rahimi E, Ghasemian Safaei H. Detection of *Helicobacter pylori* in City Water, Dental Unit's Water and Bottled Mineral Water in Isfahan, Iran. Scientific World Journal 2013.

[17] Marshall BJ, Warren JR. Unidentified curved bacilli in the stomach of patients with gastritis and peptic ulceration. Lancet 1984; 1(8390): 1311-1315.

[18] Ahmed N, Sechi LA. *Helicobacter pylori* and gastroduodenal pathology. New threats of the old friend. Annals of Clinical Microbiology and Antimicrobials 2005; 4:1-10.

[19] International Agency for Research on Cancer. Schistosomes, liver flukes and *Helicobacter pylori*. IARC Working Group on the Evaluation of Carcinogenic Risks to Humans. IARC monographs on the evaluation of carcinogenic risks to humans. World Health Organization, International Agency for Research on Cancer 1994; 61: 1-241.

[20] Capurso G, Lahner E, Marcheggiano A, Caruana P, Carnuccio A, Bordi C, Delle Fave G, Annibale B. Involvement of the corporal mucosa and related changes in gastric acid secretion characterize patients with iron deficiency anemy associated with *Helicobacter pylori* infection. Alimentary Pharmacology & Therapeutics 2001; 15(11): 1753-1761.

[21] Pelicano R, Franceschi F, Saracco G, Fagoonee S, Roccarina D, Gasbarrini A. *Helicobacters* and extragastric diseases. Helicobacter 2009; 14(Suppl 1): 58-68.

[22] Arnold DM, Bernotas A, Nazi I, Stasi R, Kuwana M, Liu Y, Kelton JG, Crowther MA. Platelet count response to *H. pylori* treatment in patients with immune thrombocytopenic purpura with and without *H. pylori* infection: a systematic review. Haematologica 2009; 94(6): 850-856.

[23] Franceschi F, Navarese EP, Mollo R, Giupponi B, De Marco G, Merra G, Gasbarrini G, Silveri NG. *Helicobacter pylori* and atherosclerosis. A review of the literature. Recenti Progressi in Medicina 2009; 100(2): 91-96.

[24] Rogha M, Nikvarz M, Poumoghaddas Z, Shirneshan K, Dadkhah D, Poumoghaddas M. Is *Helicobacter pylori* infection a risk factor for coronary heart disease? ARYA Atherosclerosis 2012; 8(1): 5-8.

[25] Isaeva GSh, Abuzarova ER, Valeeva IuV, Pozdeev OK, Murav′eva EV. *Helicobacter pylori* in patients with disorders of hepatobiliary system. Zh Mikrobiol Epidemiol Immunobiol 2009; 2: 96-101.

[26] Pirouz T, Zounubi L, Keivani H, Rakhshani N, Hormazdi M. Detection of *Helicobacter pylori* in paraffin-embedded specimens from patients with chronic liver diseases, using the amplification method. Digestive Diseases and Sciences 2009; 54(7): 1456-1459.

[27] Zhou X, Zhang C, Wu J, Zhang G. Association between *Helicobacter pylori* infection and diabetes mellitus: a meta-analysis of observational studies. Diabetes Research and Clinical Practice 2013; 99(2): 200-208.

[28] Blaser MJ, Berg DE. *Helicobacter pylori* genetic diversity and risk of human disease. The Journal of Clinical Investigation 2001; 107(7): 767-773.

[29] Suerbaum S, Michetti P. *Helicobacter pylori* infection. New England Journal of Medicine 2002; 347(15): 1175-1186.

[30] Megraud F, Neman-Simha, Brugmann D. Further evidence of the toxic effect of ammonia produced by Helicobacter pylori urease on human epithelial cells. Infection and Immunity 1992; 60(5): 1858-1863.

[31] Suzuki M, Miura S, Suematsu M, Fukumura D, Kurose I, Suzuki H, Kai A, Kudoh Y, Ohashi M, Tsuchiya M *Helicobacter pylori*-associated ammonia production enhances neutrophil-dependent gastric mucosal cell injury. American Journal of Physiology 1992; 263 (5 Pt 1): G719-725.

[32] Montecucco C, Rapuolli R. Living dangerously: how *Helicobacter pylori* survives in the human stomach. Nature Reviews. Molecular Cell Biology 2001; 2(6): 457-466.

[33] Harris PR, Mobley HL, Perez-Perez GI, Blaser MJ, Smith PD. *Helicobacter pylori* urease is a potent stimulus of mononuclear phagocyte activation and inflammatory cytokine production. Gastroenterology 1996; 111(2): 419-425.

[34] Leunk RD, Johnson PT, David BC, Kraft WG, Morgan DR. Cytotoxic activity in broth-culture filtrates of *Campylobacter pylori*. Journal of Medical Microbiology 1988; 26(2): 93-99.

[35] Amieva MR, El-Omar EM. Host-bacterial interactions in *Helicobacter pylori* infection. Gastroenterology 2008; 134(1): 306-323.

[36] Atherton JC, Cao P, Peek RMJr, Tummuru MK, Blaser MJ, Cover TL. Mosaicism in vacuolating cytotoxin alleles of *Helicobacter pylori*. Association of specific vacA types

with cytotoxin production and peptic ulceration. *Journal of Biological Chemistry 1995; 270(30): 17771-17777.*

[37] Covacci A, Rappuoli R. Tyrosine-phosphorylated bacterial proteins: Trojan horses for the host cell. Journal of Experimental Medicine 2000; 191(4): 587-592.

[38] Backert S, Selbach M. Role of type IV secretion in *Helicobacter pylori* pathogenesis. Cellular Microbiology 2008; 10(8): 1573-1581.

[39] Hatakeyama M. Oncogenic mechanisms of the *Helicobacter pylori* CagA protein. Nature Reviews. Cancer 2004; 4(9): 688-694.

[40] Higashi H, Tsutsumi R, Muto S, Sugiyama T, Azuma T, Asaka M, Hatakeyama M. SHP-2 tyrosine phosphatase as an intrancellular target of *Helicobacter pylori* CagA protein. Science 2002; 295(5555): 683-686.

[41] Murata-Kamiya N, Kurashima Y, Teishikata Y, Yamahashi Y, Saito Y, Higashi H, Aburatani H, Akiyama T, Peek RMJr, Azuma T, Hatakeyama M. *Helicobacter pylori* CagA interacts with E-cadherin and deregulates the β-catenin signal that promotes intestinal transdifferentiation in gastric epithelial cells. Oncogene 2007; 26(32): 4671-4626.

[42] Amieva MR, Vogelmann R, Covacci A, Tompkins LS, Nelson WJ, Falkow S. Disruption of the epithelial apical-junctional complex by *Helicobacter pylori* CagA. Science 2003; 300(5624): 1430-1434.

[43] Suzuki M, Mimuro H, Suzuki T, Park M, Yamamoto T, Sasakawa C. Interaction of CagA with Crk plays an important role in *Helicobacter pylori*-induced loss of gastric epithelial cell adhesion. Journal of Experimental Medicine 2005; 202(9): 1235-1247.

[44] Brandt S, Kwok T, Hartig R, Konig W, Backert S. NF-kappaB activation and potentiation of proinflammatory responses by the *Helicobacter pylori* CagA protein. Proceedings of the National Academy of Sciences of the United States of America 2005; 102(26): 9300-9305.

[45] Blaser MJ, Perez-Perez GI, Kleanthous H, Cover TL, Peek RM, Chyou PH, Stemmermann GN, Nomura A. Infection with *Helicobacter pylori* strains possessing cagA is associated with an increased risk of developing adenocarcinoma of the stomach. Cancer Research 1995; 55(10): 2111-2115.

[46] Parsonnet J, Friedman GD, Orentreich N, Vogelman H. Risk for gastric cancer in people with CagA positive or CagA negative *Helicobacter pylori* infection. Gut 1997; 40(3): 297-301.

[47] Figueiredo C, van Doorn LJ, Nogueira C, Soares JM, Pinho C, Figueira P, Quint WG, Carneiro F. *Helicobacter pylori* genotypes are associated with clinical outcome in Portuguese patients and show a high prevalence of infections with multiple strains. Scandinavian Journal of Gastroenterology 2001; 36(2): 128-135.

[48] Roesler BM, Costa SCB, Zeitune JMR. Virulence factors of *Helicobacter pylori* and their relationship with the development of early and advanced distal intestinal type gastric adennocarcinoma. In: Paola Tonino (ed.). Gastritis and gastric cancer. New insights in gastroprotection, diagnosis and treatments. Rijeka: InTech; 2011.

[49] Lu H, Hsu P, Graham DY, Yamaoka Y. Duodenal ulcer promoting gene of *Helicobacter pylori.* Gastroenterology 2005; 128(4): 833-848.

[50] Zhang Z, Zheng Q, Chen X, Xiao S, Liu W, Lu H. The *Helicobacter pylori* duodenal ulcer promoting gene, dupA in China. BMC Gastroenterology 2008; 8: 49-54.

[51] Yamaoka Y. Roles of the plasticity regions of *Helicobacter pylori* in gastroduodenal pathogenesis. Journal of Medical Microbiology 2008; 57(5): 545-553.

[52] Douraghi M, Mohammadi M, Oghalaie A, Abdirad A, Mohagheghi MA, Hosseini ME, Zeraati H, Ghasemi A, Esmaieli M, Mohajerani N. dupA as a risk determinant in *Helicobacter pylori* infection. Journal of Medical Microbiology 2008; 57 (Pt.5): 554-562.

[53] Argent RH, Burette A, Miendje Deyi VY, Atherton JC. The presence of dupA in *Helicobacter pylori* is not significantly associated with duodenal ulceration in Belgium, South Africa, China or North America. Clinical Infectious Diseases 2007; 45(9): 1204-1206.

[54] Schimidt HMA, Andres S, Kaakoush NO, Engstrand L, Eriksson L, Goh KL, Fock KM, Hilmi I, Dhamodaran S, Forman D, Mitchell H. The prevalence of the duodenal ulcer promoting gene (dupA) in *Helicobacter pylori* isolates varies by ethnic group and is not universally associated with disease development: a case-control study. Gut Pathogens 2009; 1(1): 5-13.

[55] Roesler BM, Oliveira TB, Costa SCB, Zeitune JMR. Is there any relationship between *Helicobacter pylori* dupA gene and the development of early and advanced gastric cancer in Brazilian patients? Journal of Medical Research and Science 2011; 2(1): 15-24.

[56] Arachchi HSJ, Kalra V, Lal B, Bhatia V, Baba CS, Chakravarthy S, Rohatgi S, Sarma PM, Mishra V, Das B, Ahuja V. Prevalence of duodenal ulcer promoting gene (dupA) of *Helicobacter pylori* in patients with duodenal ulcer in North Indian population. Helicobacter. 2007; 12(6): 591-597

[57] Gressmann H, Linz B, Ghai R, Pleissner KP, Schlapbach R, Yamaoka Y, Kraft C, Suerbaum S, Meyer TF, Achtman M. Gain and loss of multiple genes during the evolution of *Helicobacter pylori.* PLoS Genetics 2005; 1(4): e43.

[58] Siegel R, Ward E, Brawley O, Jemal A. Cancer statistics, 2011. The impact of eliminating socioeconomic and racial disparities on premature cancer deaths. CA. a cancer journal for clinicians 2011; 61(4): 212-236.

[59] Bray F, Jemal A, Grey N, Ferlay J, Forman D. Global cancer transition according to the Human Development Index (2008-2030): a population-based study. Lancet Oncology 2012, 13(8): 790-801.

[60] World Health Organization. Global action against cancer. Global cancer control. WHO Library Cataloguing-in-Publication Data. Switzerland 2005. http://www.who.int/cancer/media/en/GlobalActionCancerEnglfull.pdf (accessed 01 december 2013).

[61] Malfertheiner P, Bornschein J, Selgrad M. Role of *Helicobacter pylori* infection in gastric cancer pathogenesis: a chance for prevention. Journal of Digestive Diseases 2010; 11(1): 2-11.

[62] Nardone G, Rocco A, Malfertheiner P. Review article: *Helicobacter pylori* and molecular events in precancerous gastric lesions. Alimentary pharmacology & therapeutics 2004; 20(3): 261-270.

[63] Hoehnberger P, Gretschel S. Gastric cancer. Lancet 2003; 362(9380): 305-315.

[64] Bowles MJ, Benjamin IC. ABC of the upper gastrointestinal tract. Cancer of the stomach and pancreas. BMJ 2001; 323(7326): 1413-1416.

[65] Verdecchia A, Mariotto A, Gatta G, Bustamante-Teixeira MT, Ajiki W. Comparison of stomach cancer incidence and survival in four continents. European Journal of Cancer 2003; 39(11): 1603-1609.

[66] Guerra MR, Gallo CVM, Mendonça GAS. The risk of cancer in Brazil: tendencies and recent epidemiologic studies. Revista Brasileira de Cancerologia 2005; 51(3): 227-234.

[67] Ministério da Saúde. Instituto Nacional do Câncer José Alencar Gomes da Silva. Estimativa 2014 – Incidência de Câncer no Brasil. MS: http://www2.inca.gov.br (accessed 29 November 2013).

[68] Lauren P. The two histological main types of gastric carcinoma: Diffuse and so-called intestinal type carcinoma. Acta Pathologica et Microbiologica Scandinavica 1975; 64: 31-49.

[69] Sugiyama T, Asaka M. *Helicobacter pylori* infection and gastric cancer. Medical Electron Microscopy 2004; 37(3): 149-157.

[70] Yoshimura T, Shimoyama T, Fukuda S, Tanaka M, Axon AT, Munakata A. Most gastric cancer occurs on the distal side of the endoscopic atrophic border. Scandinavian Journal of Gastroenterology 1999; 34(11): 1077-1081.

[71] Polk DB; Peek Jr RM. *Helicobacter pylori*: gastric cancer and beyond. Nature Reviews. Cancer 2010; 10(6): 403-414.

[72] Correa P, Haenszel W, Cuello C, Tannenbaum S, Archer M. A model for gastric cancer epidemiology. Lancet 1975; 2(7924): 58-60.

[73] Correa P. A human model of gastric carcinogenesis. Cancer Research 1988; 48(13): 3554-3560.

[74] Correa P. Human gastric carcinogenesis: a multistep and multifactorial process – First American Cancer Society Award lecture on cancer epidemiology and prevention. Cancer Research 1992; 52(24): 6735-6740.

[75] Correa P, Piazuelo MB. The gastric precancerous cascade. Journal of Digestive Diseases 2012; 13(1): 2-9.

[76] Mera R, Fontham ET, Bravo LE, Bravo JC, Piazuelo MB, Camargo MC, Correa P. Long term follow up of patients treated for *Helicobacter pylori* infection. Gut 2005; 54(11): 1536-1540.

[77] Cheung TK, Xia HH, Wong BCY. *Helicobacter pylori* eradication for gastric cancer prevention. Journal of Gastroenterology 2007; 42(Suppl. 17): 10-15.

[78] Yang Y, Deng CS, Peng JZ, Wong BC, Lam SK, Xia HH. Effect of *Helicobacter pylori* on apoptosis and apoptosis related genes in gastric cancer cells. Molecular Pathology 2003; 56(1): 19-24.

[79] Kuipers EJ. Review article: relationship between *Helicobacter pylori*, atrophic gastritis and gastric cancer. Alimentary pharmacology & therapeutics 1998; 12(Suppl 1): 25-36.

[80] Forman D, Newell DG, Fullerton F, Yarnell JW, Stacey AR, Wald N, Sitas F. Association between infection with *Helicobacter pylori* and risk of gastric cancer: evidence from a prospective investigation. BMJ 1991; 302(6788): 1302-1305.

[81] Danesh J. *Helicobacter pylori* infection and gastric cancer: systemic review of the epidemiological studies. Alimentary pharmacology & therapeutics 1999; 13(7): 851-856.

[82] Herrera V, Parsonnet J. *Helicobacter pylori* and gastric adenocarcinoma. Clinical Microbiology and Infection 2009; 15(11): 971-976.

[83] de Vries AC, Haringsma J, Kuipers EJ. The detection, surveillance and treatment of premalignant gastric lesions related to *Helicobacter pylori* infection. Helicobacter 2007; 12(1): 1-15.

[84] Correa P, Houghton J. Carcinogenesis of *Helicobacter pylori*. Gastroenterology 2007; 133(2): 659-672.

[85] Filipe MI, Potet F, Bogomoletz WV, Dawson PA, Fabiani B, Chauveinc P, Fenzy A, Gazzard B, Goldfain D, Zeegen R. Incomplete sulphomucin-secreting intestinal metaplasia for gastric cancer. Preliminary data from a prospective study from three centres. Gut 1985; 26(12): 1319-1326.

[86] Rugge M, Correa P, Dixon MF, Haltori T, Leandro G, Lewin K, Riddeli RH, Sipponen P, Watanabe H. Gastric dysplasia: the Padova international classification. The American journal of surgical pathology 2000; 24(2): 167-176.

[87] Lauwers GY, Srivastava A. Gastric preneoplastic lesions and epithelial dysplasia. Gastroenterology clinics of North America 2007; 36(4): 813-829.

[88] Hirota WK, Zuckerman MJ, Adler DG, Davila RE, Egan J, Leighton JA, Qureshi WA, Rajan E, Fanelli R, Wheeler-Harbaugh J, Baron TH, Faigel DO. ASGE guideline: the role of endoscopy in the surveillance of premalignant conditions of the upper GI tract. Gastrointestinal Endoscopy 2006; 63(4): 570-580.

[89] Everett SM, Axon ATR. Early gastric cancer: disease or pseudo-disease? Lancet 1998; 351(9112): 1350-1352.

[90] Goelz SE, Hamilton SR, Vogelstein B. Purification of DNA from formaldehyde fixed and paraffin embedded human tissue. Biochemical and Biophysical Research Communications 1985; 130(1): 118-126.

[91] Saiki RK, Gelfand DH, Stoffel S, Scharf SJ, Higuchi R, Horn GT, Mullis KB, Erlich HA. Primer-directed enzymatic amplification of DNA with a termostable DNA polymerase. Science 1988; 239(4839): 487-491.

[92] Lage AP, Godfroid P, Fauconnier A, Burette A, Butzler JP, Bollen A, Glupczynski Y. Diagnosis of *Helicobacter pylori* infection by PCR: comparison with other invasive techniques and detection of cagA gene in gastric biopsy specimens. Journal of Clinical Microbiology 1995; 33(10): 2752-2756.

[93] Atherton JC, Peek RM, Tham KT, Cover TL, Blaser MJ. Clinical and pathological importance of heterogenicity in vacA, the vacuolating cytotoxin gene of *Helicobacter pylori*. Gastroenterology 1997; 112(1): 92-97.

[94] Atherton JC, Cover TL, Twells RJ, Morales MR, Hawkey CJ, Blaser MJ. Simple and accurate PCR-based system for typing vacuolating cytotoxin alleles of *Helicobacter pylori*. Journal of Clinical Microbiology 1999; 37(9): 2979-2982.

[95] Thomazini CM, Pinheiro NA, Pardini MI, Naresse LE, Rodrigues MAM. Infecção por *Helicobacter pylori* e câncer gástrico: freqüência de cepas patogênicas cagA e vacA em pacientes com câncer gástrico. Jornal Brasileiro de Patologia e Medicina Laboratorial 2006; 42(1): 25-30.

[96] Faundez G, Troncoso M, Figueroa G. cagA and vacA in strains of *Helicobacter pylori* from ulcer and non-ulcerative dyspepsia patients. BMC Gastroenterology 2002; 2:20-24.

[97] Mattar R, Marques SB, Monteiro MS, Santos AF, Iriya K, Carrilho FJ. *Helicobacter pylori* cag pathogenicity island genes: clinical relevance for peptic ulcer disease development in Brazil. Journal of Medical Microbiology 2007; 56(1): 9-14.

[98] Foxman B, Riley L. Molecular Epidemiology: Focus on Infection. American Journal of Epidemiology 2001; 153(12): 1135-1141.

[99] Nozaki K, Shimizu N, Inada K, Tsukamoto T, Inoue M, Kumagai T, Sugiyama A, Mizoshita T, Kaminishi M, Tatematsu M. Synergistic promoting effects of *Helicobacter*

pylori infection and high-salt diet on gastric carcinogenesis in Mongolian gerbils. Japanese Journal of Cancer Research 2002; 93(10): 1083-1089.

[100] Humar B, Blair V, Charlton A, More H, Martin I, Guilford P, E-cadherin deficiency initiates gastric signet-ring cell carcinoma in mice and man. Cancer Research 2009; 69(5): 2050-2056.

[101] Fukayama M, Hino R, Uozaki H. Epstein-Barr vírus and gastric carcinoma: vírus-host interactions leading to carcinoma. Cancer Science 2008; 99(9): 1726-1733.

[102] Suzuki H, Hibi T, Marshall BJ. *Helicobacter pylori:* present status and future prospects in Japan. Journal of Gastroenterology 2007; 42(1): 1-15.

[103] Xia HH, Yu Wong BC, Talley NJ, Lam SK. Alternative and rescue treatment regimens for *Helicobacter pylori* eradication. Expert Opinion of Pharmacotherapy 2002; 3(9): 1301-1311.

[104] Parsonnet J, Harris RA, Hack HM, Owens DK. Modelling cost-effectiveness of *Helicobacter pylori* screening to prevent gastric cancer: a mandate for clinical trials. Lancet 1996; 348(9021): 150-154.

[105] Fendrick AM, Chernew ME, Hirth RA, Bloom BS, Bandekar RR, Scheiman JM. Clinical and economic effects of population-based *Helicobacter pylori* screening to prevent gastric cancer. Archives of Internal Medicine 1999; 159(2): 142-148.

[106] Roderick P, Davies R, Raftery J, Crabbe D, Pearce R, Patel P et al. Cost-effectiveness of population screening for *Helicobacter pylori* in preventing gastric cancer and peptic ulcer disease, using simulation. Journal of Medical Screening 2003; 10(3): 148-156.

[107] Fuccio L, Zagari RM, Minardi ME, Bazzoli F. Systematic review. *Helicobacter pylori* eradication for the prevention of gastric cancer. Alimentary Pharmacology & Therapeutics 2007; 25(2): 133-141.

[108] Uemura N, Okamoto S, Yamamoto S, Matsumura M, Yamaguchi S, Yamakido M, Taniyama K, Sasaki N, Schlemper RJ. *Helicobacter pylori* infection and the development of gastric cancer. New England Journal of Medicine 2001; 345(11): 784-789.

[109] Leung WK, Lin SR, Ching JY, To KF, Ng EK, Chan FK, Lau JY, Sung JJ. Factors predicting progression of gastric intestinal metaplasia. Results of a randomized trial on *Helicobacter pylori* eradication. Gut 2004; 53(9): 1244-1249.

[110] Zhou L, Sung JJ, Lin S, Jin Z, Ding S, Huang X, Xia Z, Guo H, Liu J, Chao W. A five-year follow-up study on the pathological changes of gastric mucosa after *H. pylori* eradication. Chinese Medical Journal 2003; 116(1): 11-14.

[111] Correa P, Fontham ET, Bravo JC, Bravo LE, Ruiz B, Zarama G, Realpe JL, Malcom GT, Li D, Johnson WD, Mera R. Chemoprevention of gastric dysplasia: randomized trial of antioxidant supplements and anti-*Helicobacter pylori* therapy. Journal of the National Cancer Institute 2000; 92(23): 1881-1888.

[112] Genta RM, Lew GM, Graham DY. Changes in the gastric mucosa following eradication of *Helicobacter pylori*. Modern Pathology 1993; 6(3): 281-289.

[113] Ciok J, Dzieniszewski J, Lucer C. *Helicobacter pylori* eradication and antral intestinal metaplasia – two years follow-up study. Journal of Physiology and Pharmacology 1997; 48(Suppl. 4): 115-122.

[114] Uemura N, Mukai T, Okamoto S, Yamaguchi S, Mashiba H, Taniyama K, Sasaki N, Haruma K, Sumii K, Kajiyama G. Effect of *Helicobacter pylori* eradication on subsequent development of cancer after endoscopic resection of early gastric cancer. Cancer Epidemiology, Biomarkers & Prevention 1997; 6(8): 639-642.

[115] Kim N, Lim SH, Lee KH, Choi SE, Jung HC, Song IS, Kim CY. Long-term effects of *Helicobacter pylori* eradication on intestinal metaplasia in patients with duodenal and benign gastric ulcers. Digestive Diseases and Sciences 2000; 45(9): 1754-1762.

[116] Ohkusa T, Fujiki K, Takashimizu I, Kumagai J, Tanizawa T, Eishi Y, Yokoyama T, Watanabe M. Improvement in atrophic gastritis and intestinal metaplasia in patients in whom *Helicobacter pylori* was eradicated. Annals of Internal Medicine 2001; 134(5): 380-386.

[117] Kokkola A, Sipponen P, Rautelin H, Härkönen M, Kosunen TU, Haaapiainen R, Puolakkainen P. The effect of *Helicobacter pylori* eradication on the natural course of atrophic gastritis with dysplasia. Alimentary Pharmacology & Therapeutics 2002; 16(3): 515-520.

[118] Ito M, Haruma K, Kamada T, Mihara M, Kim S, Kitadai Y, Sumii M, Tanaka S, Yoshihara M, Chayama K. *Helicobacter pylori* eradication therapy improves atrophic gastritis and intestinal metaplasia: a 5-year prospective study of patients with atrophic gastritis. Alimentary Pharmacology & Therapeutics 2002; 16(8): 1449-1456.

[119] You WC, Brown LM, Zhang L, Li JY, Jin ML, Chang YS, Ma JL, Pan KF, Liu WD, Hu Y, Crystal-Mansour S, Pee D, Blot WJ, Fraumeni JF Jr, Xu GW, Gail MH. Randomized double-blind factorial trial of three treatments to reduce the prevalence of precancerous gastric lesions. Journal of the National Cancer Institute 2006; 98(14): 974-983.

[120] Ley C, Mohar A, Guarner J, Herrera-Goepfert R, Figueroa LS, Halperin D, Johnstone I, Parsonnet J. *Helicobacter pylori* eradication and gastric preneoplastic conditions: a randomized, double-blind, placebo-controlled trial. Cancer Epidemiology, Biomarkers & Prevention 2004; 13(1): 4-10.

[121] Witteman EM, Mravunac M, Becx MJ, Hopman WP, Verschoor JS, Tytgat GN, de Koning RW. Improvement of gastric inflammation and resolution of epithelial damage one year after eradication of *Helicobacter pylori*. Journal of Clinical Pathology 1995; 48(3): 250-256.

[122] Forbes GM, Warren JR, Glaser ME, Cullen DJ, Marshall BJ, Collins BJ. Long-term follow-up of gastric histology after *Helicobacter pylori* eradication. Journal of Gastroenterology and Hepatology 1996; 11(7): 670-673.

[123] van der Hulst RW, van der Ende A, Dekker FW, Ten Kate FJ, Weel JF, Keller JJ, Kruizinga SP, Dankert J, Tytgat JN. Effect of *Helicobacter pylori* eradication on gastritis in relation to cagA: a prospective 1-year follow-up study. Gastroenterology 1997; 113(1): 25-30.

[124] Satoh K, Kimura K, Takimoto T, Kihira K. A follow-up study of atrophic gastritis and intestinal metaplasia after eradication of *Helicobacter pylori*. Helicobacter 1998; 3(4): 236-240.

[125] Kyzekova J, Mour J. The effect of eradication therapy on histological changes in the gastric mucosa in patients with non-ulcer dyspepsia and *Helicobacter pylori* infection. Prospective randomized intervention study. Hepatogastroenterology 1999; 46(27): 2048-2056.

[126] Annibale B, Aprile MR, D'Ambra G, Caruana P, Bordi C, Delle Fave G. Cure of *Helicobacter pylori* infection in atrophic body gastritis patients does not improve mucosal atrophy but reduces hypergastrinemia and its related effects on body ECL-cell hyperplasia. Alimentary Pharmacology & Therapeutics 2000; 14(5): 625-634.

[127] Sung JJ, Lin SR, Ching IY, Zhou LY, To KF, Wang RT, Leung WK, Ng EK, Lau JY, Lee YT, Yeung CK, Chao W, Chung SC. Atrophy and intestinal metaplasia one year after cure of *H. pylori* infection: a prospective, randomized study. Gastroenterology 2000; 119(1): 7-14.

[128] Kamada T, Haruma K, Hata J, Kusunoki H, Sasaki A, Ito M, Tanaka S, Yoshihara M. The long-term effect of *Helicobacter pylori* eradication therapy on symptoms in dyspeptic patients with fundic atrophic gastritis. Alimentary Pharmacology & Therapeutics 2003; 18(2): 245-252.

[129] Kuipers EJ, Nelis GF, Klinkenberg-Knol EC, Snel P, Goldfain D, Kolkman JJ, Festen HP, Dent J, Zeitoun P, Havu N, Lamm M, Walan A. Cure of *Helicobacter pylori* infection in patients with reflux oesophagitis treated with long term omeprazole reverses gastritis without exacerbation of reflux disease: results of a randomised controlled trial. Gut 2004; 53(1): 12-20.

[130] Ruiz B, Garay J, Correa P, Fontham ET, Bravo JC, Bravo LE, Realpe JL, Mera R. Morphometric evaluation of gastric antral atrophy: improvement after cure of *Helicobacter pylori* infection. American Journal of Gastroenterology 2001; 96(12): 3281-3287.

[131] Fukase K, Kato M, Kikuchi S, Inoue K, Uemura N, Okamoto S, Terao S, Amagai K, Hayashi S, Asaka M, Japan Gast Study Group. Effect of eradication of *Helicobacter pylori* on incidence of metachronous gastric carcinoma after endoscopic resection of early gastric cancer: an open-label, randomized controlled trial. Lancet 2008; 372(9636): 350-352.

[132] Ito M, Takata S, Tatsugami M, Wada Y, Imagawa S, Matsumoto Y, Takamura A, Kitamura S, Matsuo T, Tanaka S, Haruma K, Chayama K. Clinical prevention of gastric cancer by *Helicobacter pylori* eradication therapy: a systematic review. Journal of Gastroenterology 2009; 44(5): 365-371.

[133] Takata S, Ito M, Yoshihara M, Tanaka S, Imagawa S, Haruma K, Chayama K. Host factors contributing to the discovery of gastric cancer after successful eradication therapy of *Helicobacter pylori:* preliminary report. Journal of Gastroenterology and Hepatology 2007; 22(4): 571-576.

[134] Wong BC, Lam SK, Wong WM, Chen JS, Zheng TT, Feng RE, Lai KC, Hu WH, Yuen ST, Leung SY, Fong DY, Ho J, Ching CK, Chen JS, China Gastric Cancer Study Group. *Helicobacter pylori* eradication to prevent gastric cancer in a high-risk region of China: a randomized controlled trial. JAMA 2004; 291(2): 187-194.

[135] Kabir S. Effect of *Helicobacter pylori* eradication on incidence of gastric cancer in human and animal models: underlying biochemical and molecular events. Helicobacter 2004; 14(3): 159-171.

[136] Rogers AB, Fox JG. Inflammation and Cancer. Rodent models of infectious gastrointestinal and liver cancer. American Journal of Physiology. Gastrointestinal and Liver Physiology 2004; 286(3): G361-G366.

[137] Romero-Gallo J, Harris EJ, Krishna U, Washington MK, Perez-Perez GI, Peek Jr RM. Effect of *Helicobacter pylori* eradication on gastric carcinogenesis. Laboratory Investigation 2008; 88(3): 328-336.

[138] Oda T, Murakami K, Nishizono A, Kodama M, Nasu M, Fujioka T. Long-term *Helicobacter pylori* infection in Japanese monkeys induces atrophic gastritis and accumulation of mutations in the *p53* tumor suppressor gene. Helicobacter 2002; 7(3): 143-151.

[139] Hirayama F, Takagi S, Kusuhara H, Iwao E, Yokoyama Y, Ykeda Y. Induction of gastric ulcer and intestinal metaplasia in mongolian gerbils infected with *Helicobacter pylori*. Journal of Gastroenterology 1996; 31(5): 755-757.

[140] Shimizu N, Inada K, Nakanishi H, Tsukamoto T, Ikehara Y, Kaminishi M, Kuramoto S, Sugiyama A, Katsuyama T, Tatematsu M. *Helicobacter pylori* infection enhances glandular stomach carcinogenesis in Mongolian gerbils treated with chemical carcinogens. Carcinogenesis 1999; 20(4): 669-676.

[141] Sugiyama A, Maruta F, Ikeno T, Ishida K, Kawasaki S, Katsuyama T, Shimizu N, Tatematsu M. *Helicobacter pylori* infection enhances N-methyl-N-nitrosourea-induced stomach carcinogenesis in the Mongolian gerbil. Cancer Research 1998; 58(10): 2067-2069.

[142] Tokieda M, Honda S, Fujioka T, Nasu M. Effect of *Helicobacter pylori* infection on the N-methyl-N-nitro-N-nitrosoguanidine-induced gastric carcinogenesis in Mongolian gerbils. Carcinogenesis 1999; 20(7): 1261-1266.

[143] Franco AT, Israel DA, Washington MK, Krishna U, Fox JG, Rogers AB, Neish AS, Collier-Hyams L, Perez-Perez GI, Hatakeyama M, Whitehead R, Gaus K, O'Brien DP, Romero-Gallo J, Peek RM Jr. Activation of beta-cateninby carcinogenic *Helicobacter pylori*. Proceedings of the National Academy of Sciences of the United States of America 2005; 102(30): 10646-10651.

[144] Cai X, Carlson J, Stoicov C, Li H, Wang TC, Houghton J. *Helicobacter felis* eradication restores normal architecture and inhibits gastric cancer progression in C57BL/6 mice. Gastroenterology 2005; 128(7): 1937-1952.

[145] Ono H, Kondo H, Gotoda T, Shirao K, Yamaguchi H, Saito D, Hosokawa K, Shimoda T, Yoshida S. Endoscopic mucosal resection for treatment of early gastric cancer. Gut 2001; 48(2): 225-229.

9

Immune Response to *Helicobacter pylori*

Batool Mutar Mahdi

1. Introduction

Helicobacter pylori (H. pylori) is a Gram-negative microaerophilic spiral bacterium previously known Campylobacterpylori. It has a significant attention since its isolation and characterisation in 1983 [1]. It colonizes the gastrointestinal mucosa of its host in spite of a strong persistent humoral and cellular immune response to *H. pylori* at the local and systemic level, the organism persists for the lifetime of its host.

It is a pathogen, playing an important role in the aetiology of gastritis (especially active antral gastritis). Gastritis is a histopathologic term characterized by chronic inflammation of the stomach mucosa. It is classification based on the underlying cause (eg, *H. pylori,* that cause atrophic gastritis, bile reflux, nonsteroidal anti-inflammatory drugs [NSAIDs], autoimmunity, or allergic response) [2]. Gastritis is also classified as erosive or nonerosive based on the severity of mucosal injury by endoscopy. Other classification is according to the site of involvement (cardia, body, antrum). Histological classification is acute or chronic based on the inflammatory cell type. Acute gastritis is characterized by PMN infiltration of the mucosa of the antrum and body. Chronic gastritis implies some degree of atrophy or metaplasia. It predominantly involves the antrum with subsequent loss of G cells and decreased gastrin secretion or the corpus with loss of oxyntic glands, leading to reduced acid, pepsin, and intrinsic factor [3, 4, 5].

H. pylori causes more than half of peptic ulcers worldwide. The bacterium causes peptic ulcers by damaging the mucous membrane of the stomach and duodenum. Damage to the mucous membrane causing stomach acid to get through to the sensitive lining layer. Together, the stomach acid and *H. pylori* irritate the lining of the stomach or duodenum and cause an ulcer [6].Ulcers in the stomach and duodenum result when the consequences of inflammation allow stomach acid and the digestive enzyme pepsin to overwhelm the mechanisms that protect the stomach and duodenal mucous membranes. The location of colonization of *H. pylori,* which affects the location of the ulcer, depends on the acidity of the stomach [7].The majority of patients with duodenal ulcer (DU) are infected with *H. pylori* [8].

H. pylori infection is a major cause of gastric adenocarcinoma, specifically non-cardia gastric cancer. H. pylori infection also causes gastric mucosa-associated lymphoid tissue (MALT) lymphoma [9]. Some *H. pylori* bacteria had a toxin produced by a gene called cytotoxin-associated gene A (*cagA*) injected into the junctions where cells of the stomach lining. This toxin (known as CagA) alters the structure of stomach cells and allows the bacteria to attach to them more easily. Long-term exposure to the toxin causes chronic inflammation [10]. Other type of cancer is gastric MALT lymphoma is a rare type of non-Hodgkin lymphoma that is characterized by the slow multiplication of B lymphocytes. Normally, the lining of the stomach lacks lymphoid tissue, but growth of this tissue is often stimulated in response to colonization of *H. pylori* [11]. Nearly all patients with gastric MALT lymphoma show signs of *H. pylori* infection, and the risk of developing this tumor is more than six times higher in infected people than in uninfected people [12]

The prevalence of gastric cancers among *H. pylori*-infected patients varies between individuals, countries, and geographic areas, *H. pylori* disease-related outcomes are believed to be determined by interaction between host factors, bacterial factors, and their *interaction* with the *environment* [13] produces different diseases in different persons. High and low acid secretion rates probably contribute to duodenal ulceration and gastric carcinogenesis, respectively. *H. pylori*products and certain cytokines released in gastritis release gastrin from G-cells but inhibit parietal cells. Also tumour necrosis *factor* alpha inhibits somatostatin-cells and interleukin 1 beta inhibits enterochromaffin-like cells. The net result is that antral gastritis tends to increase, whilst corpus gastritis tends to decrease acid secretion. Corpus atrophy further lowers acid through loss of parietal cells. Factors postulated to increase corpus gastritis include: *host* genetics, early acquisition of bacteria, more aggressive strains, poor general health and diets high in salt or lacking in antioxidant vitamins [14]. *Other factor is environmental* factors that play an important role in the manifestation, course, and prognosis of diseases of *H. pylori*-induced gastritis. This disease is the outcome of allelic group of a *host* and the microbial (microflora) and physical environments. *Host* alleles predisposing to a disease in one genomic and/or *environmental* surroundings may not be deleterious in other group, in addition to that microbes can have different effects in different hosts and under different *environmental* conditions [15]. *H. pylori* eradication may not eliminate the risk of gastric cancer. Therapy of this bacteria may be used in high-risk populations to reduce gastric cancer incidence. It can reverse many biochemical, genetic, and epigenetic changes that *H. pylori* infection induces in the stomach [16]. The major factors playing a pathogenic role in *H. pylori*-related non-cancer diseases are host polymorphisms in genes involved in inflammation and protection against oxidative damage, host exposure to dietary genotoxic agents, and bacterial genetic polymorphisms [17]. The study of *host*-bacterial *interaction* is key to detection the molecular and cellular pathways involved and will lead to developing preventive and therapeutic modules against this pathogen [18].

Gastric inflammation nearly always precedes the development of peptic ulceration, and is a critical component in initiating the multi-step progression towards gastric carcinogenesis due to this interaction between these three factors [19].

H. pylori is spread from person to person by two routes, oral-oral and faecal-oral route [20].Food prepared under less ideal conditions or exposed to contaminated water or soil may increase the risk. Inadequate sanitation practices, low social class, and crowded or high-density living conditions seem to be related to a higher prevalence of *H. pylori* infection. Therefore poor hygiene and crowded conditions may facilitate transmission of infection among family members Understanding the route of *H. pylori* transmission is important if public health measures to prevent its spread. Iatrogenic transmission of *H. pylori* following endoscopy is the only proven mode. The person-to-person mode of transmission is supported by the higher incidence of infection among institutionalized children and adults and detection of *H. pylori* DNA in vomitus, saliva, dental plaque, gastric juice, and feces. Waterborne transmission, probably due to fecal contamination or contaminated well water, may be an important source of infection, especially in parts of the world in which untreated water is common. *H. pylori* has been isolated in domestic cats, housefly. However, evidence is lacking that H. *pylori* can be transmitted to humans from flies that have been in contact with *H. pylori*-infected feces. Mode of transmission of *H. pylori* is important to prevent its spread and identifying high-risk populations [21, 22].

The pathogenesity of this bacterium depend on the production of several virulence factors. The most important ones are CagA (cytotoxic associated gene A) and VacA (vacuolizating cytotoxin A). The immunodominant CagA protein is encoded by genes called the cagA-PAI (pathogenicity island), a 40 kb genomic fragment containing ORFs (open reading frames) encoding approximately 31 genes that forms a type IV secretion system, which is found in 60–70% of *H pylori* strains and can be divided into two regions, cag I and cag II, according to a novel insertion sequence [23] This secretion system (T4SS) forms a pilus that delivers CagA, an oncoprotein, into the cytosol of gastric epithelial cells through a rigid needle structure covered by CagY, a VirB10-homologous protein and CagT, a Virb7-homologous protein, at the base [24]. This is accomplished by a specialized adhesin of the pilus surface, the CagL protein, which binds to and activates host cell integrins for subsequent delivery of CagA across the host cell membrane. Injected CagA becomes tyrosine-phosphorylated by Src and Abl family kinases and mimics a host cell protein in binding and activation of multiple signalling factors. After the induction of membrane dynamics, actin cytoskeletal rearrangements and the disruption of cell-to-cell junctions as well as proliferative, pro-inflammatory and anti-apoptotic nuclear responses. All these signalling cascades contribute in *H. pylori* pathogenesis [25]. Therefore, CagA remains the only identified effector mechanism that is translocated by the T4SS of *H. pylori* into gastric epithelial cells where it induces host cell kinases that phosphorylate tyrosine residues in CagA adjacent to the site of bacterial adhesion on the host gastric epithelial cells, which in turn activate eukaryotic signal transduction pathways and cytoskeletal plasticity [26]. Wild-type *H pylori* (not phosphorylation-resistant CagA)induced a growth factor-like response in gastric epithelial cells. CagA formed a physical complex with the SRC homology 2 domain (SH2)-containing tyrosine phosphatase SHP-2 in a phosphorylation-dependent manner and stimulated the phosphatase activity. On the other hand, the CagA effect on cells was reproduced by constitutively active SHP-2. Thus, upon translocation, CagA perturbs cellular functions by deregulating SHP-2 [27]. Injected CagA associates with the epithelial tight-junction scaffolding protein ZO-1 and the transmembrane protein junctional adhesion molecule, causing an ectopic assembly of tight-junction components at sites of bacterial attachment, and altering the composition and function of the apical-junctional complex. Long-term CagA delivery to polarized epithelia caused a disruption of the epithelial barrier function and dysplastic alterations in epithelial cell morphology [28].

Regarding VacA, there is a significant polymorphism in this gene (vacA s, vacA i and vacA m). There are two types of the s (s1 and s2), i (i1 and i2), and m (m1 and m2) regions of *vacA* [29]. Three polymorphic subtypes, namely m1T, m1Tm2 and m2. The s1a/i1/m1Tm2 genotype had a higher frequency of lymphoid follicle formation in the corpus than the s1a/i1/m1T and s1a/i1/m2 strains while *vacA* s1/m1 strains are most closely associated with gastric carcinoma [30]. The method PCR- genotyping from gastric biopsy had advantages over routine diagnostic tools such as histological *H. pylori* detection, which has high interobserver variation, very much depending on the experience of the pathologist, and over *H. pylori* culture, which is more time-consuming, requires expertise, and is not always successful. In general, PCR-based techniques show high sensitivity for *H. pylori* detection and permit further characterization of bacteria virulence-associated genotypes. In archive materials, the genotyping of the *vacA* i region allows the analysis of the *H. pylori* strains in the same biopsy specimen that can also be used for histopathological evaluation, conferring a more reliable measurement of the effects of local infecting strains. Another advantage of the use of archive materials is that it permits retrospective studies to be performed without the need of *H. pylori* isolation from fresh biopsy specimens [31].

In most cases, the infection is asymptomatic and clinical manifestation appears in only 10-15% of infected individuals. This is due to virulence of *H. pylori* strains and host immune response to this bacterium [32]. The different clinical outcomes may be explained by bacterial factors and the host immune responses. *H. pylori* induce a strong immune response with infiltration of neutrophils, B- and T-cells into the gastroduodenal mucosa that fails to clear the infection. Several virulence factors have been associated with the development of gastroduodenal disease, e.g. the cytotoxin-associated gene A (CagA) and a vacuolating toxin [33] individuals infected with strains lacking these genetic markers may still develop peptic ulcers, and that many individuals infected with bacterial strains bearing these genotypes do not develop any symptoms [34]. On other hand, the lower epithelial cytokine responses may be of importance for the pathogenesis of *H. pylori*-induced ulcers, most likely can be explained by host factors, i.e. mainly a decreased ability of the epithelium to produce cytokines, but possibly partly also down-regulation by regulatory T cells [35]. *H. pylori*infection induces strong antibody responses in the human gastric mucosa, both in asymptomatic carriers and in ulcer patients [36].

This will shed a light on the immune response to *H. pylori* colonization and its effect on clinical outcomes.

2. Host immune response to *H. pylori*

The immune response towards bacterial pathogens can be divided into an innate and an adaptive response.

2.1. Innate immune response to *H. pylori*

Recognition of bacterial antigenic molecules is mediated by TLRs (Toll-like receptors) that are expressed by distinct cell types throughout the gastrointestinal tract, and play an important role in regulation of the innate immune response especially TLR4 It is expressed on antigen-presenting cells such as monocytes and dendritic cells. Bacterial contact with monocytes and other APCs leads to the secretion of proinflammatory cytokines such as TNF-α (tumour necrosis factor-α), IL (interleukin)-1β and IL-8. *H. pylori* infection has been shown to be associated with increased levels of these cytokines which, in turn, act as local chemoattractants, inducing granulocytic infiltration [37]. The gastric epithelia of children respond to *H. pylori* infection by increasing the expression of TLR2, TLR4, TLR5, TLR9 and the cytokines IL-8, IL-10 and TNF-α that participate actively in innate immune responses [38]. Their role in the progression of gastric lesions leading to cancer is associated with decreasing levels of TLRs inhibitors and elevated TLRs levels throughout all the spectrum of lesions [39].

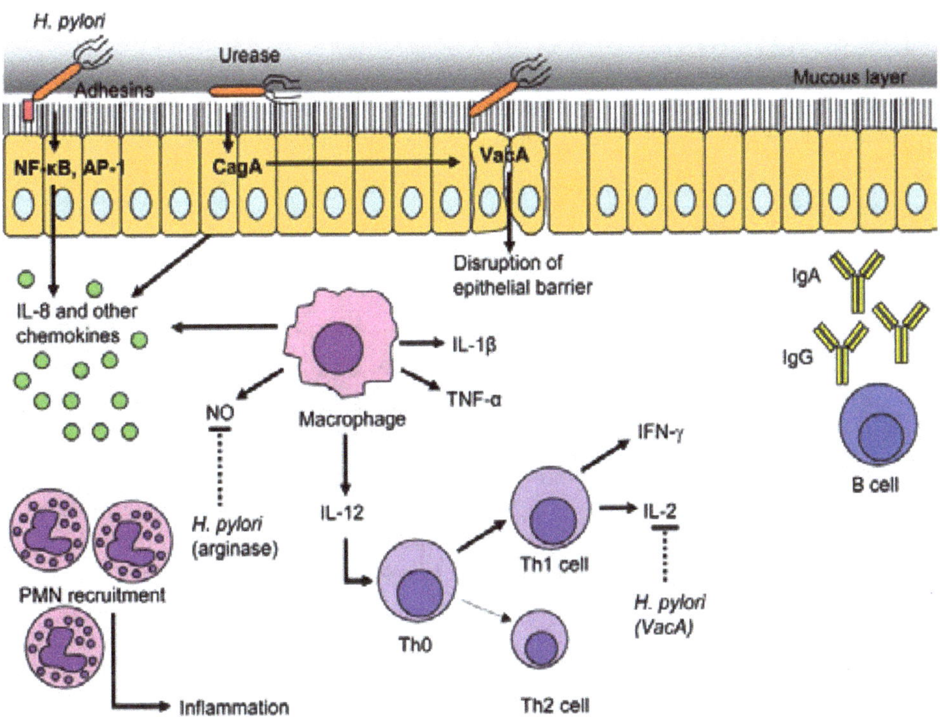

Figure 1. *H. pylori* pathogenesis, the inflammatory immune response and some of escape mechanisms [54].

2.2. Adaptive immunity: cellular immune response and humoral response

2.2.1. Cellular immune response

Adaptive immune responses towards *H. pylori* infection have been developed after failure of innate immune response to eliminate the pathogen. The immune response to *Helicobacter pylori* is a versatile group of mechanisms involving responses that are both protective and damaging to the host. The innate and the adaptive immune responses lead to damaging inflammatory responses allowing for persistence of many infections [40]. *H. pylori* associated inflammatory reaction is characterized by a mucosal infiltration of different cells like polymorphonuclear leukocytes (PMN), T cells, macrophages, and plasma cells [41] in addition to that *H. pylori* adheres to the cells of gastric mucosa and secretes different molecules that can change gastric epithelial cell function [42]. Chronic active gastritis is associated with an increased CD4/CD8 T-cell ratio within the gastric mucosa and accumulation of CD4+ T-helper lymphocytes in the lamina propia of the gastric mucosa. *H. pylori* infection results in a Th1-predominant host immune response in the gastric mucosa and induction of IFN- γ (interferon-γ) and IFN-γ -related genes. A Th1-predominant immune response is associated with elevated levels of the pro-inflammatory cytokines IL-12, IL-18 and TNF-α([43]. Other cell that infiltrates the gastric mucosa was Th17 which are $CD4^+$ T cells associated with infections and inflammation. Th17 are induced during both *H. pylori* infection and gastric cancer in the inflammatory process of gastric stroma and may be an important link between inflammation and carcinogenesis [44]. The host genetic milieu contributes to the inflammatory response to *H. pylori* infection is IL-1B. The *IL-1B* gene encodes the expression of IL-1β, a potent pro-inflammatory cytokine and powerful inhibitor of gastric acid secretion that had a most important responsibility in initiating and amplifying the inflammatory response to *H. pylori* infection [45]. It had been that IL-1 polymorphism had an effect on IL-1 production in gastric mucosa infected with *H. pylori* [46]. This indicate that individual genetic polymorphism had an effect on disease expression.

Yuceyar etal 2002 [47] found that there is no alteration in total T and B lymphocytes and CD4+ T, CD8+ T lymphocytes and natural killer cells of both duodenal ulcer and chronic antral gastritis patients compared to normal persons. Although there was a slight increase in the proportion of active T lymphocytes in duodenal ulcer and chronic antral gastritis groups comparing to healthy subjects the difference was not statistically significant. This indicate that there is no systemic alteration in the specific immune system in response to *H. pylori* in patients with duodenal ulcer and chronic antral gastritis. Other study confirmed the systemic immune response to helicobacters at the cellular level in patients with *Helicobacter pylori* infection by leukocyte migration inhibition test was performed and a highly significant inhibitory effect on leukocyte migration was found in patients with *Helicobacter pylori* infection [48].

2.2.2. Humoral immune response

H. pylori induce a strong specific systemic and local antibody response and infected individual had antibodies against whole bacteria or part of it [49]and increase in plasma cells in gastric mucosa which produce IgA [50]. Other important antibody was IgG that binds to *H. pylori* and enhance phagocytosis [51].This antibodies lead to complement activation by either classical or alternative pathways [52]. In addition to that, the role of the secretory IgA is important in neutralizing urease and VacA as well as inhibiting adherence of *H. pylori* to gastric mucosa [53].The immune response to *H. pylori* can be summarized by figure -1- [54]. There is high seroprevalence of *H. pylori* antibodies undervalue of past infection, the relation of the *H. pylori* cytotoxin to gastric precancerous lesions is warranted. There is a strong mucosal IgA response to *H. pylori* in non-neoplastic antral mucosa of gastric cancer patients irrespective of the biopsy urease results [55].

2.2.2.1. Evasion of immune response by H. pylori

Helicobacter pylori is a gastric bacterial pathogen that evades host immune responses in vivo by different mechanisms like inducing apoptosis of macrophages in association with alterations in the mitochondrial pathway [56].

Elimination of this key immunomodulatory cell may represent a *mechanism* employed by the bacterium to evade host immune responses. It can survive intracellularly within macrophages by interfering with lysosomal proteins, similar to *Mycobacterium tuberculosis* [57]. *H. pylori* like many other pathogen escape the immune system by production an enzyme arginase that prevent nitrous oxide production [58].

Vacuolating cytotoxin secreted by *H. pylori* has turned out to be a potent immunomodulatory toxin. VacA-deficient *H. pylori* induced significantly higher expression of integrin-linked kinase (ILK) and endothelial nitric oxygen synthase (eNOS), and significantly more production of reactive oxygen species (ROS) in monocyte/macrophage-like U937 cells, as compared with isogenic vacA+ *H. pylori*. Thus, vacA-deficient *H. pylori* appears to upregulate ILK expression, which modulates the expression of eNOS and as a result, stimulates the production of ROS. It is VacA that prevents such a process by inhibiting ILK expression, helping *H. pylori escape* host immunoreaction and persist in gastric mucosa [59].

In addition to that, *H. pylori* LPS exhibits a reduced endotoxic potency in terms of pyrogenicity, lethality, toxicity, mitogenicity and the lower immune response elicited by *H. pylori* LPS in comparison with other enterobacterial LPS may represent an *escape mechanism* from the host [60]. *H. pylori*, possess flagellin molecules that cannot be recognized by TLR5 that is important for its survival [61]. *H. pylori* infection could alter cellular gene expression processes that evade host immune mechanism by activating NF-κB and Wnt/β-catenin signaling pathway, disturb metal ion homeostasis, and induce carcinogenesis [62].

VacA of *H pylori* act as an immunomodulator by interfering with the IL-2 signalling pathway in T-cells by blocking Ca2+ mobilization and the activity of the Ca2+/calmodulin-dependent phosphatase calcineurin [63]. It also interferes with antigen presentation mediated by MHC class II [64]. VacA by itself act as immunosuppressive by a direct action on T-cells rather than APCs [65]. *VacA* is a crucial element for *H. pylori* to *escape* from host immune defense by means of differentially regulating the expression of some related genes by altering their mRNA expression at different times [66].

2.2.2.2. *Vaccination against H. pylori infection*

Helicobacter pylori can persist in the gastric mucosa of infected individuals for life, in the face of chronic inflammation and low pH. Efforts to develop vaccines have largely failed and, in the wake of emerging antibiotic resistance, novel therapeutic approaches have developed [67].

There is a consent that vaccines are essential to limit the severity of this infection. Great development has been made since its detection 25 years ago the virulence factors and several aspects of the pathogenesis of the *H. pylori* gastric diseases. Several key bacterial factors have been identified: urease, vacuolating cytotoxin, cytotoxin-associated antigen, the pathogenicity island, neutrophil-activating protein, and among others. These proteins, in their native or recombinant forms, have been shown to confer protection against infectious challenge with *H. pylori* in animal models. However, a quantity of clinical trials in healthy volunteers have been conducted using urease given orally as a soluble protein or expressed in bacterial vectors with limited results or a mixture of *H. pylori* antigens was reported to be highly immunogenic in *H. pylori*-negative volunteers following intramuscular administration of the vaccine with aluminium hydroxide as an adjuvant [69].

H. pylori is a mucosa-associated organism, it was initially thought that an IgA type anti-*Helicobacter* antibody response would be essential for protective immunity [69]. An adjuvant is an important component of any oral/mucosal vaccine as it is responsible for stimulating immune system, but due to toxicities associated with these agents, there are currently no suitable and safe adjuvants available for use in humans. Another important limitation to effective oral immunization is that it requires multiple doses and a large amount of antigen administration. These studies showed that mucosal immunity can be induced by oral or intranasal routes of immunization. The intranasal route of immunization is similar to the oral route in that it also requires the administration of bacterial antigen in conjunction with an adjuvant multiple times [70].

Considering the side effects of oral adjuvants, researches have focused attention on making oral immunization safe and effective for human usage. Thus, *E. coli LT* heat-labile toxin that was used as an oral adjuvant in humans did show a significant decrease in gastric *H. pylori* density but was associated with cramping and diarrhea [71]. Another approach is to use other mucosal routes such as the nasal mucosa and the rectal mucosa for effective immunization. When mice were immunized orally, rectally and intranasally in combination with *E. coli* heat-labile toxin (LT) and subsequently challenged with purified *H. pylori* antigen, mice immunized by either of the routes were found to be protected against this challenge compared with controls. These studies showed that mucosal immunity can be induced by oral or intranasal routes of immunization. The intranasal route of immunization is similar to the oral route in that it also requires the administration of bacterial antigen in conjunction with an adjuvant multiple times [72].

Although the intransal route of immunization seems the most efficient and effective route of mucosal immunization, it still has some disadvantages histologic inflammation in the olfactory bulb and cause paralysis of facial nerves [72]. Intranasal route could also result in oral ingestion thus exposing the subject to various side effects and toxicities. Eriksson et al. [73] found that

CTA1-DD adjuvant was to be safe for intranasal administration without any accumulation in the nervous tissue.

Other modalities of administering vaccines such as the intraperitoneal (i.p.) and subcutaneous (s.c.) routes are also being done. Mice were vaccinated i.p. using *H. pylori* antigen in combination with aluminum hydroxide and upon rechallenge with *H. pylori* were found to confer protection that was shown by absence of bacteria, both histologically and in culture of gastric biopsy tissues. This immunity was noted to be antibody independent and achieved by IL-5-secreting T cells [74]. The results of these experiments suggest that until a safe, effective, and inexpensive mucosal (oral/nasal) vaccine becomes available, systemic immunizations should be a consideration.

Urease is important as a vaccine antigen has been confirmed by numerous studies in mice, ferrets, and non-human primates [75]. Urease conferred protection against helicobacter infection when delivered either as a native protein or as an enzymatically inactive recombinant protein [76]. Therapeutic immunisation with urease has recently been reported in ferrets naturally infected with *H. mustelae*. [77]. Infection with *H. mustelae*occurs in ferrets soon after weaning, persists for life, induces active chronic gastritis, and is associated with the development of ulceration in a subgroup of infected animals [78]. Thus, therapeutic immunisation is possible in a natural setting of helicobacter infection, confirming that the inability of the natural immune response to clear helicobacter infection can be overcome.

Other method of delivery of the antigen used in mice by immunisation with genetically engineered bacteria expressing *H. pylori* antigens elicits a protective immune response against gastric helicobacter infections. Immunisation with live bacterial vaccines usually requires only one or two doses, does not depend on the addition of extra mucosal adjuvant, and the vaccine can be produced at very low cost. Additional improvements to the vaccine should result from a better understanding of the natural immune responses to helicobacter infection and of the mechanisms by which vaccination restores protection [79].

Zhang etal, 2013 [80] used recombinant technology, Lactococcus lactis (L. lactis) could serve as an antigen-delivering vehicle for the development of edible *vaccine*. They produced edible UreB (urease B) *vaccine* derived from L. lactis against H. *pylori*. The UreB subunit is the most effective and common immunogen of all strains of H. *pylori*. The UreB was produced as a chimeric protein fused with IL-2 (human interleukin 2) as the mucosal adjuvant. Mucosal immunization of mice with recombinant L. lactis NZ9000 containing the UreB-IL-2 protein elicited more anti-UreB antibody that specifically bounded to the purified bacterial UreB protein and more cytokines such as IFN-γ, IL-4, and IL-17, and had a lower H. *pylori* burden and urease activity than control mice. These results suggest that the recombinant L. lactis expressing UreB-IL-2 can be potentially used as an edible *vaccine* for controlling H. *pylori* infection.

Altman etal, 2013 [81] demonstrated that synthetic glycoconjugates based on delipidated lipopolysaccharide (LPS) of *Helicobacter pylori* and containing an α(1-6)-glucan chain induced broadly cross-reactive functional antibodies in immunized animals. Thus, they prepared glycoconjugates based on dextrans produced by lactic acid bacteria Leuconostoc mesenteroides B512F and consisting of linear α(1-6)-glucan chains with limited branching. Three dextrans with averaged molecular masses of 5, 000 Da, 3, 500 Da and 1, 500 Da, respectively, were modified with a diamino group-containing linker and conjugated to a carrier protein, tetanus toxoid (TT) or diphtheria toxoid (DT. The conjugates were immunogenic in both rabbits and mice and induced specific IgG responses against α(1-6)- glucan -expressing H. *pylori* LPS. Studies performed with post-immune sera of mice and rabbits immunized with dextran-based conjugates demonstrated cross-reactivity with LPS from typeable and non-typeable strains of H. *pylori* and selected mutants. The post-immune sera from rabbits that received the conjugates exhibited functional activity against α(1-6)-glucan-positive strains of *H. pylori*. These data provide evidence that dextran-based conjugates may offer a simplified approach to the development of carbohydrate-based *vaccines* against *H. pylori*.

Helicobacter pylori neutrophil-activating protein (NAP) is a toll-like receptor 2 (TLR2) agonist and potent immunomodulator inducing Th1-type immune response. Iankov etal 2013 [82]studied the humoral immune response against NAP-tagged antigens, encoded by attenuated measles virus (MV) vector platform, in MV infection susceptible type I interferon receptor knockout and human CD46 transgenic (Ifnarko-CD46Ge) mice. Immunogenicity of MV expressing a full-length human immunoglobulin lambda light chain (MV-lambda) was compared to that of MV expressing lambda-NAP chimeric protein (MV-lambda-NAP). MV-lambda-NAP immunized Ifnarko-CD46Ge mice developed significantly higher (6-20-fold) anti-lambda ELISA titers as compared to the MV-lambda-immunized control animal group, indicating that covalently-linked NAP co-expression significantly enhanced lambda immunogenicity. In contrast, ELISA titers against MV antigens were not significantly different between the animals vaccinated with MV-lambda or MV-lambda-NAP. NAP-tagged antigen expression did not affect development of protective anti-measles immunity. Both MV-lambda and MV-lambda-NAP-immunized groups showed strong virus neutralization serum titers in plaque reduction microneutralization test. They concluded that MV-encoded lambda-NAP is highly immunogenic as compared to the unmodified full-length lambda chain. Boost of immune response to poor immunogens using live vectors expressing NAP-tagged chimeric antigens is an attractive approach with potential application in immunoprophylaxis of infectious diseases and cancer immunotherapy.

An important consideration in the development of subunit *vaccines* is the loss of activity caused by physical instability of the protein. CagL is a protein present in strains of *H. pylori*. It contributes to bacterial adherence via $\alpha5\beta1$ integrin, thereby making it an attractive subunit *vaccine* candidate. Choudhari etal, 2013 [83] used CagL in different pH and temperature conditions using a variety of spectroscopic techniques. Stability was assessed in terms of transition temperature with the accumulated data, and then incorporated into an empirical phase diagram (EPD) that provided an overview of CagL physical stability. These analyses indicated maximum CagL stability at pH 4-6 up to 40°C in the absence of excipient. Using this EPD analysis, aggregation assays were developed to screen a panel of excipients with some found to inhibit CagL aggregation. These analyses will help in the formulation of a stable *vaccine* against H.*pylori*.

Helicobacter pylori is a major human pathogen that colonizes the stomach and is the lead etiological agent for several pathologies. Sutton P and Chionh YT 2013 [84] demonstrated that effective *vaccine* against these bacteria would be invaluable for protecting against gastric adenocarcinoma. However, the development of such a *vaccine* has stalled and the field has progressed little in the last decade. The key problems that are preventing the development of a *H. pylori vaccine*. Primarily, this involves the inability to produce a completely protective immune response. The knock-on effects of this include a loss of industry investment. Overcoming these problems will likely involve defeating the immune-evasion defenses of *H. pylori*, in particular the mechanism(s) by which it evades antibody-mediated attack.

Chronic *H. pylori* infection can be successfully eradicated by intragastric vaccination with *H. pylori* antigens such as recombinant VacA and CagA, which were administered together with a genetically detoxified mutant of the heat-labile enterotoxin of Escherichia coli (referred to as LTK63), in which the serine in position 63 was replaced by a lysine. The therapeutic vaccination confers efficacious protection against reinfection [85]. Vaccines against *Helicobacter pylori* could circumvent the problem of increasing antibiotic resistance. They would be particularly useful in developing countries, where re-infection rates are high following standard eradication regimes. The vaccine could be given orally with an *H. pylori* whole cell sonicate preparation and cholera toxin adjuvant. Protection was associated with increased serum *H. pylori* IgG antibodies. In this type of vaccine the levels of gastric IL-12p40 and IFN-gamma transcripts were significantly decreased. Gastric IL-10 and TGF-beta transcripts were found only at relatively low levels [86]. Other type of vaccines were used a recombinant antigen ureB138 (a segment of the beta-subunit of urease) against *Helicobacter pylori* infection [87]. Using mucosal vaccination with *H. pylori* antigens when given together with cholera toxin (CT) adjuvant, but not without adjuvant, can induce protective immune responses against *H. pylori* infection. However, the toxicity of CT prevents its use as a mucosal adjuvant in humans. The using a nontoxic double mutant Escherichia coli heat-labile toxin, LT(R192G/L211A) (dmLT), as a mucosal adjuvant in an experimental H. pylori vaccine and compared it to CT in promoting immune responses and protection against *H. pylori* infection. Immunization via the sublingual or intragastric route with *H. pylori* lysate antigens and dmLT resulted in a significant decrease in bacterial load after challenge. Cellular immune responses in the sublingually route resulting in enhanced *in vitro* proliferative and cytokine responses from spleen and mesenteric lymph node cells to *H. pylori* antigens. Thus, dmLT is an attractive adjuvant for inclusion in a mucosal vaccine against *H. pylori* infection [88].

3. Conclusions

Helicobacter infection is an important cause of cancer development. Immune response to this bacterial infection is playing an important role in gastric inflammation. The infection may be innocent or subclinical. Therefore, frequent patients screening for this bacteria and eradication of *Helicobacter* spp. is very crucial. Researches about these bacteria are very essential starting from laboratory animal to application of the researches from lab bench to clinic. Innate and adaptive immune responses of the host are seriously significant for the development of new plans to prevent the development of *H. pylori*-induced gastroduodenal disease and production a vaccine to eradicate this infection. It will be necessary to determine the feasibility of using different epitopes extracted from *H. pylori* in a vaccine design.

Author details

Batool Mutar Mahdi

Clinical Immunology, Department of Microbiology, HLA Research Unit, Al-Kindy College of Medicine, Baghdad University, Baghdad, Iraq

References

[1] Marshall BJ, Warren JR. Unidentified curved bacilli in the stomach of patients with gastritis and peptic ulceration. Lancet 1984; i: 1311-5.

[2] Gao L, Weck MN, Stegmaier C, Rothenbacher D, Brenner H. Alcohol consumption and chronic atrophic gastritis: Population-based study among 9, 444 older adults from Germany. *Int J Cancer*. Jun 2 2009;

[3] Weck MN, Gao L, Brenner H. Helicobacter pylori infection and chronic atrophic gastritis: associations according to severity of disease. *Epidemiology*. 2009;20(4):569-74.

[4] Dixon MF, Genta RM, Yardley JH, Correa P. Classification and grading of gastritis. The updated Sydney System. International Workshop on the Histopathology of Gastritis, Houston 1994. *Am J Surg Pathol*. 1996;20(10):1161-81.

[5] Blaser MJ, Atherton JC. "*Helicobacter pylori* persistence: biology and disease". *J. Clin. Invest.* 2004;113 (3): 321–33.

[6] *Helicobacter pylori* and peptic ulcer disease; economics of peptic ulcer disease and *H. pylori* infection. Centers for Disease Control and Prevention website. www.cdc.gov/ulcer/economic.htm.

[7] Dixon MF. "Patterns of inflammation linked to ulcer disease".Baillieres Best Pract Res Clin Gastroenterol.2000;14 (1): 27–40.

[8] Ciociola AA, McSorley DJ, Turner K, et al. *Helicobacter pylori* infection rates in duodenal ulcer patients in the United States may be lower than previously estimated. Am J Gastroenterol 1999; 94:1834.

[9] Parsonnet J, Friedman GD, Vandersteen DP et al. *Helicobacter pylori* infection and gastric lymphoma. N. Engl. J. Med. 1994;330, 1267–1271.

[10] Wen S, Moss SF. Helicobacter pylori virulence factors in gastric carcinogenesis. Cancer Letters2009; 282(1):1–8.

[11] Kusters JG, van Vliet AH, Kuipers EJ. Pathogenesis of Helicobacter pylori infection. *Clinical Microbiology Reviews* 2006; 19(3):449–490.

[12] Sagaert X, Van Cutsem E, De Hertogh G, Geboes K, Tousseyn T. Gastric MALT lymphoma: A model of chronic inflammation-induced tumor development. Nature Reviews Gastroenterology & Hepatology 2010; 7(6):336–346.

[13] Menaker RJ, Sharaf AA, Jones NL. *Helicobacter pylori* infection and gastric cancer: host, bug, environment, or all three? Curr Gastroenterol Rep. 2004 ;6(6):429-35.

[14] Calam J.Host mechanisms: are they the key to the various clinical outcomes of *Helicobacter pylori* infection? Ital J Gastroenterol Hepatol. 1997 ;29(4):375-82.

[15] Bleich A, Mahler M. Environment as a critical factor for the pathogenesis and outcome of gastrointestinal disease: experimental and human inflammatory bowel disease and helicobacter-induced gastritis. Pathobiology. 2005;72(6):293-307.

[16] Kabir S. Effect of *Helicobacter pylori* eradication on incidence of gastric cancer in human and animal models: underlying biochemical and molecular events. Helicobacter 2009; 14(3): 159-171.

[17] Izzotti A, Durando P, Ansaldi F, Gianiorio F, Pulliero A. Interaction between *Helicobacter pylori,* diet, and genetic polymorphisms as related to non-cancer diseases. Mutat Res. 2009 ; 10;667(1-2):142-57.

[18] McNamara D, El-Omar E.*Helicobacter pylori* infection and the pathogenesis of gastric cancer: a paradigm for host-bacterial interactions. Dig Liver Dis. 2008 ;40(7):504-9.

[19] Correa P. Human gastric carcinogenesis: a multistep and multifactorial process-First American Cancer Society Award Lecture on Cancer Epidemiology and Prevention. Cancer Res 1992; 52: 6735-6740.

[20] Brown LM. *Helicobacter pylori*: epidemiology and routes of transmission. Epidemiol. Rev. 2000;22, 283–297.

[21] Brown LM.*Helicobacter pylori*: epidemiology and routes of transmission. Epidemiol Rev. 2000;22(2):283-97.

[22] Mégraud F.Transmission of *Helicobacter pylori*: faecal-oral versus oral-oral route. Aliment Pharmacol Ther. 1995;9 Suppl 2:85-91.

[23] Mobley HL. Defining *Helicobacter pylori* as a pathogen: strain heterogeneity and virulence. Am. J. Med1996;100, 2S–9S, discussion 9S–11S.

[24] Rohde M, Puls J, Buhrdorf R, Fischer W, Haas R. A novel sheated surface organelle of the *Helicobacter pylori* cag type IV secretion system. Molecular Microbiology 2003; 49(1): 219-234.

[25] Backert S, Selbach M. Role of type IV secretion in *Helicobacter pylori* pathogenesis. Cellular Microbiology 2008; 10(8): 1573-1581.

[26] Odenbreit S, Puls J, Sedlmaier B, Gerland E, Fisher W, Haas R. Translocation of *Helicobacter pylori* CagA into gastric epithelial cells by type IV secretion. Science 2000; 287(5457): 1497-1500.

[27] Higashi H, Tsutsumi R, Muto S, Sugiyama T, Azuma T, Asaka M, Hatakeyama M. SHP-2 tyrosine phosphatase as na intracellular target of *Helicobacter pylori* CagA protein. Science 2002; 295: 683-686.

[28] Amieva MR, Vogelmann R, Covacci A, Tompkins LS, Nelson WJ, Falkow S. Disruption of the epithelial apical-junctional complex by *Helicobacter pylori* CagA. Science 2003; 300(5624): 1430-1434.

[29] Portal-Celhay C and Perez-Perez GI. Immune responses to *Helicobacter pylori* colonization: mechanisms and clinical outcomes. Clin. Sci. 2006;110, 305–314.

[30] Miehlke, S., Kirsch, C., Agha-Amiri, K. et al. The *Helicobacter pylori* vacA s1 m1 genotype and cagA is associated with gastric carcinoma in Germany. Int. J. Cancer.2000. 87, 322–327.

[31] Ferreira RM, Machado JC, Letley D, Atherton JC, Pardo ML, Gonzalez CA, Carneiro F, Figueiredo C. A novel method for genotyping the *Helicobacter pylori* vacA intermediate region directly in gastric biopsy specimens. J Clin Microbiol 2012, 50(12): 3893-9.

[32] Stromberg E, Edebo A, Svennerholm AM, Lindholm C.Decreased epithelial cytokine responses in the duodenal mucosa of *Helicobacter pylori*-infected duodenal ulcer patients. Clin Diagn Lab Immunol. 2003; 10:116-124.

[33] Hamlet A, Thoreson AC, Nilsson O, et al. Duodenal Helicobacter pylori infection differs in cagA genotype between asymptomatic subjects and patients with duodenal ulcers. *Gastroenterology*.1999;116:259–68.

[34] van Doorn LJ, Figueiredo C, Sanna R, et al. Clinical relevance of the cagA, vacA, and iceA status of Helicobacter pylori. *Gastroenterology*.1998;115:58–66.

[35] Stromberg E, Edebo A, Lundin S, Bergin P, Brisslert M, Svennerholm A and Lindholm C.Down-regulation of epithelial IL-8 responses in *Helicobacter pylori*-infected duodenal ulcer patients depends on host factors, rather than bacterial factors.Clin Exp Immunol. 2005 ; 140(1): 117–125.

[36] Mattsson A, Quiding-Jarbrink M, Lonroth H, Hamlet A and Ahlstedt I.Antibody-Secreting Cells in the Stomachs of Symptomatic and Asymptomatic *Helicobacter pylori*-Infected Subjects Infect. Immun. June 1998 vol. 66 no. 6 2705-2712

[37] Crabtree, J. E. Immune and inflammatory responses to *Helicobacter pylori* infection. Scand. J. Gastroenterol. 1996;215: 3S–10S.

[38] Lagunes-Servin H, Torres J, Maldonado-Bernal C, Pérez-Rodríguez M, Huerta-Yépez S, Madrazo de la Garza A, Muñoz-Pérez L, Flores-Luna L, Ramón-García G, Camorlinga-Ponce M. Toll-Like Receptors and Cytokines are Upregulated during *Helicobacter pylori* Infection in Children. Helicobacter. 2013 Jul 22. doi: 10.1111/hel.12067. [Epub ahead of print]

[39] Pimentel-Nunes P, Gonçalves N, Boal-Carvalho I, Afonso L, Lopes P, Roncon-Albuquerque R, Henrique R, Moreira-Dias L, Leite-Moreira A and Dinis-Ribeiro M.*Helicobacter pylori* Induces Increased Expression of Toll-Like Receptors and Decreased Toll-Interacting Protein in Gastric Mucosa that Persists Throughout Gastric Carcinogenesis.Helicobacter2013;18:22-32.

[40] Ihan A, Pinchuk IV, Beswick EJ. Inflammation, immunity, and vaccines for *Helicobacter pylori* infection.Helicobacter. 2012 Sep;17 Suppl 1:16-21.

[41] Avilés-Jiménez F, Reyes-Leon A, NietoPatlán E, Hansen LM, Burgueño J, Ramos IP et al. In vivo expression of *Helicobacter pylori* virulence genes in patients with gastritis, ulcer, and gastric cancer. Infect Immun 2012;80:594-601.

[42] Chatterjee A, Chatterjee S, Bandyopadhyay SK. *H pylori*-induced gastric ulcer: pathophysiology and herbal remedy. Int J Biol Med Res 2012;3:1461-5.

[43] Tummala, S., Keates, S. and Kelly, C. P. Update on the immunologic basis of *Helicobacter pylori* gastritis. Curr. Opin. Gastroenterol.2004; 20, 592–597.

[44] Irina V. Pinchuk, Katherine T. Morris, Robert A. Nofchissey, Rachel B. Earley, Jeng-Yih Wu, Thomas Y. Ma, and Ellen J. Beswick. Stromal Cells Induce Th17 during *Helicobacter pylori* Infection and in the Gastric Tumor Microenvironment.*PLoS One.* 2013; 8: e53798.

[45] Noach, L. A., Bosma, N. B., Jansen, J., Hoek, F. J., van Deventer, S. J. and Tygat, G. N. Mucosal tumor necrosis factor-α, interleukin-1β, and interleukin-8 production in patients with *Helicobacter pylori* infection. Scand. J. Gastroenterol. 1994;29, 425–429.

[46] Hwang, I. R., Kodama, T., Kikuchi, S. et al. (2002) Effect of interleukin 1 polymorphisms on gastric mucosal interleukin 1beta production in *Helicobacter pylori* infection. Gastroenterology 123, 1793–1803

[47] Yuceyar H, Saruc M, Kokuludag A, Terzioglu E, Goksel G, Isisag A. The systemic cellular immune response in the *Helicobacter pylori*-associated duodenal ulcer and chronic antral gastritis" Hepatogastroenterology 2002, 49(46): 1177-9.

[48] Fixa B, Komárková O, Krejsek J, Nozicka Z, Bures J. Specific cellular immune response in patients with *Helicobacter pylori* infection. Hepatogastroenterology 1990, 37(6):606-7.

[49] Nessa J, Chart H, Owen RJ and Drasar B. Human serum antibody response to *H pylori* whole cell antigen in an institutionalized Bangaladish population. J Appl microb. 2001;90:68-72.

[50] Mattsson A, Quiding-Jabrink M, Lonroth H, Hamlet A, Ahlstedt I and Svennerholm A. Antibody secreting cells in the stomach of symptomatic and asymptomatic *H pylori* infected subjects. 1998; 66:2705-2712.

[51] Tosi, M. F. and Czinn, S. J. Opsonic activity of specific human IgG against *Helicobacter pylori*. J. Infect. Dis.1990; 162, 156–162.

[52] Berstad, A. E, Holbjorn, K., Bukholm, G., Moran, A. P. and Brandtzaeg, P Complement activation directly induced by *Helicobacter pylori.* Gastroenterology;2001 120, 1108–1116.

[53] Cover TL. The vaculating cytotoxin of *H pylori*. Mol 241-246.

[54] Portal-Celhay C and Perez-Perez G. Immune responses to *Helicobacter pylori* colonization: mechanisms and clinical outcomes.Clinical Science.2006; 110: 305–314.

[55] Crabtree JE, Wyatt JI, Sobala GM.Systemic and mucosal humoral responses to *Helicobacter pylori* in gastric cancer.. Gut1993, 34:1339-43.

[56] Menaker RJ, Ceponis PJ, Jones NL. *Helicobacter pylori* induces apoptosis of macrophages in association with alterations in the mitochondrial pathway. Infect Immun. 2004 ;72:2889-98.

[57] Ramarao, N. and Meyer, T. F. *Helicobacter pylori* resists phagocytosis by macrophages: quantitative assessment by confocal microscopy and fluorescenceactivated cell sorting. Infect. Immun. 2001; 69, 2604–2611

[58] Gobert, A. P., McGee, D. J., Akhtar, M. et al. *Helicobacter pylori* arginase inhibits nitric oxide production by eukaryotic cells: a strategy for bacterial survival. Proc. Natl. Acad. Sci. 2001; 98:13844–13849.

[59] Yuan J, Li P, Tao J, Shi X, Hu B, Chen H, Guo X. H. pylori escape host immunoreaction through inhibiting ILK expression by VacA. Cell Mol Immunol. 2009;6:191-197.

[60] Perez-Perez, G. I., Shepherd, V. L., Morrow, J. D. and Blaser, M. J. Activation of human THP-1 cells and rat bone marrow-derived macrophages by *Helicobacter pylori* lipopolysaccharide. Infect. Immun. 1995;63, 1183–1187

[61] Andersen-Nissen, E., Smith, K. D., Strobe, K. L. et al. Evasion of Toll-like receptor 5 by flagellated bacteria. Proc. Natl. Acad. Sci.2005; 102:9247–9252.

[62] Yang ZM, Chen WW, Wang YF. Gene expression profiling in gastric mucosa from *Helicobacter pylori*-infected and uninfected patients undergoing chronic superficial gastritis. PLoS One. 2012;7:e33030.

[63] Boncristiano, M., Paccani, S. R., Barone, S. et al. The *Helicobacter pylori* vacuolating toxin inhibits T cell activation by two independent mechanisms. J. Exp. Med. 2003;198: 1887–1897.

[64] Molinari, M., Salio, M., Galli, C. et al. Selective inhibition of Ii-dependent antigen presentation by *Helicobacter pylori* toxin VacA. J. Exp. Med. 1998;187 :135–140

[65] Gebert, B., Fischer, W., Weiss, R., Hoffmann, R. andHaas, R. *Helicobacter pylori* vacuolating cytotoxin inhibits T-lymphocyte activation. Science.2003; 301: 1099–1102.

[66] Yuan JP, Li T, Li ZH, Yang GZ, Hu BY, Shi XD, Shi TL, Tong SQ, Guo XK. mRNA expression profiling reveals a role of *Helicobacter pylori* vacuolating toxin in escaping host defense. World J Gastroenterol. 2004 ;10:1528-32.

[67] Every AL. Key host-pathogen interactions for designing novel interventions against *Helicobacter pylori*. Trends Microbiol. 2013;21(5):253-9.

[68] Del Giudice G, Malfertheiner P, Rappuoli R. Development of vaccines against *Helicobacter pylori*. Expert Rev Vaccines. 2009 ;8(8):1037-49.

[69] Sutton P. Progress in vaccination against *Helicobacter pylori. Vaccine* 2001;19:2286–90.

[70] Kleanthous H, Myers GA, Georgakopoulos KM, et al. Rectal and intranasal immunizations with recombinant urease induce distinct local and serum immune responses in mice and protect against *Helicobacter pylori* infection. Infect Immun 1998;66:2879–86.

[71] Michetti P, Kreiss C, Kotloff KL, et al. Oral immunization with urease and *Escherichia coli* heat-labile enterotoxin is safe and immunogenic in*Helicobacter pylori*-infected adults. *Gastroenterology* 1999;116:804–12.

[72] Blanchard TG, Eisenberg JC, Matsumoto Y. Clearance of *Helicobacter pylori* infection through immunization: the site of T cell activation contributes to vaccine efficacy. Vaccine 2004;22:888–97.

[73] Eriksson AM, Schon KM, Lycke NY. The cholera toxin-derived CTA1-DD vaccine adjuvant administered intranasally does not cause inflammation or accumulate in the nervous tissues. J Immunol 2004;173:3310–9.

[74] Gottwein JM, Blanchard TG, Targoni OS, et al. Protective anti-Helicobacter immunity is induced with aluminum hydroxide or complete Freund's adjuvant by systemic immunization. J Infect Dis 2001;184:308–14.

[75] Stadtlander CTKH, Gangemi JD, Khanolvar SS, Kitsos CM, Farris HE, Fulton LK, et al. Immunogenicity and Safety of recombinant *Helicobacter pylori* urease in a nonhuman primate. Dig Dis Sci;1996 41:1853–1862.

[76] Michetti P, CorthésyTheulaz I, Davin C, Haas R, y AC, Heitz M, et al.Immunization of BALB/c mice against Helicobacter felis infection with H. pylori urease. Gastroenterology.1994;107:1002–1011.

[77] Cuenca R, Blanchard TG, Czinn SJ, Nedrud JG, Monath TP, Lee CK, et al. Therapeutic immunization against Helicobacter mustelae in naturally infected ferrets. Gastroenterology.1996; 110:1770–1775.

[78] Kreiss C, Buclin T, Cosma M, CorthésyTheulaz I, Michetti PSafety of oral immunization with recombinant urease in patients with *Helicobacter pylori* infection. Lancet. 1996; 347:1630–1631.

[79] Corthésy-Theulaz I, Bachmann D, Hopkins S, Kraehenbuhl J-P, Michetti P, Blum AL Mucosal immunization against *Helicobacter pylori* in mice via attenuated recombinant Salmonella. Gastroenterology.1997; 112:A953.

[80] Zhang HX, Qiu YY, Zhao YH, Liu M, Yu AL. Immunogenicity of oral vaccination with Lactococcus lactis derived vaccine candidate antigen (UreB) of*Helicobacter pylori* fused with the human interleukin 2 as adjuvant.Mol Cell Probes. 2013 Sep 13. pii: S0890-8508(13)00048-0. doi: 10.1016/j.mcp.2013.08.003. [Epub ahead of print]

[81] Altman E, Chandan V, Harrison B. The potential of dextran-based glycoconjugates for development of *Helicobacter pylori* vaccine.Glycoconj J. 2013 Aug 30. [Epub ahead of print].

[82] Iankov ID, Federspiel MJ, Galanis E. Measles virus expressed *Helicobacter pylori* neutrophil-activating protein significantly enhances the immunogenicity of poor immunogens.Vaccine. 2013;31(42):4795-801.

[83] Choudhari SP, Pendleton KP, Ramsey JD, Blanchard TG, Picking WD. A systematic approach toward stabilization of CagL, a protein antigen from *Helicobacter pylori* that is a candidate subunit vaccine. J Pharm Sci. 2013 ;102(8):2508-19.

[84] Sutton P, Chionh YT.Why can't we make an effective vaccine against *Helicobacter pylori*? Expert Rev Vaccines. 2013 ;12(4):433-41.

[85] Ghiara P, Rossi M, Marchetti M, Di Tommaso A, Vindigni C, Ciampolini F et al. Therapeutic intragastric vaccination against Heliconbacter pylori in mice eradicates an otherwise chronic infection and confers protection against reinfection. Infect Immun 1997, 65(12): 4996-5002.

[86] Jeremy AH, Du Y, Dixon MF, Robinson PA, Crabtree JE. Protection against *Helicobacter pylori* infection in the Mongolian gerbil after prophylatic vaccination.Microbes Infect 2006, 8(2):340-6.

[87] Morihara F, Fujii R, Hifurni E, Nishizono A, Uda T. Effects of vaccination by a recombinant antigen ureB138 (a segment of the beta-subunit of urease) against *Helicobacter pylori* infection. J Med Microbiol 2007, 56(6):847-53.

[88] Sjökvist Ottsjö L, Flach CF, Clements J, Holmgren J, Raghavan S. A double mutant heat-labile toxin from Escherichia coli, LT(R192G/L211A), is an effective mucosal adjuvant for vaccination against *Helicobacter pylori* infection. Infect Immun 2013, 81(5): 1532-40.

10

Helicobacter pylori and Liver – Detection of Bacteria in Liver Tissue from Patients with Hepatocellular Carcinoma Using Laser Capture Microdissection Technique (LCM)

Elizabeth Maria Afonso Rabelo-Gonçalves,
Bruna Maria Röesler and
José Murilo Robilotta Zeitune

1. Introduction

Hepatocellular carcinoma (HCC) is the most common primary tumor of the liver in humans [1]. It is the fifth most common cancer in men (523,000 cases per year, 7.9% of all cancers) and the seventh among women (226,000 cases per year, 3.7% of all cancers) [2], with over a half of million new cases diagnosed annually. It is the second leading cause of the cancer related mortality in the world [3,4,5] and its prevalence differs according to geographic location, gender, age and ethnicity [6].

In general, the distribution of HCC cases presents great geographic variation, with higher incidence in Easter Asia and sub-Saharan Africa where infection with hepatitis B virus (HBV) is endemic with rates of over 20 per 100,000 individuals. Mediterranean countries such as Italy, Spain and Greece have intermediate rates of 10 to 20 per 100,000 individuals. The North and South America have a relatively low incidence (< 5 per 100,000 individuals) [4], although a rising incidence was observed in the USA, probably associated with the rise in hepatitis C virus (HCV) infection. Recent decreases in the incidence of HCC were reported among Chinese populations in Hong Kong, Shangai and Singapore; the incidence in Japan is also decreasing [3].

In Brazil, there are few reports on the prevalence of HCC [7]. It was suggested that the prevalence was considered low according to epidemiologic and retrospective studies [8]. In

1997, Brazilian researchers showed that HVB was the most common cause of liver disease in patients with HCC [9]. After that, another survey demonstrated that in Southeastern and Southern Brazil, HCV accounted for over 55% of cases. In the Northeast and North, HCV accounted for less than 50% and HBV accounted for 22-25% of cases; hepatitis B was more prevalent in the Northern than in the Southern regions [10].

The development of HCC has been attributed to several risk factors. In general, chronic viral infection with HBV and HCV is considered the major cause of HCC in 75-80% of cases [1], although HBV is globally considered the leading risk factor responsible for 50% of cases [11]. Furthermore, cirrhosis [12], exposure to the carcinogenic fungal aflatoxin B1 [13], inherited diseases [14], Wilson's disease [15] and heavy alcohol consumption [16] are also risk factors attributed to its development. Recently, upcoming risk factors for HCC include obesity, diabetes and related nonalcoholic fatty liver disease [3].

In 1994, researchers described the infectious agent *Helicobacter (H.) hepaticus* and its role in causing active hepatitis and associated liver tumors in mice [17]. Since then, several studies related to *H. hepaticus* experimental infection have demonstrated that this bacterium may induce a strong inflammatory change in the liver leading to HCC. Considering that *H. pylori* was classified as a class I carcinogen [18] and *Helicobacter* spp. DNA was detected in hepatic tissue from patients with different hepatobiliary diseases, it has been proposed that in humans, as in animals, *Helicobacter* spp. may also colonize and induce chronic hepatic diseases mainly HCC.

In fact, studies related to the possible association between *H. pylori* and hepatobiliary diseases have been developed since 1998, when Helicobacter DNA was identified in Chilean patients with chronic cholecystitis [19]. After that, a variety of researches have been conducted to verify the role of *H. pylori* in the development of HCC [20, 21, 22, 23, 24, 25, 26 e 27]. Considering the role of chronic inflammation and infection in the development of cancer, in the case of HCC, future studies should be performed to verify the role of *Helicobacter* infection in the liver pathophisiology [28]. However, whether this bacterium causes liver tumor or acts as a cofactor in the process of carcinogenesis needs to be confirmed.

The mechanism by which *H. pylori* colonizes the human liver is not totally enlightened. The *H. pylori* DNA detected in the liver tissue may result from bacterial translocation from the stomach into the blood through the portal system, especially in the later stages of chronic liver disease when portal hypertension occurs [1, 29, 30]. In addition, the bacteria may reach the liver by phagocytes and macrophages or circulating retrograde transfer from the duodenum [31]. However, the studies involving the growth of *H. pylori* from the HCC liver reinforce the bacterial colonization ruling out the possibility of retrograde contamination [32, 33]. Additionally, no other bacteria from the digestive tract are associated with human hepatocarcinogenesis [23, 34].

Several researchers have suggested that *H. pylori* may damage hepatocytes in vitro by a cytopathic effect in a liver and HCC cell lines [35, 36]. Furthermore, it was demonstrated in a HCC cell line (Huh7) that an inoculum of *H. pylori* was able to adhere and internalize into hepatocytes and this result was also dependent on virulence factors of bacteria [37]. Proteomic analysis of human hepatic cell line (HepG2) co-cultured with *H. pylori* have revealed that bacteria may exert the pathological effect on HepG2 cells by up-regulating the expression of some proteins enrolled in transcription regulation, signal transduction and metabolism [38].

In most pathology laboratories, archives of formalin-fixed paraffin-embedded (FFPE) tissues represent the only tissue specimens available for routine diagnostics. A major advantage of such archives is that long-term clinical data is often available [39]. Furthermore, another benefit of using FFPE tissues is that they are the easiest to store and transport [40]. Because of this, FFPE tissues have been used in PCR-based studies related to cancer research, genetics, infectious diseases and molecular epidemiology [41]. Additionally, the use of FFPE tissue also allows employing modern transcriptomic and epigenomic methods with nucleic acids [39].

However, isolating high-quality genomic DNA from FFPE sections remains a challenge for researchers. Formalin is the most commonly used tissue fixative worldwide because it offers the best compromise between cost, practicality and morphological fixative properties [39, 42]. However, the fixation of tissue in formalin leads to extensive protein-DNA cross-linking of all tissue components and nucleic acids isolated from these specimens are highly fragmented [43]. This is particularly troublesome when long DNA regions are amplified, old paraffin blocks are used or fixation time is over three days [41, 44]. Because of this, FFPE tissue requires special protocols in order to extract small amounts of DNA suitable for amplification [45]. Nevertheless, methods of DNA extraction from FFPE tissue are generally laborious and time consuming.

Although studies on the role of the *H. pylori* in the development of HCC were more frequent in the last decade [46], most of them presents a prospective nature. This probably occurs because the retrospective studies frequently employ FFPE liver tissue and DNA extraction is a limiting factor in this type of sample. However, several researchers have detected *H. pylori* and its virulence factors (vacA genes and 26 kDa) in paraffin embedded liver samples [21, 27, 34, 47, 48].

Laser capture microdissection (LCM) is a technique that has recently become available for isolation of individual or groups of cells from a heterogeneous tissue sections by microscopic visualization. The technique was first described in 1996 by researchers of the National Institutes of Health (NIH) in Bethesda, MD [49] and allows the isolation of cells reducing the interference from nontarget cell population. The method allows selection of unmixed starting material for DNA, RNA or protein extraction for further downstream analyses [50].

The LCM system is based on an inverted light microscope fitted with a laser device to facilitate the visualization and procurement of cells [51]. The PALM MicroBeam System (Carl Zeiss, MicroImaging GmbH, Göottingen, Germany) was used in this study and it is based on the Laser Microdissection and Pressure Catapulting technology. This system consists of an inverted microscope with a motorized stage and a pulsed "cold" nitrogen ultra-violet (UV) laser. The laser is focused through the objective lenses to a micron-sized spot diameter. The narrow laser focal spot allows the ablation of the material while the surrounding tissue remains fully intact. The microscope stage and UV laser are controlled by a PC, and a video camera allows for tissue sections to be displayed on the PC screen. Cells or regions of interest are then identified and manually delineated on the computer screen using the software program. The microscope is then instructed to collect delineated regions. The noncontact capture of homogeneous tissue samples or individual cells is achieved by means of catapulting using PALM's patented Laser Pressure Catapulting technology. With the same laser, the separated cells, or the selected tissue area, can be directly catapulted into the eppendorf cap containing a depressed lid [52, 53]. The Figure 1 shows the LCM technology employed in this study.

LCM has been used in a wide variety of applications, including pathology [54, 55], organ transplantation [56, 57], gene expression [52, 58] and molecular characterization of cancer cells [59, 60, 61]. LCM is compatible with most stains and tissue preservation techniques including frozen sections, FFPE tissues, cytology preparations and cultured cells [52, 62]. Because of its high precision and accuracy LCM has been successfully employed to isolation of bacterial cells in FFPE tissues including *H. pylori* [48, 61, 62, 64, 65].

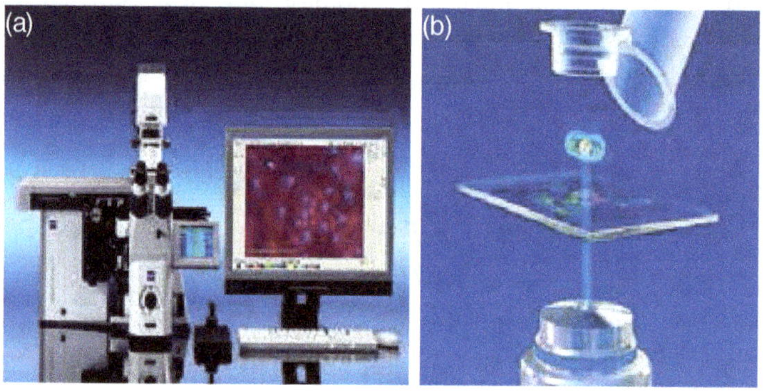

Figure 1. Images of LCM technology used in the study. In A is represented the complete PALM MicroBeam system. In B is illustrated the path of the laser beam passing through the objective lens to reach the tissue slice and the catapulting process for capturing the cells of interest into the Eppendorf cap. Source of the images: www.zeiss.de.

2. Clinical samples, methods and results

2.1. Clinical samples

This study was carried out utilizing six cases of FFPE liver tissue from patients with HCC from Department of Anatomic Pathology, Faculty of Medical Sciences, State University of Campinas (UNICAMP), Campinas, São Paulo, Brazil. The mean ages of patients was 56.0 years, with 4 male cases (66,6%) and 2 female cases (33,4%). All the fragments of liver were obtained during hepatic surgery (either transplantation or partial hepatectomy). These samples were *H. pylori* positive previously detected by polymerase chain reaction (PCR) with *H. pylori* specific 16S rRNA primers [27]. The selection criteria for the paraffin blocks included specimens archived for 5 years (2008 to 2012). The present study was approved by the Ethics Committee of the Faculty of Medical Sciences, UNICAMP (CEP 616/2009).

2.2. Methods

2.2.1. Tissue preparation for LCM

Six *H. pylori* positive samples were cut into 10μm-thick sections and mounted on 0.17mm PEN membrane-covered slides (Carl Zeiss, MicroImaging GmbH, Göttingen, Germany). After slicing, the sections were placed at 60°C for 30 minutes, then deparaffinized in 3 xylene baths (3x1min), rehydrated in decreasing alcohols (100%, 95% e 70%, each for 30 seconds) and washed for 30 seconds in tap water. Further, the routine staining with carbol fuchsin was performed [66]. At this step the sections have remained in the dye for at most 15 seconds. The stained sections were observed under the microscope for the identification of bacteria.

2.2.2. Bacterial microdissection

Stained bacteria were microdissected using a PALM MicroBeam system (Carl Zeiss, MicroImaging GmbH, Göttingen, Germany) (Figure 1A). The areas with target bacteria were traced around and microdissected together with the pieces of thin membrane by laser microbeam and then ejected into the Eppendorf tube cap by a single laser shot (Figure 1B). The tube was stored at -80°C until DNA extraction.

2.2.3. DNA extraction

After microdissection, the cap was inserted into an Eppendorf tube containing 100μl digestion buffer, prepared with 10mM Tris-HCl (pH 8.0), 1mM EDTA, 1% Tween 20 and 0.3% proteinase K. After that, samples remained in a water bath at 56°C for 3 hours and the tube was heated to 95°C for 5 min to inactivate proteinase K. The crude lysate was directly employed as template for PCR. All of these procedures were previously described with minor modifications [48].

2.2.4. PCR amplification

The samples were further amplified by PCR using *H. pylori* 16S rRNA primers. The sequence of the sense primer (JW21) was 5′-GCGACCTGCTGGAACATTAC-3′(position 691-710) and the antisense primer (JW22) was 5′-CGTTAGCTCCATTACTGGAGA-3′ (position 829-809) and they amplified a product of approximately 129bp [27]. Briefly, 1μl of DNA extracted was added to 25μl PCR mix containing deoxynucleoside triphosphates (dNTPs) at concentrations of 200 μM each, 2.0μl of 25mM MgCl2, 0.25 μl of GoTaq Hot Start Polymerase (Promega Corp., Madison, WI, USA), 4.0 μl of 5X GoTaq Flexi Buffer (supplied with the enzyme) and 20 pmol each primer (Life Technologies, Carlsbed, CA, USA). Amplification reactions included an initial 2-minute denaturation step at 94ºC, followed by 40 cycles of 30 seconds at 94ºC, 30 seconds at 55ºC and 45 seconds at 72ºC. A final extension step for 7 minutes at 72ºC was performed. The DNA extracted from *H. pylori* from FFPE gastric tissue was used as positive control and distilled water in place of the DNA samples was used as negative control for PCR assays.

2.2.5. Detection of PCR products

For analysis of the amplified products, 5µl of the amplicons were put on 1,5% agarose gels containing 1µg of ethidium bromide per ml. The amplicons were visualized by UV transillumination.

2.2.6. Sequence analysis

The 16S rRNA amplicons were further identified by sequence analysis using ABI Prism Dye Terminator sequencing kit with AmpliTaq DNA polymerase and the ABI 3500xL Sequencer (Applied Biosystems, Foster City, CA, USA). Sequence comparison was then carried out using the Blast program and GenBank databases.

2.3. Results

Analyzing the tissue sections stained with carbol fuchsin, we visualized microorganisms resembling *H. pylori* mainly in hepatic sinus from HCC samples. The number of cocci was greater than of bacilli (Figure 3).

Our PCR results showed that all six microdissected samples were positive for 16S rRNA gene (Figure 2) and showed 98% similarity to *H. pylori* 16S rRNA gene by sequence analysis (GeneBank accession number CP003419.1) (Figure 4).

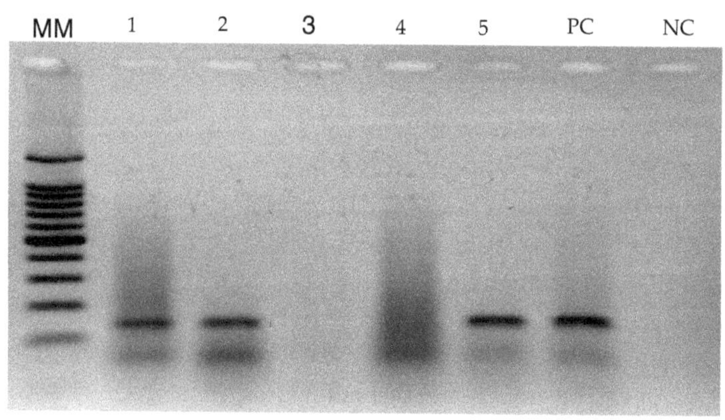

Figure 2. Results of amplification of *H. pylori* 16S rRNA gene. 1, 2 and 5 are positive samples; 3 and 4 are negative samples. MM: molecular marker, PC: positive control and NC: negative control.

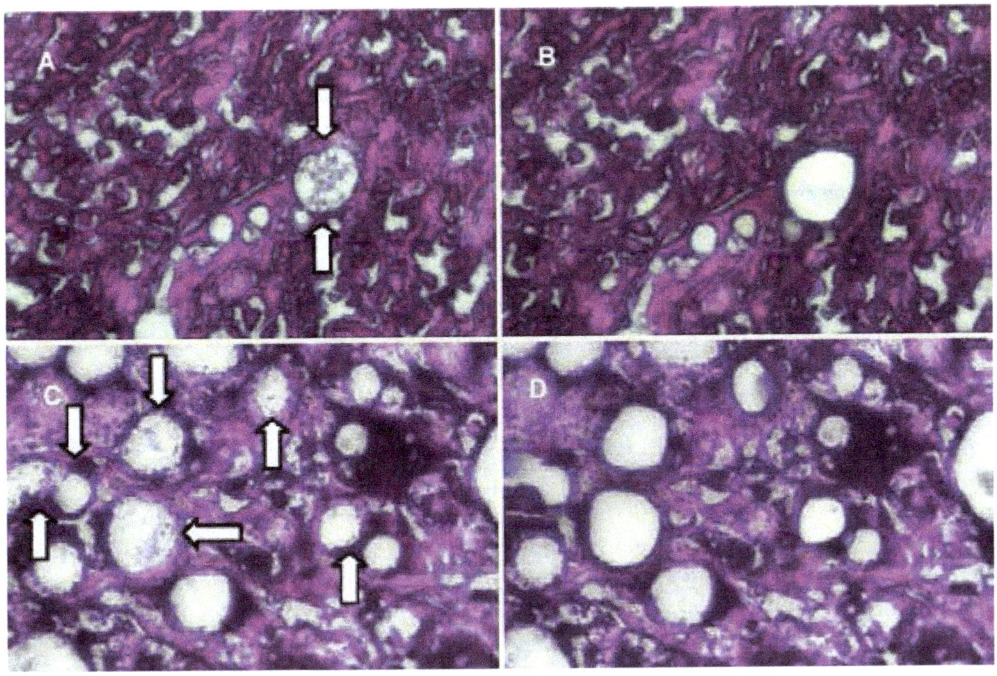

Figure 3. Optical microscopy of FFPE liver fragments of HCC patients with PCR-positive *H. pylori* 16S rRNA and stained with carbol fuchsin. In (A) and (C) bacteria are represented within sinusoid (arrows) before microdissection (magnification: 610X). In (B) and (D) the same samples are represented after bacterial microdissection (magnification: 610X).

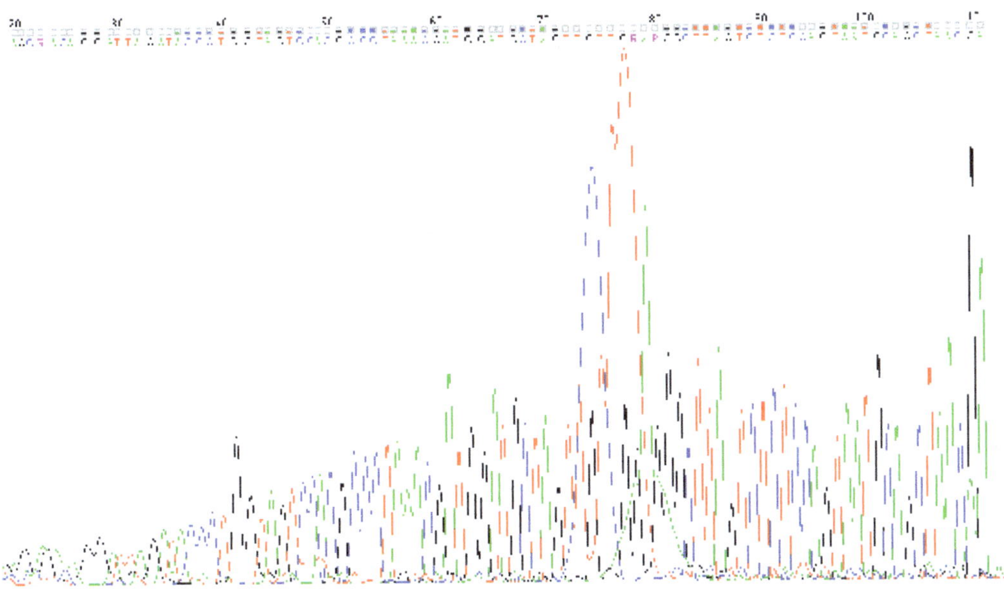

Figure 4. Electropherogram sequence of *H. pylori* 16S rRNA gene and alignment results of the BLAST databases.

3. Conclusion

The results described here confirm the identification of *H. pylori* in FFPE liver tissue from patients with HCC. Although specific primers were used for amplification of the *H. pylori* 16S rRNA gene, we cannot exclude the possibility of cross-reaction of these primers with other *Helicobacter* spp [65].

Considering the difficulty of DNA extraction from paraffin embedded samples, the use of LCM simplified the achievement of specific DNA because the DNA extraction process was reduced to a single digestion step of bacterial cells without further purification. Consequently, the crude lysate was used directly as template for PCR amplification. This is particularly advantageous when compared to traditional methods of DNA extraction that are generally laborious, toxic and time consuming [67].

Another advantage of using LCM is that it allowed the exact location of *H. pylori* in the liver, since bacteria were mainly found in the peritumoral tissue. Considering that our samples presented tumoral and peritumoral tissue in the same paraffin block, the technique was highly effective for obtaining a target bacterial population within a selected area in the HCC tissue. This is very important when we consider that the necrotic state and nuclease content of tissues may influence in recovering intact DNA specially when performing traditional methods for DNA extraction [68].

Furthermore, LCM was useful to reduce the interference from nontarget cell population considering that bacteria were found in small quantities in the liver tissue (Figure 3). In relation to nontarget cell population, it is important to consider that the major obstacle in the analysis of tumoral tissue is that it is composed by different cell types including stroma and inflammatory cells [69, 70, 71] and there is a potential dilution effect of the larger quantities of nontarget DNA found in whole tissue sections [64]. Thus, the employment of LCM was very efficient in isolating *H. pylori* despite of the reduced bacterial quantity in the HCC tissue.

In summary, we suggest that LCM can be extensively applied for identification of *H. pylori* in FFPE liver tissue. Further studies will be performed in order to amplify virulence genes of bacteria as well as to isolate *H. pylori* from other tissues using LCM technique.

Acknowledgements

This work was supported by grants from FAPESP (2009/09889-5) and FAEPEX 101/2011.

Author details

Elizabeth Maria Afonso Rabelo-Gonçalves*, Bruna Maria Röesler and José Murilo Robilotta Zeitune

*Address all correspondence to: elizabeth.goncalves@gc.unicamp.br

Department of Internal Medicine, Center of Diagnosis of Digestive Diseases, Faculty of Medical Sciences, State University of Campinas, Campinas, São Paulo, Brazil

References

[1] Tu QV, Okoli AS, Kovach Z, Mendz GL. Hepatocellular carcinoma: prevalence and molecular pathogenesis of *Helicobacter* spp. Future Microbiology 2009;4(10) 1283-1301.

[2] GLOBOCAN. International Agency for Research on Cancer (IARC). 2008. http://www-dep.iarc.fr. (accessed may 2013).

[3] El-Seragh HB. Epidemiology of viral hepatitis and hepatocellular carcinoma. Gastroenterology 2012;42(6) 1264-1273.

[4] Mittal S & El-Seragh HB. Epidemiology of hepatocellular carcinoma. Consider the population. Journal of Clinical Gastroenterology 2013;47 Suppl S2-6.

[5] World Health Organization. Mortality Database. WHO Statistical Information System. 2008. http://www.who.int/whosis (accessed may 2013).

[6] Hall AJ & Wild CP. Liver cancer in low and middle income countries. British Medical Journal 2003;326(7397) 994-995.

[7] Carvalho FM, Pereira TA, Gonçalves PL, Jarske RD, Pereira FEL, Louro ID. Hepatocellular carcinoma and liver cirrhosis TP53 mutation analysis reflects a moderate dietary exposure to aflatoxins in Espírito Santo State, Brazil. Molecular Biology Reports 2013; 40(8) 4883-4887.

[8] Bosch FX, Ribes J, Cléries R, Diaz M. Epidemiology of hepatocellular carcinoma. Clinical Liver Diseases 2005;9(2) 191-211.

[9] Gonçalves S, Pereira FF, Gayotto LC. Hepatocellular carcinoma in Brazil: report of a national survey (Florianopolis, SC, 1995). Revista do Instituto de Medicina Tropical de São Paulo 1997;39(3) 165-170.

[10] Carrilho FJ, Kikuchi L, Branco F, Gonçalves CS, Mattos AA. Brazilian HCC Study Group. Clinics 2010;65(12) 1285-1290.

[11] Parkin DM. The global health burden of infection-associated cancers in the year of 2002. International Journal of Cancer 2002;118(12) 3030-3044.

[12] Gao J, Xie L, Yang W, Zhang W, Gao S, Wang J, Xiang Y. Risk factors of hepatocellular carcinoma - current status and perspectives. Asian Pacific Journal of Cancer Prevention 2012;13(3) 743-750.

[13] Soman NR & Wogan GN. Activation of the c-Kis-ras oncogene in aflatoxin B1-induced hepatocellular carcinoma and adenoma in the rat: detection by denaturating gradient gel electrophoresis. Proceeding of the National Academy of Sciences 1993;90(5) 2045-2049.

[14] Taddei T, Mistry P, Schilsky ML. Inherited metabolic disease of the liver. Current Opinion in Gastroenterology 2008; 24(3) 278-286.

[15] Kumagi T, Horiike N, Abe M, Kurose K, Iuchi H, Masumoto T, Joko K, Akbar SF, Michitaka K, Onji M. Small hepatocellular carcinoma associated with Wilson's disease. Internal Medicine 2005;44(5) 493-443.

[16] La Vecchia C. Alcohol and liver cancer. European Journal of Cancer Prevention 2007;16(6) 497-495.

[17] Ward JM, Fox JG, Anver MR, Haines DC, George CV, Collins MJ Jr, Gorelick PL, Nagashima K, Gonda MA, Gilden RV. Chronic active hepatitis and associated liver tumors in mice caused by a persistent bacterial infection with a novel *Helicobacter species*. Journal of the National Cancer Institute 1994;86(16) 1222-1227.

[18] IARC: Working group on the evaluation of carcinogenic risks to human *Helicobacter pylori*. IARC Monography Evaluation Carcinogenic Risks Human 1994;61 177-240.

[19] Fox JG, Dewhirst FE, Shen Z, Feng Y, Taylor NS, Paster BJ, Ericson RL, Lau CN, Correa P, Araya JC, Roa I. Hepatic *Helicobacter species* identified in bile and gallbladder tissue from Chileans with chronic cholecystitis. Gastroenterology 1998;114(4) 755-763.

[20] Ponzetto A, Pellicano R, Leone N, Cutufia MA, Turrini F, Grigioni WF, D'Errico A, Mortimer P, Rizzetto M, Silengo L. *Helicobacter* infection and cirrhosis in hepatitis C virus carriage: is it an innocent bystander or a troublemaker? Medical Hypotheses 2000;54(2) 275-277.

[21] Dore MP, Realdi G, Mura D, Graham DY, Sepulveda AR. *Helicobacter* infection in patients with HCV-related chronic hepatitis, cirrhosis, and hepatocellular carcinoma. Digestive Diseases and Sciences. 2002;47(7) 1638-1643.

[22] Fan XG, Peng XN, Huang Y, Yakoob J, Wang ZM, Chen YP. *Helicobacter species* ribosomal DNA recovered from the liver tissue of Chinese patients with primary hepatocellular carcinoma. Clinical and Infectious Diseases 2002;35(12) 1555-1557.

[23] Verhoef C, Pot RG, de Man RA, Zondervan PE, Kuipers EJ, IJzermans JN, Kusters JG. Detection of identical *Helicobacter* DNA in the stomach and in the non-cirrhotic liver of patients with hepatocellular carcinoma. European Journal of Gastroenterology and Hepatology 2003;15(11) 1171-1174.

[24] Pellicano R, Mazzaferro V, Grigioni WF, Cutufia MA, Fagoonee S, Silengo L, Rizzetto M, Ponzetto A. *Helicobacter species* sequences in liver samples from patients with and without hepatocellular carcinoma. World Journal of Gastroenterology 2004;10(4) 598-601.

[25] Ito K, Nakamura M, Toda G, Negishi M, Torii A, Ohno T. Potential role of *Helicobacter pylori* in hepatocarcinogenesis. International Journal of Molecular Medicine 2004;13(2) 221-227.

[26] Rocha M, Avenaud P, Ménard A, Le Bail B, Balabaud C, Bioulac-Sage P, de Magalhães Queiroz DM, Mégraud F. Association of *Helicobacter species* with hepatitis C cirrhosis with or without hepatocellular carcinoma. Gut 2005;54(3) 396-401.

[27] Pirouz T, Zounubi L, Keivani H, Rakhshani N, Hormazdi M. Detection of *Helicobacter pylori* in paraffin-embedded specimens from patients with chronic liver diseases, using the amplification method. Digestive Diseases and Sciences 2009;54(7) 1456-1459.

[28] Gonciarz M, Wloch M, Gonciarz Z. *Helicobacter pylori* in liver diseases. Journal of Physiology and Pharmacology 2006;57(3) 155-161.

[29] Casafont F, Martin L, Pons-Romero F. Bacterial overgrowth in the small intestine in chronic liver disease. In: Blum HE, Bode JC, Bode Ch, Sartor RB(ed). Gut and the liver. London: Kluwer Academic Publishers; 1998. p 332-337.

[30] Tsunneyama K, Harada K, Kono N, Hiramatsu K, Zen Y, Sudo Y, Gershwin ME, Ikemoto M, Arai Y, Nakanuma Y. Scavenger cells with Gram-positive bacterial lipoteichoic acid infiltrate around the damaged interlobular bile ductus of primary biliary cirrhosis. Journal of Hepatology 2001;35(2) 156-163.

[31] Queiroz DMM & Santos A. Isolation of a *Helicobacter* strain from the human liver. Gastroenterology 2001;121(4) 1023-1024.

[32] Xuan SY, Qiang X, Zhou RR, Shi YX, Jiang WJ. *Helicobacter* infection in hepatocellular carcinoma tissue. World Journal of Gastroenterology 2006; 12(15) 2335-2340.

[33] Leelawat K, Suksumek N, Leelawat S, Lek-Uthai U. Detection of VacA gene specific for *Helicobacter pylori* in hepatocellular carcinoma and cholangiocarcinoma specimens of Thai patients. Southeast Asian Journal of Tropical Medicine and Public Health 2007;38(5) 881-885.

[34] Al-Soud AW, Stenram U, Ljungh A, Tranberg KG, Nilsson HO, Wadstrom T. DNA of *Helicobacter* spp. and common gut bacteria in primary liver carcinoma. Digestive and Liver Diseases 2008;40(2) 126-131.

[35] Taylor NS, Fox JG, Yan L. In vitro hepatotoxic factor in *Helicobacter hepaticus. H. pylori* and other *Helicobacter species.* Journal of Medical Microbiology 1995;42(1) 48-42.

[36] Chen R, Fan XG, Huang Y, Li N, Chen CH. In vitro cytotoxicity of Helicobacter pylori on hepatocarcinoma HepG2 cells. Al Zheng 2004; 23(1) 44-49.

[37] Ito K, Yamaoka Y, Ota H, El-Zimaity H, Graham DY. Adherence, internalization and persistence of *Helicobacter pylori* in hepatocytes. Digestive Diseases and Sciences 2008; 53(9) 2541-2549.

[38] Zhang Y, Fan XG, Chen R, Xiao ZQ, Feng XP, Tian XF, Chen ZH. Comparative proteome analysis of untreated and *Helicobacter pylori*-treated HepG2. World Journal of Gastroenterology 2005;11(22) 3485-3489.

[39] Frankel A. Formalin fixation in the '-omics' era: a primer for the surgeon-scientist. ANZ Journal of Surgery 2012;82(6) 395-402.

[40] Rivero ERC, Neves AC, Silva-Valenzuela MG, Sousa SOM, Nunes FD. Simple salting-out method for DNA extraction from formalin-fixed, paraffin-embedded tissues. Pathology Research and Practice 2006;202(7) 523-529.

[41] Greer CE, Wheeler CM, Manos MM. Sample preparation and PCR amplification form paraffin-embedded tissues. PCR Methods and Application Journal 1994;3(6) S113-S122.

[42] Klopfleisch R, Weiss AT, Gruber AD. Excavation of a buried treasure - DNA, mRNA, miRNA and protein analysis in formalin fixed, paraffin embedded tissues. Histology and Histopathology 2011;26(6) 797-810.

[43] Wu L, Pattern N, Yamashiro CT, Chui B. Extraction and amplification of DNA from formalin-fixed, paraffin-embedded tissues. Applied Immunohistochemistry and Molecular Morphology 2002; 10(3) 269-274.

[44] Karlsen F, Kalantari M, Chitemerere M, Johansson B, Hagmar B. Modifications of human and viral deoxyribonucleic acid by formaldehyde fixation. Laboratory Investigation 1994;71(4) 604-11.

[45] Muñoz-Cadavid C, Rudd S, Zaki SR, Patel M, Moser SA, Brandt ME, Gómez BL. Improving Molecular Detection of fungal DNA in formalin-fixed paraffin-embedded tissues: comparison of five tissue DNA extraction methods using parafungal PCR. Journal of Clinical Microbiology 2010;48(6) 2147-2153.

[46] Bulajic M, Panic N, Stimec B, Isaksson B, Jesenofsky R, Schneider-Brachert W, Löhr JM. PCR in *Helicobacter* spp. diagnostic in extragastric malignancies of digestive system. European Journal of Gastroenterology and Hepatology 2012; 24(2) 117-125.

[47] Nilsson HO, Mulchandani R, Tranberg KG, Stenram U, Wadström T. *Helicobacter species* identified in liver from patients with cholangiocarcinoma and hepatocellular carcinoma. Gastroenterology 2001;120(1) 323-324.

[48] Tian XF, Fan XG, Huang Y, Dai H, Ying RS. Procuration and identification of bacteria in paraffin-embedded liver tissues of hepatocellular carcinoma by laser-assisted microdissection technique. Acta Pathologica, Microbiologica et Imunologica Scandinavica 2008;116(1) 10-15.

[49] Emmer-Buck MR, Bonner RF, Smith PD, Chuaqui RF, Zhuang Z, Goldstein SR, Weiss RA, Liotta LA. Laser capture microdissection. Science 1996; 274(1274) 998-1001.

[50] Aaltonen KE, Ebbesson A, Wigerup C, Hedenfalk I. Laser capture microdissection (LCM) and whole genome amplification (WGA) of DNA from normal breast tissue - optimization for genome wide array analyses. BMC Research Notes 2011;4(3) 1-7.

[51] Liu A. Laser capture microdissection in the tissue biorepository. Journal of Biomolecular Techniques 2010; 21(3) 120-125.

[52] Esposito G. Complimentary techniques: laser capture microdissection - increasing specificity of gene expression profiling of cancer specimens. Advances in Experimental Medicine and Biology 2007; 593: 54-65.

[53] Sluka P, O'Donnell L, McLachlan R, Stanton PG. Application of laser-capture microdissection to analysis of gene expression in the testis. Progress in Histochemistry and Cytochemistry 2007; 42(2008) 173-201.

[54] Agar NS, Halliday GM, Barnetson RS, Jones A.M. A novel technique for the examination of skin biopsies by laser capture microdissection. Journal of Cutaneous Pathology 2003; 30(4) 265-270.

[55] Okuduku AF, Hahne JC, Von Deimling A, Wernert N. Laser-assisted microdissection, techniques and applications in pathology. International Journal of Molecular Medicine 2005; 15(5) 763-769.

[56] Kleheergher W, Rothämel T, Glöckner S, Lehmann U, Kreipe H. Laser-assisted microdisscetion and short tandem repeat PCR for the investigation of graft chimerism after solid organ transplantation. Pathobiology 2000;68(4-5)196-201.

[57] Lehmann U, Versmold A, Kreipe H. Combined laser-assisted microdissection and short tandem repeat analysis for detection of in situ microchimerism after solid organ transplantation. Methods in Molecular Biology 2005; 293: 113-123.

[58] Wang L, Zhu JS, Song MQ, Chen GQ, Chen JL. Comparison of gene expression profiles between primary tumor and metastatic lesions in gastric cancer patients using laser microdissection and cDNA microarray. World Journal of Gastroenterology 2006;12(43) 6949-6954.

[59] Jensen LH, Cruger DG, Lindebjerg J, Byriel L, Bruun-Petersen G, Jakobsen A. Laser microdissection and microsatellite analysis of colorectal adenocarcinomas. Anticancer Research 2006;26(3A) 2069-2074.

[60] Pai CY, Hsieh LL, Tsai CW, Chiou FS, Yang CH, Hsu BD. Allelic alterations at the STR markers in the buccal tissue cells of oral cancer patients and the oral epithelial cells of healthy betel quid-chewers: an evaluation of forensic applicability. Forensic Science International 2002;129(3) 158-67.

[61] Huang C, Yang L, Li Z, Yang J, Zhao J, Dehui X, Liu L, Wang Q, Song T. Detection of CCND1 amplification using laser capture microdissection coupled with real-time polymerase chain reaction in human esophageal squamous cell carcinoma. Cancer Genetics and Cytogenetics 2007;175(1) 19-25.

[62] Cheng L, Zhang S, MacLennan GT, Williamson SR, Davidson DD, Wang M, Jones TD, Lopez-Beltran A, Montironi R. Laser-assisted microdissection in translational re-

search: theory, technical considerations, and future applications. Applied Immunohistochemistry and Molecular Morphology 2013;21(1) 31-47.

[63] Ryan P, Kelly RG, Lee G, Collins JK, O'Sullivan GC, O'Conell J, Shanahan F. Bacterial DNA within granulomas of patients with Crohn's disease: detection by laser capture microdissection and PCR. American Journal of Gastroenterology 2004;99(8) 1539-1543.

[64] Klitgaard K, Molbak L, Jensen TK, Lindboe CF, Boye M. Laser capture microdissection of bacterial cells targeted by fluorescence in situ hybridization. BioTechniques 2005;39(6) 864-868.

[65] Rabelo-Gonçalves EM, Sgardioli IC, Lopes-Cendes I, Escanhoela CA, Almeida JR, Zeitune JM. Improved detection of *Helicobacter pylori* DNA in formalin-fixed paraffin-embedded (FFPE) tissue of patients with hepatocellular carcinoma using laser capture microdissection (LCM). *Helicobacter* 2013;18(3) 244-245.

[66] Rocha GA, Queiroz DMM, Mendes EN, Lage AP, Barbosa A. Simple carbolfuchsin staining for showing C. pylori and other spiral bacteria in gastric mucosa. Journal of Clinical Pathology 1989;42(9) 1004-1005.

[67] Steinau M, Patel SS, Unger ER. Efficient DNA extraction for HPV genotyping in formalin-fixed, paraffin-embedded tissues. Jounal of Molecular Diagnostic 2011;13(4) 377-381.

[68] Goelz SE, Hamilton SR, Vogelstein B. Purification of DNA from formaldeyde fixed and paraffin-embedded tissues. Biochemical and Biophysical Research Communications 1985;130(1) 118-126.

[69] Hanahan D, Weinberg RA. The hallmarks of cancer. Cell 2000;100(1) 57-70.

[70] Cheng L, Zhang S, Wang M, Davidson DD, Morton MJ, Huang J, Zheng S, Jones TD, Beck SD, Foster RS. Molecular genetic evidence supporting the neoplastic nature of stromal cells in 'fibrosis' after chemotherapy for testicular germ cell tumours. Journal of Pathology 2007;213(1) 65-71.

[71] Hanahan D, Weinberg R.A. Hallmarks of cancer: the next generation. Cell 2011; 144(5) 646-674.

Permissions

All chapters in this book were first published by InTech Open; hereby published with permission under the Creative Commons Attribution License or equivalent. Every chapter published in this book has been scrutinized by our experts. Their significance has been extensively debated. The topics covered herein carry significant findings which will fuel the growth of the discipline. They may even be implemented as practical applications or may be referred to as a beginning point for another development.

The contributors of this book come from diverse backgrounds, making this book a truly international effort. This book will bring forth new frontiers with its revolutionizing research information and detailed analysis of the nascent developments around the world.

We would like to thank all the contributing authors for lending their expertise to make the book truly unique. They have played a crucial role in the development of this book. Without their invaluable contributions this book wouldn't have been possible. They have made vital efforts to compile up to date information on the varied aspects of this subject to make this book a valuable addition to the collection of many professionals and students.

This book was conceptualized with the vision of imparting up-to-date information and advanced data in this field. To ensure the same, a matchless editorial board was set up. Every individual on the board went through rigorous rounds of assessment to prove their worth. After which they invested a large part of their time researching and compiling the most relevant data for our readers.

The editorial board has been involved in producing this book since its inception. They have spent rigorous hours researching and exploring the diverse topics which have resulted in the successful publishing of this book. They have passed on their knowledge of decades through this book. To expedite this challenging task, the publisher supported the team at every step. A small team of assistant editors was also appointed to further simplify the editing procedure and attain best results for the readers.

Apart from the editorial board, the designing team has also invested a significant amount of their time in understanding the subject and creating the most relevant covers. They scrutinized every image to scout for the most suitable representation of the subject and create an appropriate cover for the book.

The publishing team has been an ardent support to the editorial, designing and production team. Their endless efforts to recruit the best for this project, has resulted in the accomplishment of this book. They are a veteran in the field of academics and their pool of knowledge is as vast as their experience in printing. Their expertise and guidance has proved useful at every step. Their uncompromising quality standards have made this book an exceptional effort. Their encouragement from time to time has been an inspiration for everyone.

The publisher and the editorial board hope that this book will prove to be a valuable piece of knowledge for researchers, students, practitioners and scholars across the globe.

List of Contributors

Florica Nicolescu
Toxicology Department, "Carol Davila" University of Medicine and Pharmacy, Bucharest, Romania

Rajinikanth Siddalingam and Kumarappan Chidambaram
Department of Pharmaceutical Technology, School of Pharmacy, Taylor's University, Subang Jaya, Kuala Lumpur, Malaysia

Aleksandra Sokic-Milutinovic, Dragan Popovic, Tamara Alempijevic, Sanja Dragasevic, Snezana Lukic and Aleksandra Pavlovic-Markovic
School of Medicine, University of Belgrade, Belgrade, Serbia
Clinic for Gastroenterology and Hepatology, Clinical center of Serbia, Belgrade, Serbia

Yousef Javadzadeh and Sanaz Hamedeyazdan
Biotechnology Research center, Tabriz University of Medical Sciences, Iran

Malgorzata Plonka
University School of Physical Education, Cracow, Poland
Department of Physiology Jagiellonian University Medical College, Cracow, Poland

Aneta Targosz and Tomasz Brzozowski
Department of Physiology Jagiellonian University Medical College, Cracow, Poland

Elżbieta Karczewska, Karolina Klesiewicz, Paweł Nowak, Iwona Skiba and Alicja Budak
Department of Pharmaceutical Microbiology, Jagiellonian University Medical College, Krakow, Poland

Edward Sito
Falck Medycyna Outpatient Clinic of Gastroenterology, Krakow, Poland

Małgorzata Zwolińska-Wcisło and Tomasz Mach
Chair of Gastroenterology, Hepatology and Infectious Diseases, Jagiellonian University Medical College, Krakow, Poland

Carolina Negrei
Department of Toxicology, "Carol Davila" University of Medicine and Pharmacy, Bucharest, Romania

Daniel Boda
Dermato-oncology Excellence Research Center "Carol Davila" University of Medicine and Pharmacy, Bucharest, Romania

Batool Mutar Mahdi
Clinical Immunology, Department of Microbiology, HLA Research Unit, Al-Kindy College of Medicine, Baghdad University, Baghdad, Iraq

Bruna Maria Roesler and José Murilo Robilotta Zeitune
Department of Internal Medicine, Center of Diagnosis of Digestive Diseases, Faculty of Medical Sciences - State University of Campinas - UNICAMP, Campinas, São Paulo, Brazil

Elizabeth Maria Afonso Rabelo-Gonçalves
Department of Internal Medicine, Center of Diagnosis of Digestive Diseases, Faculty of Medical Sciences, State University of Campinas, Campinas, São Paulo, Brazil

Index

www.ingramcontent.com/pod-product-compliance
Lightning Source LLC
La Vergne TN
LVHW080615210926
848485LV00003B/160